IoT and Cloud Computing-Based Healthcare Information Systems

Biomedical Engineering: Techniques and Applications Book Series

IoT and Cloud Computing-Based Healthcare Information Systems

Edited by

Anand Sharma, PhD

Hiren Kumar Deva Sarma, PhD

S. R. Biradar, PhD

AAP | APPLE ACADEMIC PRESS

First edition published 2023

Apple Academic Press Inc.
1265 Goldenrod Circle, NE,
Palm Bay, FL 32905 USA

760 Laurentian Drive, Unit 19,
Burlington, ON L7N 0A4, CANADA

CRC Press
6000 Broken Sound Parkway NW,
Suite 300, Boca Raton, FL 33487-2742 USA

4 Park Square, Milton Park,
Abingdon, Oxon, OX14 4RN UK

Library and Archives Canada Cataloguing in Publication

Title: IoT and cloud computing-based healthcare information systems / edited by Anand Sharma, PhD, Hiren Kumar Deva Sarma, PhD, S.R. Biradar, PhD.
Names: Sharma, Anand (Lecturer in information technology), editor. | Sarma, Hiren Kumar Deva, editor. | Biradar, S. R., editor.
Series: Biomedical engineering (Apple Academic Press)
Description: First edition. | Series statement: Biomedical engineering: techniques and applications | Includes bibliographical references and index.
Identifiers: Canadiana (print) 20230142079 | Canadiana (ebook) 20230142125 | ISBN 9781774911228 (hardcover) | ISBN 9781774911235 (softcover) | ISBN 9781003304630 (ebook)
Subjects: LCSH: Medicine—Information technology. | LCSH: Information storage and retrieval systems—Medical care. | LCSH: Internet of things. | LCSH: Cloud computing.
Classification: LCC R858 .I58 2023 | DDC 610.285—dc23

Library of Congress Cataloging-in-Publication Data

CIP data on file with US Library of Congress

ISBN: 978-1-77491-122-8 (hbk)
ISBN: 978-1-77491-123-5 (pbk)
ISBN: 978-1-00330-463-0 (ebk)

ABOUT THE BOOK SERIES BIOMEDICAL ENGINEERING: TECHNIQUES AND APPLICATIONS

This new book series covers important research issues and concepts of the biomedical engineering progress in alignment with the latest technologies and applications. The books in the series include chapters on the recent research developments in the field of biomedical engineering. The series explores various real-time/offline medical applications that directly or indirectly rely on medical and information technology. Books in the series include case studies in the fields of medical science, i.e., biomedical engineering, medical information security, interdisciplinary tools along with modern tools, and technologies used.

Coverage & Approach

- In-depth information about biomedical engineering along with applications.
- Technical approaches in solving real-time health problems
- Practical solutions through case studies in biomedical data
- Health and medical data collection, monitoring, and security

The editors welcome book chapters and book proposals on all topics in the biomedical engineering and associated domains, including Big Data, IoT, ML, and emerging trends and research opportunities.

BOOK SERIES EDITORS:

Raghvendra Kumar, PhD
Associate Professor, Computer Science & Engineering Department,
GIET University, India
Email: raghvendraagrawal7@gmail.com

Vijender Kumar Solanki, PhD
Associate Professor, Department of CSE,
CMR Institute of Technology (Autonomous), Hyderabad, India
Email: spesinfo@yahoo.com

Noor Zaman, PhD
School of Computing and Information Technology,
Taylor's University, Selangor, Malaysia
Email: noorzaman650@hotmail.com

Brojo Kishore Mishra, PhD
Professor, Department of CSE, School of Engineering,
GIET University, Gunupur, Odisha, India
Email: bkmishra@giet.edu

FORTHCOMING BOOKS IN THE SERIES

Handbook of Artificial Intelligence in Biomedical Engineering
Editors: Saravanan Krishnan, Ramesh Kesavan, and B. Surendiran

Handbook of Deep Learning in Biomedical Engineering and Health Informatics
Editors: E. Golden Julie, S. M. Jai Sakthi, and Harold Y. Robinson

High-Performance Medical Image Processing
Editors: Sanjay Saxena and Sudip Paul

The Role of the Internet of Things (IoT) in Biomedical Engineering
Editors: Sushree Bibhuprada B. Priyadarshini, PhD, Devendra Kumar Sharma, PhD, Rohit Sharma, PhD, and Korhan Cengiz, PhD

IoT and Cloud Computing-Based Healthcare Information Systems
Editors: Anand Sharma, PhD, Hiren Kumar Deva Sarma, PhD, and S. R. Biradar, PhD

ABOUT THE EDITORS

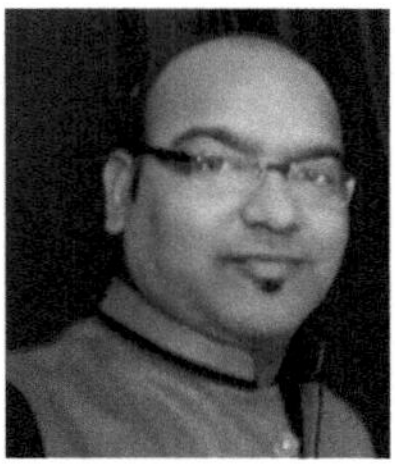

Anand Sharma, PhD
Assistant Professor, CSE, SET, MUST, Laxmangarh, Rajasthan, India, Tel.: +91-9649012214, E-mail: anand_glee@yahoo.co.in

Anand Sharma, PhD, has been working at Mody University of Science and Technology, Lakshmangarh, India, for last 10 years. He has more than 14 years of experience in teaching and research. He has been invited to several reputed institutions, including ISI-Kolkata, IIT-Mumbai, IIT-Jodhpur, IIT-Delhi, RTU-Kota, etc. He is an academician associated with the field of education and provides resources to enhance knowledge and to promote understanding of fundamental as well as applied concepts in the respective research area.

Dr. Sharma has pioneered research in areas of information security, IoT, WBAN, and machine learning. He is a member of IEEE, IET, ACM, and IE (India) and a life member of CSI and ISTE. He is serving as secretary of CSI-Lakshmangarh Chapter and as Student Branch Coordinator of CSI-MUST Student Branch. He has organized more than 15 conferences, seminars, and workshops; has chaired more than eight special sessions; and has delivered six keynote addresses at international conferences. He serves in an advisory capacity for several international journals as an editorial member and for international conferences on the technical programming and organizing committees. Dr. Sharma received his PhD degree in Engineering from MUST, Lakshmangarh, India; his MTech from ABV-IIITM, Gwalior; and BE from RGPV, Bhopal, India.

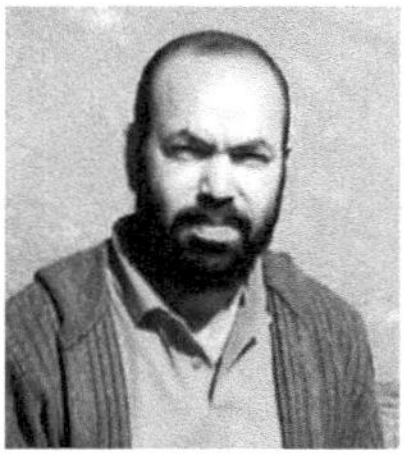

Hiren Kumar Deva Sarma, PhD
Professor and HOD, IT Department, SMIT, Sikkim, India, Tel.: +91-9733316230,
E-mail: hirenkdsarma@gmail.com

Hiren Kumar Deva Sarma, PhD, is presently working as a Professor and Head of the Department of Information Technology, Sikkim Manipal Institute of Technology, Sikkim, India. He was appointed as a Visiting Fellow by various universities, including North Eastern Hill University, Shillong; Assam University, Silchar; and Mizoram University, Aizawl, India. He has more than 23 years of teaching experience and research. He has successfully completed research projects funded by AICTE and the Department of Electronics and Information Technology, Government of India. He has received a Young Scientist Award of URSI (International Union of Radio Science) during the General Assembly of URSI in 2005, held at New Delhi, India.

Professor Sarma has more than 70 international publications in peer-reviewed journals, book chapters, and conference proceedings. He has edited books published by ACCB Publishing (England) and Springer. He has presented his research in many places outside India, including New Mexico (USA); Berkeley, California (USA); and Japan. He has served as reviewer for several journals, including Wireless Personal Communications, Neural Computing and Applications, Network and Computer Applications, and IEEE Systems Journal. He has also served as a book reviewer for Pearson Education India and Tata McGraw Hill India. Dr. Sarma received his PhD (Computer Science and Engineering) from Jadavpur University, Kolkata, India, and his MTech and BE from Tezpur University and Gauhati University, India, respectively.

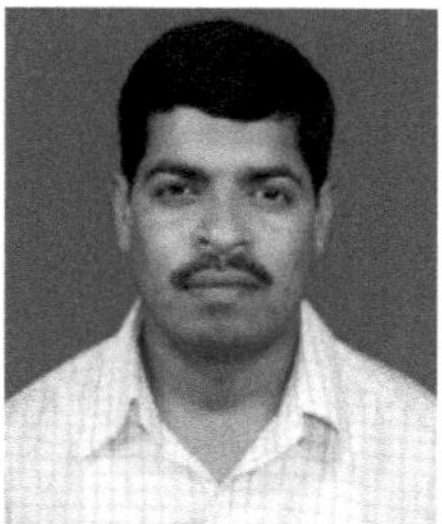

S. R. Biradar, PhD
Professor, Department ISE, SDM CET, Dharwad, Karnataka, India, Tel.: +91-9741421201,
E-mail: srbiradar@gmail.com

S. R. Biradar, PhD, is currently working as a Professor in the Information Science and Engineering Department and Deputy Dean (Academic Programs) at SDM College of Engineering and Technology, Dharwad, Karnataka, India. Previously, he has worked at the Sikkim Manipal Institute of Technology, Sikkim, India, and Mody University, Lakshmangarh, India. His research is broadly in networks, Internet of Things, and big data. He has more than 22 years of research and teaching experience. Prof. Biradar has published over 65 journal and conference papers. He has received travel grants from the Department of Science and Technology, Government of India, to visit Las Vegas, USA, to present his paper at an international conference. Dr. Biradar received his BE degree in Computer Science and Engineering (CSE) from Karnataka University, his MTech degree in CSE from MAHE Manipal, and his PhD degree in Engineering from the Jadavpur University, India.

CONTENTS

CONTRIBUTORS

Adil Aziz
Department of Internal Medicine, CKS Hospitals, Jaipur, Rajasthan, India

S. R. Biradar
Department of Information Science and Engineering, SDM College of Engineering and Technology, Dharwad, Karnataka, India

Sudipta Chakrabarty
Department of Master of Computer Application, Techno India Salt Lake, Kolkata, West Bengal, India

Biswajeet Champaty
School of Engineering, Ajeenkya DY Patil University, Pune, Maharashtra – 412105, India, E-mail: biswajeet.champaty@adypu.edu.in

Khyati Chopra
Department of Electronics and Communication Engineering, G.D. Goenka University, Gurgaon, Haryana, India, E-mail: ekta.soni@gdgoenka.ac.in

Diwaker
Assistant Professor, School of Computing, DIT University, Dehradun, Uttarakhand, India

Anita Dixit
Department of Information Science and Engineering, SDM College of Engineering and Technology, Dharwad, Karnataka, India, E-mail: anitadixit@sdmcet.ac.in

Md. Ruhul Islam
Department of Computer Science and Engineering, Sikkim Manipal Institute of Technology, Sikkim, India

Sandeep Jaiswal
Department of Biomedical Engineering, SET, Mody University, Laxmangarh, Rajasthan, India, E-mail: bmejaiswal@gmail.com

Sunil Kumar Jangir
Department of Computer Science and Engineering, School of Engineering and Technology, Mody University of Science and Technology, Laxmangarh, Rajasthan, India

S. R. Jayasimha
Department of Master of Computer Applications, RV College of Engineering, Bangalore, Karnataka, India, E-mail: jayasimhasr@rvce.edu.in

Kavita
Associate Professor, Department of CS and IT, Faculty of Engineering and Technology, Jayoti Vidyapeeth Women's University, Jaipur, Rajasthan, India

Manoj Kumar Khinchi
Mody University, Laxmangarh, Rajasthan, India

Manish Kumar
Associate Professor, Department of CSE, CEC-CGC, Landran, Mohali, Punjab, India; Department of Biomedical Engineering, Mody University of Science and Technology, Laxmangarh, Rajasthan, India, E-mail: manish.4379@cgc.edu.in

Sunil Kumar
Department of Physiotherapy, CKS Hospitals, Jaipur, Rajasthan, India

K. Mohana Lakshmi
Department of Electronics and Communication Engineering, CMR Technical Campus, Hyderabad, Telangana, India

Niranjan Lal
CSE, SET, Mody University, Laxmangarh, Sikar, Rajasthan, India,
E-mail: niranjan_verma51@yahoo.com

Bhanvi Menghani
Department of Information Technology, Jaipur Engineering College and Research Center, Jaipur, Rajasthan, India

Shivani Monga
PhD Scholar, Department of CS and IT, Faculty of Engineering and Technology, Jayoti Vidyapeeth Women's University, Jaipur, Rajasthan, India, E-mail: Shivanimonga385@gmail.com

Shweta Naik
Department of Computer Science and Engineering, Girijabai Sail Institute of Technology, Karwar, Karnataka, India

Nisha
Assistant Professor, Department of Sports Nutrition, School of Sports Sciences, CURAJ, Kishangarh, Ajmer, Rajasthan, India, E-mail: nishaduttajsr@gmail.com

Fatima Noor
Department of Home Science, F/O Agricultural Sciences, Aligarh Muslim University, Aligarh, Uttar Pradesh, India

Vibha Ojha
Government Engineering College, Ajmer, Rajasthan, India, E-mail: vibha.ojha@gmail.com

Nandita Sanjay Pal
Institute of Technology, Nirma University, Ahmedabad, Gujarat, India

Suneetha Rikhari
Department of Electronics and Communication Engineering, Mody University of Science and Technology, Laxmangarh, Rajasthan, India, E-mail: suneetha.rikhari@gmail.com

Angana Saikia
Department of Biomedical Engineering, SET, Mody University, Laxmangarh, Rajasthan, India

Hiren Kumar Deva Sarma
Department of Information Technology, Sikkim Manipal Institute of Technology, Sikkim, India, E-mail: hirenkdsarma@gmail.com

Anand Sharma
CSE Department SET, School of Engineering and Technology, Mody University of Science and Technology, Laxmangarh, Rajasthan, India

Pooja Sharma
IPEM, Ghaziabad, Uttar Pradesh, India

Raghav Sharma
Department of Information Technology, Jaipur Engineering College and Research Center, Jaipur, Rajasthan, India

Rahul Sharma
Department of Computer Science and Engineering, Chandigarh University, Mohali, Punjab, India, E-mail: prof.rahuls@gmail.com

Vishal Sharma
Research Scholar, CSE, SET, Mody University, Laxmangarh, Sikar, Rajasthan, India

Aadita Soni
Mody University of Science and Technology, Laxmangarh, Rajasthan, India

Arin Soni
Indian Institute of Technology, Mumbai, Maharashtra, India

Ekta Soni
Department of Electronics and Communication Engineering, G.D. Goenka University, Gurgaon, Haryana, India, E-mail: ekta.soni@gdgoenka.ac.in

Sunita
Assistant Professor, Department of Biosciences, Mody University of Science and Technology, Sikar, Rajasthan, India, E-mail: sunita.sos@modyuniversity.ac.in

Anirudhi Thanvi
Department of Information Technology, Jaipur Engineering College and Research Center, Jaipur, Rajasthan, India, E-mail: anil2thanvi@gmail.com

Ritika Upadhyay
School of Engineering, Ajeenkya DY Patil University, Pune, Maharashtra – 412105, India

J. Usha
Department of Master of Computer Applications, RV College of Engineering, Bangalore, Karnataka, India

Amit Kumar Verma
Faculty, Department of Pharmacy, MJP Rohilkhand University, Bareilly, Uttar Pradesh, India, E-mail: professoramitmjpuniversity@gmail.com

Jai Prakash Verma
Institute of Technology, Nirma University, Ahmedabad, Gujarat, India, E-mail: jaiprakash.verma@nirmauni.ac.in

Meenakshi Yadav
Sirifort Institute of Management Studies, Rohini, New Delhi, India

Rajesh Yadav
School of Engineering and Technology, Mody University of Science and Technology, Laxmangarh, Rajasthan, India, E-mail: yadav.rajesh27@gmail.com

ABBREVIATIONS

2D	two-dimensional
3D	three-dimensional
ACI	availability, confidentiality, and reliability
AES	advanced encryption standard
AHRQ	Agency for Healthcare Research and Quality
AI	artificial intelligence
AKS	Amazon Kinesis stream
AMA	American Medical Association
ANNs	artificial neural networks
AR	augmented reality
ATM	asynchronous transfer mode
BLAST	basic local alignment search tool
BP	back-propagation
BP	blood pressure
BPNN	back-propagation neural network
BSN	body sensor network
BSR	blood sample reader
CAD	computer-assisted diagnosis
CD	cosine distance
CFR	case fatality rate
CGHS	Central Government Health Scheme
CMR	crude mortality rate
CNN	convolution neural network
CPU	central processing unit
CSS	critical societal services
CT	computed tomography
DARPA	Defense Advanced Research Projects Agency
DISHA	Digital Information Security in Healthcare Act
DoS	denial of service
DRS	dynamic recommender system
DSA	design for social acceptance
DWT	discrete wavelet transform
EHRs	electronic health records

ELM	extreme learning machine
eMBB	enhanced mobile broadband
EMD	earth mover's distance
EMG	electromyography
EMR	elastic map-reduce
EMR	electronic medical records
eVIN	e-hospital, electronic vaccine intelligence network
FAME	foundation for African medicine and education
FCM	fuzzy C-means
FDA	Food and Drug Administration
FIFO	first in, first out
FNN	forward neural network
FPR	false positive rate
GA	genetic algorithm
GCE	global consistency error
GLCM	gray level co-occurrence matrix
GPS	global position system
GPU	graphics processing unit
GT	ground truth
GTSSE	game theory with Stackelberg security equilibrium
H2H	hospital-to-home
HAI	hospital-acquired infections
HAL	hybrid assistive limb
HEI	healthy eating index
HER	electronic healthcare records
HHS	health and human services
HMIS	health management information system
HMM	hidden Markov models
HR	heart rate
IaaS	infrastructure-as-a-service
ICM	Indian classical music
IDE	integrated development environment
IDSP	integrated disease surveillance program
IFR	infection fatality rate
IGA	interactive genetic algorithm
IGMSY	Indira Gandhi Matritva Sahyog Yojna
IHIP	integrated health information platform
IIoMT	intelligent internet of medical things

IMIA	International Medical Information Association
IoHT	internet of health things
IoMT	internet of medical things
$IoMusT^2$	internet of musical therapy things
IoT	internet of things
IR	infrared
ISS	integrated surgical system
IT	information technology
IWD	intelligent wearable devices
JSY	Janani Suraksha Yojana
KDD	knowledge discovery database
KNN	K-nearest neighbor
LBP	local binary pattern
LDA	latent Dirichlet allocation
LDA	linear discriminant analysis
MAC	medium access control
MERS	middle east respiratory syndrome
MIR	music information retrieval
ML	machine learning
MLP	multi-layer perception
MR	magnetic resonance
MRF	Markov random field
MRI	magnetic resonance imaging
MRS	music recommendation system
NASA	National Aeronautics and Space Administration
NAT	nucleic acid test
NeHA	national e-health authority
NFC	near-field communication
NHP	National Health Portal
NIME	new interfaces for musical expression
NIN	national identification number
NIST	National Institute of Standards and Technology
NMCN	National Medical College Network
NN	nearest neighbor
NNP	National Nutrition Policy
NRHM	National Rural Health Mission
ONS	object-naming service
OrBAC	organization-based access control

ORS	online registration system
PaaS	platform as a service
PACS	picture archiving and communication system
PCA	principal component analysis
PDA	personal digital assistants
PHI	personal health information
PLC	physical layer component
PNN	probabilistic neural network
PP	possession and privacy
PSO	particle swarm optimization
QoS	quality of service
RCH	reproductive child healthcare
RFID	radio-frequency identification
RI	random index
RoI	region of interest
RPM	remote patient monitoring
RR	respiration rate
SaaS	software-as-a-service
SARS	severe acute respiratory syndrome
SARS-CoV	SARS-associated coronavirus
SCL	serial clock line
SD	secure digital
SDA	serial data line
SLFN	single-layer feed-forward neural network
ST	Slantlet transform
SVM	support vector machine
TMC	Tello mobile clinic
uRLLC	ultra-low-latency communications
VA	voice assistants
VOI	variance of information
VR	virtual reality
WHO	World Health Organization
WLAN	wireless local area network
WPAN	wireless personal area network
WSN	wireless sensor network

PREFACE

The utilization of information and communication advances in health and medical services can be used to improve medical service quality in many ways. E-health is the utilization of information and communication innovations to fortify health and medical care. It include types of anticipation and training, diagnostics, treatment, and care conveyed through advanced innovation, free of time and place.

A healthcare information system refers to a framework intended to oversee medical services data. A healthcare information system provides the underpinning solutions and has many key capacities: data generation, compilation, age of information, arrangement, examination and synthesis, communication, and use. This incorporates frameworks that gather, store, oversee, and transmit a patient's electronic medical record (EMR), that details a clinic's operational administration, and that provides information for supporting medical services strategy choices. Additionally, the system incorporates the structure that handles information identified with the exercises of suppliers and health associations.

The usage of IoT and cloud computing in healthcare provides more powerful patient considerations around the globe. As more offices begin to incorporate IoT and distributed cloud computing into their healthcare information systems, it is necessary to inspect the new patterns and advancements in the field.

IoT and cloud computing can potentially develop a situation for effectively observing patient health and well-being as well as for improving how doctors convey care. IoT and cloud computing in health are can likewise support patient commitment and patient compliance by permitting them access to their health details and instructions in the solace of their own homes and to connect with their care centers and habitats whenever needed.

This book highlights inventive examination and research on the effect that IoT and cloud innovation have on healthcare information systems.

Highlighting the challenges and difficulties in implementing IoT and cloud technology into the healthcare field, this book is a critical reference source for academicians, professionals, engineers, technology designers, analysts, and students.

—*Editors*

INTRODUCTION

This book, *IoT and Cloud Computing-Based Healthcare Information Systems,* investigates the developing area of healthcare using IoT and cloud computing. It explores the various IoT and cloud computing approaches and techniques for advancement and improvement in the zone of healthcare information systems. It incorporates a combination of logical and implementation work for medical services.

This book centers around hypotheses, frameworks, techniques, calculations, algorithms, and applications in medical services, biomedicine, telemedicine, and clinical correspondences. It acts as an interface between e-health and communication technologies and their contribution to medical fields. The IoT and cloud computing-based healthcare information systems have a large domain that includes e-health, telehealth, telemedicine, e-doctors, and e-pharmacy, IoT for remote health monitoring, IoHT, adaptation of cloud computing healthcare, cloud security and privacy in healthcare, patient tracking and monitoring medical image extraction for tumor detection.

We have edited this book for technocrats at all career levels. Whether you are a medical professional working as a manager, administrator, or policymaker at a hospital or medical institution, or as an information architect interested in IoT and cloud computing for healthcare information systems, or as a biomedical expert or a technical software developer, you will find this book useful. If you are a researcher, academician, or graduate looking to build a career in the healthcare industry, then this book will give you real insights related to these topics.

Chapter 1 of this book gives the description of digi-health. The technological dynamics of e-health, m-health, telemedicine, remote care, and mobile health are explained. It shows that the development of modern sanitization, penicillin, anesthesia, and imaging equipment has been an essential component in maintaining and managing human health.

In continuation of Chapter 1, Chapter 2 discusses "Role of Telemedicine and e-Doctors for the Betterment of Future Medical Facilities in India." This chapter focuses on the adaptation of telehealth with the help of the technology access model.

In Chapter 3, a framework based on IoT using cloud computing for healthcare information systems has been given that will provide a better solution for the medical industry. In addition, it examines different advantages, difficulties, openings, and security for IoT-based healthcare systems.

Chapter 4 presents "A Study on Uninterrupted Security in IoT-Based Healthcare System." Many attacks are perceived that can jeopardize these healthcare monitoring systems and applications. These attacks are inclusive of timing-based and fingerprint snooping, denial of service (DoS) attacks, selecting and forwarding attacks, replay attacks, and sensor attacks. This chapter discusses the end-to-end data security system required for IoT healthcare schemes.

In Chapter 5, IoHT has been discussed. Associating medical services with IT is, as of now, encouraging for individuals. Further, we can join more than one healthcare device/sensor together and then to connect to the internet to transfer the real-time status of the patient to the monitoring end. This is known as the internet of health things (IoHT), and it is a way to make the healthcare system more automatized by virtue of helping elderly and disabled people.

Chapter 6 describes "Cloud Computing in Healthcare." This defines the services provided by hardware and software within the services provided by data centers over the internet. This chapter shows the continuous development in technology to build new and innovative systems that must be analyzed using comprehensive and integrative research.

In continuation with Chapter 6, Chapter 7 expands on the effect of conscious assets (cloud computing) to sustain the smart and preventive health ecosystem. This chapter re-proposes the idea of using remotely voluntary resources, those donated by end-user hosts, to form clouds—more dispersed, less managed clouds.

In this sequence of cloud computing in healthcare, Chapter 8 focuses on security issues, mainly authentication. The two-way authentication framework has been proposed by using the watermarking technique in cloud computing.

Chapter 9 discusses the development of a low-power Bluetooth-based pulse-oxy tracker for determining oxygen saturation and its monitoring to detect concerning symptoms and abnormalities at a very early stage so as to save lives, especially the lives of old aged and low-immune patients with chronic or infectious diseases.

After the pulse-oxy tracker for patient monitoring, the application development has been discussed in Chapter 10 for patient tracking. The application will notify the location information of the patient through the GPS connections and sends information to the administrator. Doctors can prescribe the necessary treatment protocol to the patient and monitor the patient remotely.

Chapter 11 presents some precautionary, preventive, and control measures to decrease the threat of viable disease transmission of the deadly COVID-19 virus. In this work, a new framework is proposed to detect COVID-19 using a smartphone. The proposed framework is an inexpensive solution because people are continuously using their smartphones these days for their daily routine work. After installation of the proposed framework on a smartphone, every user will become capable of diagnosing the virus.

In Chapter 12, a tumor extraction system using ELM and modified K-means clustering has been implemented. The technique employed in this chapter has three modules. The first module is the pre-processing module, in which non-local and local smoothing techniques are engaged to take out the noise components. In the second module, classification is done by obtaining feature vectors from the extreme learning machine (ELM). The third module describes the tumor detection stage, where the tumors are segmented using a modified K-means clustering algorithm. Magnetic resonance (MR) tumor images are used in the proposed work.

Chapter 13 describes the inclusion of machine learning to detect cancerous cells with the help of image processing. Further, Chapter 14 explains the advancement from 5G to 6G in robotic telesurgery.

In Chapter 15, a music recommendation system (MRS) based on user rating has been developed as a cloud-based healthcare information system. In continuation with Chapter 15, Chapter 16 proposes an IoT-based music therapy to improve mental health.

Chapter 17 proposes the deployment of data science in healthcare systems to fight against the COVID-19 pandemic. Chapter 18 describes the role of IoT in healthcare systems.

In Chapter 19, a cloud-based machine learning model is proposed to predict an individual's health and recommend a nutrition plan for a healthy lifestyle. Through this, people could be aware of their health and can improve it.

Last but not least, the aim of Chapter 20 is to propose some of the most important capabilities and technical achievements of medical and healthcare robotics needed to improve human health and well-being. This chapter describes application areas, services provided, adaptation challenges, and different enabling technologies that should be considered in the design of medical and healthcare robots.

We feel that after reading this book, readers will gain a thorough, well-rounded understanding of IoT and cloud computing-based healthcare information systems. This book will play a major role in the development and advancement of healthcare information systems using IoT and cloud computing.

—Editors

CHAPTER 1

DIGI-HEALTH: TECHNOLOGY AND HEALTHCARE DYNAMICS

NISHA[1] and FATIMA NOOR[2]

[1]*Assistant Professor, Department of Sports Nutrition, School of Sports Sciences, CURAJ, Kishangarh, Ajmer, Rajasthan, India, E-mail: nishaduttajsr@gmail.com*

[2]*Department of Home Science, F/O Agricultural Sciences, Aligarh Muslim University, Aligarh, Uttar Pradesh, India*

ABSTRACT

E-health, m-health, telemedicine, remote care, and mobile health are helping us in delivering healthcare in rural and remote areas and thus strengthening healthcare facilities. Driven by the worldwide ubiquity of cell phones and digital technologies, the way healthcare is being managed has changed dramatically. Under the universal health coverage of WHO, several steps have been taken by the member states. m-health has been partially implemented in India since 2006 for women and child healthcare. Several sites and mobile apps have been developed and are being managed by the National Health Portal (NHP) under the ministry of health and family welfare.

1.1 INTRODUCTION

The advancement of technology over the period of its development has led to improved human health. Developments in the modern sanitization,

IoT and Cloud Computing-Based Healthcare Information Systems. Anand Sharma, PhD, Hiren Kumar Deva Sarma, PhD & S. R. Biradar, PhD (Eds.)

penicillin, anesthesia, and imaging equipment have been essential component in maintaining and managing human health. Since then, we have come a long way, and with the help of technological advancements, we continue to push away the boundaries of diseases. It's no different today. Digital health is described as a broad spectrum encompassing together e-health, m-health which are the upcoming areas in the healthcare system and can be made possible with the help of advanced computing science in big data, genomics, cloud computing, internet of things (IoT), and artificial intelligence (AI) [1]. WHO defines e-health as the use of information and communication technologies for health. The e-health unit works as a part and partner at the global, regional, and country-level to propagate, promote, support, and strengthen the use and application of ICT in health promotion, development, and management. In the cluster of healthcare systems and innovations, e-health is under the department of service delivery and safety.

1.2 ICT AND HEALTHCARE COVERAGE

With the advent of digital technologies, new arenas have opened up in numerous fields. Novel opportunities have opened up in the healthcare system as well with the introduction of information and communication technology. Several challenges and issues that hinder the smooth and complete healthcare support, coverage, practice, and services to the community could be easily overcome with the help of digital technology [2]. ICT interventions could be used in several places, such as to increase the demand for available services, facilitate targeted communication to the community or society, bridge the gaps between geographically distant patients and healthcare professionals, etc. Gaps might also be bridged by frequent reminders about the services and guidelines, which would broaden not only the demand but also the access to healthcare and information (Figure 1.1).

Since 2005, WHO has been working towards the field of e-health and prioritized it as a prime concern, after the World Health Assembly resolution WHA 58.28 was adopted. The major aim of e-health is to provide economical support of health and healthcare system such as health surveillance, health education, health literature, healthcare services, and health research with safe and secure use of ICT [3]. After the adoption of the resolution in 2005, universal health coverage and e-health has accelerated drastically. The foundation for e-healthcare are the various programs that are developed to deliver healthcare services so as to provide universal health coverage, for which it is essential to set out a vision for the country regarding the delivery, coverage, and functioning of the healthcare system. Along with the setting up of the vision proper arrangements need to be made for its monitoring and evaluation.

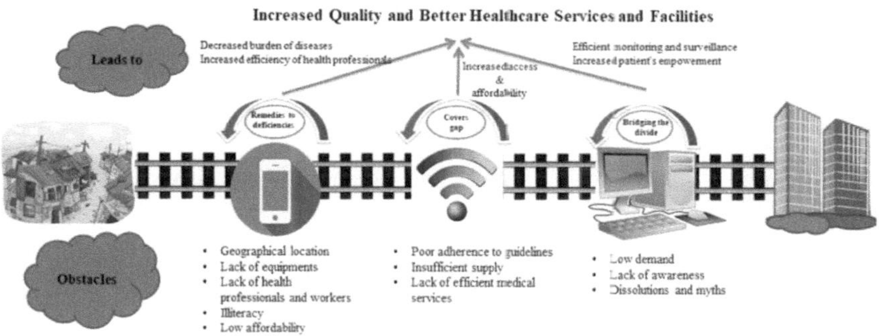

FIGURE 1.1 Digital health interventions to overcome health system challenges.

Another vital component of e-health is the delivery of goods and services that the citizens understand and value. Arranging and setting up of such a system would require involvement stakeholders, devising of standards, legislation, apt governance arrangements, technical, and financial support, etc. In several countries of the world, more than one dialect is used. Thus, it is important that anything relating to health and healthcare services is made available in vernacular language, which would make it easy for all the citizens to understand, utilize, and get benefitted. India, being a multilingual country with diverse culture, socio-economic strata, and educational levels, demands the inclusion of multilingual policy and strategy by the government to define its commitment towards the vernacular diversity and minority of the country so that it could reach people from all the walks of life.

The ability of ICT-empowered media to help the approaches and policies along with the arrangements made by the government to support the healthcare system and wellbeing through websites that furnishes data in numerous dialects. As capacities of ICT advances to deal with various media increment along with the mobile technologies that has today reached to almost all the parts of the world and to most of the communities and become quite affordable, content-based conveyance of data can be enhanced with all the more captivating audio-visual and 3D media. Moreover, as network improves, so do the open doors for offering multilingual help for all. The e-health initiatives has a vision to deliver better health outcomes in terms of:

- access;
- quality;
- affordability;
- lowering of disease burden;
- efficient monitoring of health entitlements to citizens.

The major intent of e-health is to provide healthcare support and services through ICT to the people via online medical consultation, online medical records, e-pharmacy, online medical equipment supply and management, etc. These services and facilities may be available to any individual in any geographical location of the world through web or internet services, mobile, SMS or call center services. In India, the Ministry of Health and Family Welfare is the apex body in regulating the health sector. In 2013, electronic health records standards (EHR) were notified by MoHFW. Adoption of information technology (IT) by healthcare institutions was facilitated in 2016 documents of EHR. MoHFW proposed a bill as Digital Information Security in Healthcare Act (DISHA) to govern the personal data security in the healthcare sector. Along with this National e-Health Authority (NeHA) was proposed to be set up in 2015 as a regulatory, promotional, standards setting organization, intended to be accountable for the development and smooth functioning of the healthcare system and services in the country with the major aim of attaining economical but high-quality healthcare for all through ICT.

The health sector of the country has been constantly budding with the help of some of the key emerging technologies such as m-health, telemedicine, internet of medical health, self-monitoring devices, robot-assisted surgery, e-pharmacy, AI, could computing, etc. The benefits of the e-healthcare system could be illustrated with 10E's [4]:

1. **Efficiency:** Healthcare system is required to be efficient and economical so that the entire citizen can avail the facilities. e-health

can be helpful in reducing the cost by evading the duplication of diagnostic and therapeutic interventions.

2. **Evidence-Based:** e-health system and healthcare facilities effectiveness, efficiency, proficiency, and productivity should be proven from time to time by continuous evaluation and surveillance that must be evidence-based.
3. **Empowerment:** e-health has empowered people by opening new opportunities for patient-centered medicine and by making personal medical electronic records accessible through the internet, which has enabled individuals to access patients' choice-based treatment.
4. **Enhanced Quality:** Increased efficiency, empowerment, and reduced economics for healthcare along with enhanced quality by providing the comparison between healthcare providers, which facilitates the individuals to make a clear decision among the healthcare providers to avail best quality services.
5. **Encouragement:** A better understanding and encouragement between the healthcare professional and consumer might develop, leading to enhanced quality and better health services.
6. **Education:** e-health systems and services would lead to educating healthcare professionals in remote areas. Physicians might also be able to enhance and keep themselves abreast with the latest developments in the medical field, preventive measures, etc.
7. **Enablement:** With the advent of e-healthcare systems and services, ICT would be very helpful in enabling the establishment of healthcare in a standardized way, thus ensuring quality healthcare for all.
8. **Extension:** e-healthcare would thus mean the establishment of easily assessable, quality healthcare beyond the borders of the globe. Online services would enable the extension of valuable services for medical professionals across geographical and conceptual frameworks.
9. **Equity:** e-health has the potential to make healthcare more equitable. The major challenge to this fact is the inability of a part of the population to access e-health benefits, mainly due to ICT and computer illiteracy, which could be overcome by proper government measures, regulations, and policies.
10. **Ethics:** e-health would encompass different and new ethical issues as online connections between the medical practitioner and the

patient would pose different challenges and threats such as secrecy of data, professional practice issues, equity issues, etc.

1.3 M-HEALTH

m-health, better known as mobile health, is defined as the application of mobile and wireless devices such as cellphones, personal digital assistants (PDA), patient monitoring equipment, etc., for medical healthcare services [5]. Universal health coverage is the entitlement of comprehensive health coverage and security to all individuals that could be achieved by m-health. It can be used to increase access to and provision of health services in areas where there is little infrastructure to support the internet (or other technologies) or traditional health services, but where mobile communications technology infrastructure has been prioritized. Supplying the technology for mobile communications is cheaper than providing in-person services. At the same time, mobile devices and technologies may be contributing to increasing quality of life through other initiatives such as finance, small business, and agriculture.

Reports suggest that the use of mobile phones has increased at an exponential rate all over the world in the past few years. The growth has been from about 82 per 100 people, i.e., 2.2 billion global subscriptions to more than 120 per 100 people, i.e., about 7 billion in just a decade (Figure 1.2). Maximum increment has been observed in developing countries with about 1.2 billion to 5.5 billion subscriptions in 2015 [6]. The increase in the subscription of cell phones clearly demonstrates the accessibility of mobile phones by individuals portraying its ubiquitous nature, but the major obstacle is access to smartphones along with internet facilities. Other difficulties that are to be overcome include lack of digital literacy, network infrastructure, cultural, and social acceptance, high cost of different plans and their functionality, lack of appropriate and relevant content and its understanding [2]. Though a sharp decline can be noted in the cost of smartphones and internet data plans which has rendered its use deep within the communities by the people of all the socio-economic strata present a ray of successful intervention of m-health within the country.

Implementation of m-health is a tough task and needs to overcome several hurdles, especially in low- and middle-income countries. According to WHO report, out of 37 countries under survey, 32% reported lack of funding as a major constraint while lack of legal regulation was an important constraint in implementation of m-health which was reported by 28% of the respondent countries among 32 countries under study. These two constraints were observed to be the most important barriers that need to be overcome for successful implementation of m-health. Figure 1.3 depicts the different regions of the world which use m-health programs either for accessing or providing health information and services or collecting health information. Data reveals that southeast Asian countries and western pacific regions are the regions with the least involvement in m-health technologies and programs [2].

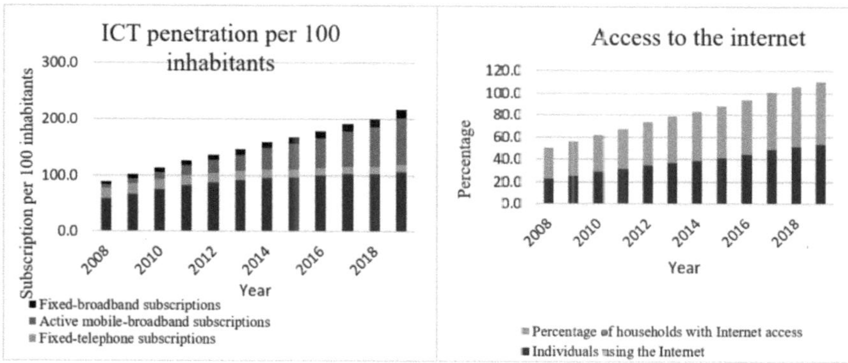

FIGURE 1.2 ICT penetration and access to the internet over time.
Source: Reports of World Development Indicators, Data Bank, The World Bank.

In India, the Ministry of Health and Family Welfare has taken this Digital India Initiative along with various e-gov initiatives as e-health India division in the healthcare sector. In a country like ours which has a huge population and the mobile phone technology entering to all the nooks and corners at an exceptionally high speed could be a great revolution. As India has a profound presence of IT and contributes approximately 8% to the GDP, integrated health information system could be a game-changer in this field [4].

Some other ongoing initiatives are: National Health Portal (NHP); reproductive child healthcare (RCH); health management information system (HMIS); integrated disease surveillance program (IDSP); integrated health information system (IHIP); integrated health information platform (IHIP); e-Shushrut, e-hospital, electronic vaccine intelligence network (eVIN); Central Government Health Scheme (CGHS); MeraAspatal (patient feedback system); National Identification Number (NIN); online registration system (ORS); and National Medical College Network (NMCN).

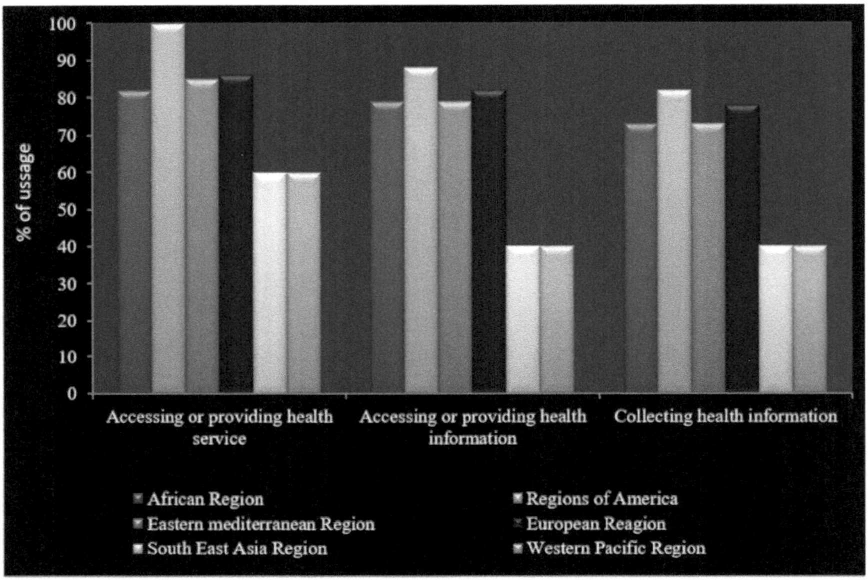

FIGURE 1.3 Usage percentage of m-health programs by different WHO regions.
Source: World Health Organization; Global Diffusion of e-Health: Making Universal Health Coverage Achievable, Report of the Third Global Survey on e-Health.

An integrated android and web-based; multimedia-empowered mobile health proposal for frontline health workers is m-Sehat [7]. It is a unique initiative by the government. It is a preloaded application that focuses on client-based tracking by keeping a real-time record and track of maternal and infant morbidity and mortality. m-Sehat was implemented in October 2015 in five districts of Uttar Pradesh. The districts that were chosen for implementation of this application were Bareilly, Faizabad, Kannauj, Mirzapur, and Sitapur as among the 25 districts of UP, these five districts were the highest priority districts in context of maternal and infant morbidity and mortality. This application is accredited to social health activists such as ASHAs Anganwadi workers, auxiliary midwives (ANMs), health program managers, etc. As these professionals are an interface between the public health system and society, they play a critical role and are essentially the first point of contact, who convince the community to adopt lifesaving health practices and to accelerate and reduce the maternal, neonatal, child mortality and total fertility rate. Several other websites and application that the Government of India is providing are listed in Table 1.1. Table 1.1 describes a few of the numerous types of website/mobile apps that are available in India for the betterment of society along with their brief description.

TABLE 1.1 List of Websites and Mobile Apps Provided by the Government of India

SL. No.	Name	Description	Portal
1.	m-Health Basics	It is designed to gain knowledge about m-health, its importance/application/ limitations.	Website
2.	Them-Health Planning and Implementation Guide	This helps in how to integrate mobile technology into health programming.	Website
3.	Frontline SMS	It is used to reach out to communities through SMS removing the barriers between the communities and NGO workers/charity payers.	Website
4.	Mobile-Family Planning Tool	CycleTel™ provides family planning tools. Women can send SMS to attain knowledge about family planning methods.	Website
5.	Mobile Alliance for Maternal Action (MAMA)	This website provides information and support to pregnant mothers and new mothers via SMS/website/social networking/voicemails.	Website
6.	Strengthen-Family-Planning-Programs	This m-health portal addresses the critical health system, such as finance, human resources, information health management system, etc., to underserved populations to strengthen family planning.	Website
7.	National Health Portal	Featured by Mobile harvest and act as a mobile extension portal of the Government of India (GoI). This app provides a single window to access services and information provided by GoI.	Mobile app

TABLE 1.1 *(Continued)*

SL. No.	Name	Description	Portal
8.	Healthy You Card	Used for: • Appointing doctors/hospitals/pharmacies/ health centers; • It also has alerts and reminders option through SMSs/e-mails for appointments/ cancellation or modification in appointments; • For Android and IOs users.	Mobile app
9.	Healthy You EHR	Patient-oriented app to maintain their medical record. It is user-friendly, cost-free, and easily accessible. For Android and IOs users	Mobile app
10.	Safe Pregnancy and Birth	This app helps in gaining knowledge in the following: • Healthy pregnancy; • Pregnancy/birth/after-birth danger signs – identify and action required; • Guidelines for community health worker; • It is multilingual; • For Android and IOs users.	Mobile app
11.	Safe Abortion App	This app helps in gaining wealth information on the following: • It helps to individual/supporters/ health-worker; • Easy calculation of pregnancy weeks; • Exploration of safe abortion methods; • Knowledge and dosage of birth-control pills and abortion pills; • FAQ section; • Multi-lingual; • For android and IOs users.	Mobile app
12.	Family Planning App	This app is designed to: • Promote counseling; • "Method choosing" tool according to individual preferences and health history; • FAQ section; • Multilingual; • For Android and IOs users.	Mobile app

TABLE 1.1 *(Continued)*

SL. No.	Name	Description	Portal
13.	Mswasthy-CDAC	It is beneficial in numerous aspects, such as BMI calculator, calorie counter, nutrition facts, hospital/doctor search, OPD scheduling, patient monitoring, etc.	Mobile app
14.	Supervision and Evidence-based Care (Comm Care App)	It supports various surveys, counseling forms. It validates data.	Mobile app
15.	TBDetect (e-MOCHA TBDetect)	It includes TB symptom, screening algorithm by WHO guidelines. It provides lectures on TB prevention and care by experts.	Mobile app
16.	m-Tikka	It is cloud-based electronic app where infants are registered, and their vaccine records are made. This also aids in surveys of vaccination.	Mobile app
17.	1 mg	It is online pharmacy app. Applicable for android users/IOs/Windows	Both mobile app and website
18.	AIIMS-WHO CC ENBC	It helps in the care unit of neonatal/newborns by following the guidelines provided by WHO for health workers. Nurses and doctors mainly use it For Android and IOs users	Both mobile app and website
19.	Mobile Technology for Water Sanitation and Health (m-Water App)	Used in the data management of water and health. It is helpful in mapping of water sources, design, and monitor surveys, data analysis, create reports.	Both mobile app and website
20.	Netmeds – India's Pharmacy	This enables the population of both rural and urban areas to have access to prescription and latest medicine, health products.	Both mobile app and website
21.	Healthcare at Home	Healthcare at home provides various services at homes, such as nursing care, ICUs at home, physiotherapy services, cancer care, and diabetes management programs.	Both mobile app and website

1.4 CONCLUSION

Both e-health and m-healthcare systems, services, and technology are evolving at a rapid speed. Therefore, there is a need to develop adequate support systems, policies, infrastructure, etc., by the government to support health professionals in both their competencies in the areas of digital health up to date. Digital health literacy is an important area of attention.

KEYWORDS

- **digital health**
- **e-health**
- **electronic health records standards**
- **m-health**
- **mobile apps**

REFERENCES

1. Michie, S., Yardley, L., West, R., Patrick, K., & Greaves, F., (2017). Developing and evaluating digital interventions to promote behavior change in health and health care: Recommendations resulting from an international workshop. *J. Med. Internet Res., 19*(6), e232.
2. World Health Organization, (2017). *Global Diffusion of e-Health: Making Universal Health Coverage Achievable: Report of the Third Global Survey on e-Health* (pp. 33–43). World Health Organization.
3. Resolution WHA58.33, (2005). Sustainable health financing, universal coverage, and social health insurance. In: *58th World Health Assembly*. Geneva. Resolutions and decisions annex. Geneva: World Health Organization; WHA58/2005/REC/1; http://apps.who.int/gb/ebwha/pdf_files/WHA58-REC1/english/A58_2005_REC1-en.pdf (accessed on 13 June 2022).
4. e-Health. https://www.nhp.gov.in/e-health-india_mty (accessed on 13 June 2022).
5. Horvath, T., Azman, H., Kennedy, G. E., & Rutherford, G. W., (2012). Mobile phone text messaging for promoting adherence to antiretroviral therapy in patients with HIV infection. *Cochrane Database of Systematic Reviews, 3,* CD009756.
6. ICT Facts and Figures. Geneva: International Telecommunications Union. https://www.itu.int/en/ITU-D/Statistics/Pages/stat/default.aspx (accessed on 13 June 2022).
7. Fletcher, R., Díaz, X. S., Bajaj, H., & Ghosh-Jerath, S., (2017). Development of smartphone-based child health screening tools for community health workers. In: *IEEE Global Humanitarian Technology Conference (GHTC)* (pp. 1–9).

CHAPTER 2

ROLE OF TELEMEDICINE AND E-DOCTORS FOR THE BETTERMENT OF FUTURE MEDICAL FACILITIES IN INDIA

ADIL AZIZ,[1] SUNIL KUMAR,[1] and SUNITA[3]

[1]*Department of Internal Medicine, CKS Hospitals, Jaipur, Rajasthan, India*

[2]*Department of Physiotherapy, CKS Hospitals, Jaipur, Rajasthan, India*

[3]*Assistant Professor, Department of Biosciences, Mody University of Science and Technology, Sikar, Rajasthan, India,*
E-mail: sunita.sos@modyuniversity.ac.in

ABSTRACT

The study is to bestow awareness about the preventive healthcare system by using the unique movable health clinic and e-doctor (doctor present at a distant location) termed as telemedicine. This is an inexpensive healthcare system for decreasing the outbreak of communicable diseases, death rate, and minimizing the number of patients eventually less overheads for medication by the rural community. The preventive healthcare system is termed as telemedicine because of four vital components: a movable clinic, healthcare worker, an application/website, server system, and e-doctors present at a distant location.

IoT and Cloud Computing-Based Healthcare Information Systems. Anand Sharma, PhD, Hiren Kumar Deva Sarma, PhD & S. R. Biradar, PhD (Eds.)

2.1 INTRODUCTION

Good health is known as the social and mental well-being of an individual, for this aspect, preventive healthcare, which means avoidance or slowing down of future disease, is a landmark achievement for the best quality of life. The good health of a person is not only important for the self-development but also a contribution to the economy by the employability and creativity for the generation of new ideas for the nation. Therefore, a healthy nation is the reflection of the quality of human capital, which is essentially the most imperative provider to the growth of any nation's economy. Indian public health system works in different clusters, sub-centers serve in villages, townships of different plain and hilly areas of the country. There could be many sub-centers under one primary health center, then comes a community health center which works under observations of district hospitals. Each district of a state has one district hospital which works in guidance of a medical college as shown in Figure 2.1. This is one face of the health system which comes under the surveillance of public sector, usually cheaper and serves the public without charging much but it has been noticed that due to lack of funding, long queues of patients and other limitation this has been found to be less efficient as compared to private hospitals those are located in urban part of country. People are likely to be attracted to private clinics as well as hospitals which charge patients monetarily higher than the government medical facilities. On average, this is a commonly seen scene that the non-affordable healthcare system is adversely affecting the budget of a common Indian. As per the data presented by UNICEF in the year 2008, 2009; the eye-opening facts came out like one-fifth more women death tolls of age group 18–30 years and one-fourth more of toddler's death in India as compared to rest of world [1, 2]. Here, we suggest the preventive healthcare can be an effective measure to reduce the death tolls and to keep an eye on the health status of a person. In accordance with this Indian government had made many remarkable efforts for 1.3 billion people [3, 4], still facing challenges addressing many diseases like AIDS (acquired immune deficiency syndrome), syphilis, hepatitis-B, and many other emerging chronic diseases [5].

India still requires major efforts for meeting the needs for nutritional requirements, newborn death toll, differences in health facility raising the inequality in the rural and urban part of the country, gender inequality and violence against women [6–8]. New strategies like e-doctor, telemedicine, and mobile clinic those are already in practice in different parts of the world, as shown in Table 2.1, can be a ray of hope for the unprivileged and rural communities across the country [9].

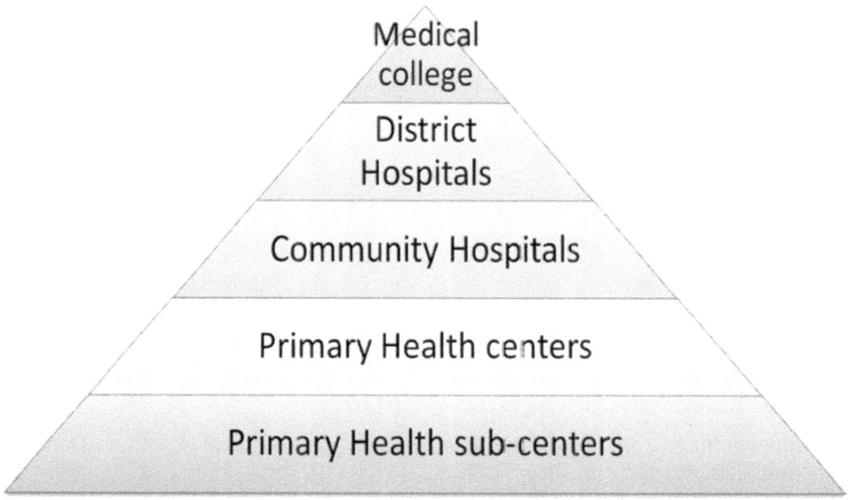

FIGURE 2.1 The health delivery system of public sector in India.

TABLE 2.1 Various World-Wide Projects for Unreached Communities

Project	Silent Features	Country
The 1,00,000 Smiles Project	Inexpensive dental healthcare	Nigeria
DoctorDial	Scheduling of doctor's visit, phone calls, text chat discussion	Nigeria
Sure, Girl Initiative	Cervical cancer awareness among female by social media	Nigeria
Dr. Recomenda	Used for health profile creation that is easy to share with a doctor	Brazil
Love on Wheels	Medical services are given by health-workers to underprivileged population	Malaysia
Flying for Life	Works for childhood development program	South Africa
Society for Family Health	AIDS awareness, health, and hygiene requirement for malaria and other ailments	Zambia

TABLE 2.1 *(Continued)*

Project	Silent Features	Country
DKT Pakistan	Educate the females contraception through social media	Pakistan
Mobile Clinic in Malawi	Community-based care in case of various diseases	Malawi
Comprehensive Community-Based Rehabilitation	Movable clinic for the health of infants, rehabilitation, prosthetics availability	Tanzania
Alcamilabs	Tuberculosis treatment	Peru, Somalia
Innopia electromechanical solutions	Development of mobile clinic for unreachable communities	Ethiopia
Biodent Clínica Dental	Online educational initiatives for dental health for students, teachers, and parents	Mexico
Samsung Solar Powered Health Center	Health Centers powered by Solar energy are serving in remote rural areas	South Africa
Foundation for African Medicine and Education (FAME)	Advancement in medicinal education for mobile medical services	Tanzania
Leprosy Control Program	Identification of patients in the rural areas and then referred to the equipped health centers or hospital	South Sudan
Medishare Africa Mobile Telemedicine Clinics Project	Utilization of satellite communications to make a connection between medical staff of mobile clinic present at rural areas of Kenya with specialized doctors in urban areas	Kenya
Children's Health and Development in Kenya	Treatment through mobile clinics by expert doctors from city to mothers and their children	Kenya
AOET Rural Health Initiative	A pharmacy and mobile clinics equipped with nurses, doctors, clinical officers	Uganda
Mwenya Uganda Mobile Clinic	Mobile dental and other medical clinics	Uganda
Tello Mobile Clinic (TMC)	Serving the marginalized and isolated communities by the help of mobile clinics	Uganda
Prosmiling Terpadu	Mobile clinic	Indonesia
Marie Stopes Bolivia	Free mobile medical services, for helping poor families	Bolivia

Source: https://healthmarketinnovations.org/programs-list/1296 [16].

A basic illustration for working model of telemedicine is made in Figure 2.2, depicting the emergence of a casualty at a remote or rural location, the person can reach to the nearest telemedicine center, where healthcare worker helps the patient to fill the consent form for treatment, after filling all the required basic data regarding body mass index, blood pressure (BP), pulse rate, blood group, etc., in an application/website which is sharable to the e-doctor present at a different location. The healthcare worker after consulting the e-doctor can give the required guidelines for further treatment and medication. Later a follow-up session can be scheduled for the patient for the next visit, by automated generated short message services.

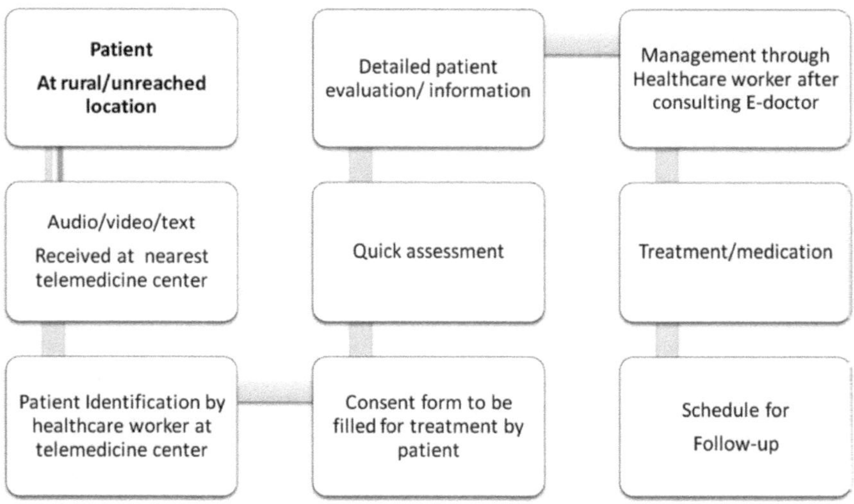

FIGURE 2.2 Process of consultation to a patient by healthcare worker with the help of e-doctor.

2.2 CAN INDIA BE AN IDEAL GROUND FOR TELEMEDICINE?

The emerging medical students holding the degree of MBBS and BDS are inclined to explore career option in mobile health (m-health) and telemedicine. Although, the technical challenge is to connect all sub-centers to either private hospitals or medical colleges through the internet. The economical terrestrial telecommunication for countrywide internet connectivity and indigenous satellites is a possible way of connectivity [11]. The government of India had launched a program through the planning commission for the 12th plan from the year 2012 to 2017, for connectivity among district hospitals and primary health centers along with sub-centers by using telemedicine or any other audio-visual media to encourage m-health. As indicated in Figure 2.3, telemedicine can be effectively divided into different forms of services given by the healthcare system by connecting the two different geographical locations by common application or website using internet service at the site of telemedicine. This cannot only treat a patient but can educate the people about the importance of preventive healthcare for good health [15].

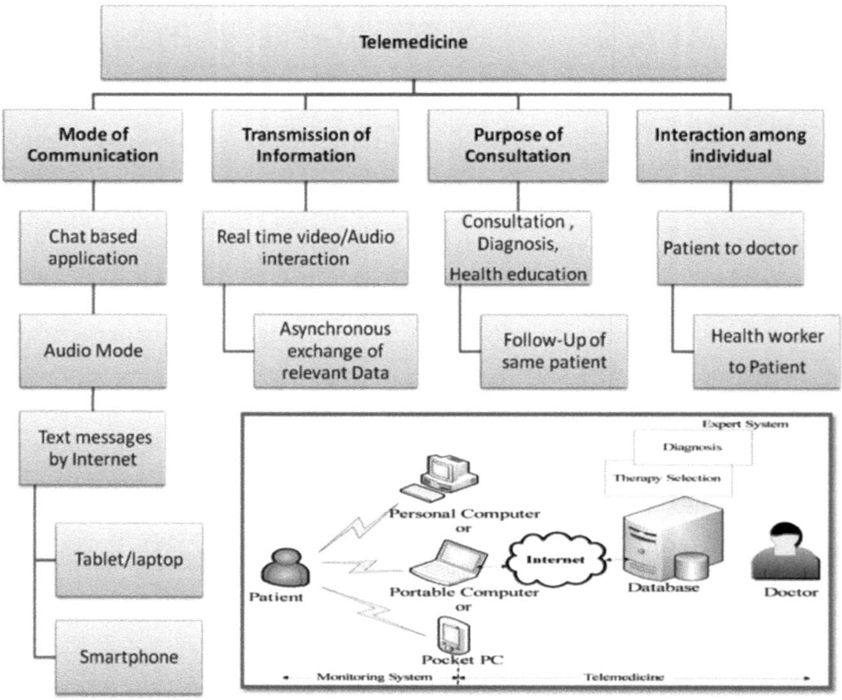

FIGURE 2.3 Classification of telemedicine on the basis of effective working model.

2.3 ROLE OF AN E-DOCTOR FOR THE SUCCESS OF TELEMEDICINE SYSTEM

Medical practitioner who is an e-doctor (not an artificial intelligence (AI) or machine learning (ML) application), entitled for providing telemedicine consultation to the person who is present at a distant location of the Indian sub-continent by the means of a website/application. The practitioner is said to be e-doctor as he/she is not present physically at the location of treatment. The e-doctor is responsible for holding the same professional and ethical guidelines as applicable to traditional doctor registered by Indian Medical Council. The foremost requirement of the e-doctor is the familiarity with the audio, video, and text mechanism of connection with a patient. The registered practitioner, who is providing consultation, must attend the online course within three years of its notification of becoming an e-doctor. After qualifying such courses, they must essentially practice telemedicine on dummy patients.

2.4 CURRENT SCENARIO

In the year 2003, the Government of India defined the National Standards on Telemedicine, later in the year 2005, government had successfully constituted a National Screening Committee for Telemedicine. Due to the widespread use of the internet by the population of all parts of the country had given hope of betterment of health by the use of different services, which was started by the year 2000 in Arragonda hospital of state Andhra Pradesh as Apollo Telehealth services included various Tele Clinics [10]. Tele radiology, tele cardiology, tele dermatology, tele pathology, tele emergency, remote condition management programs, mobile telemedicine units, tele healthcare, tele education and tele ICU (I-SEE-U a facility that enables virtual visits to ICU) has also been serving to different parts of the world like in Bangladesh, India, Kazakhstan, Maldives, Nigeria, Oman, Pakistan, Sri Lanka, Sudan, and Yemen as the hard of the non-profit organization.

Efforts for the good health of citizens of the country had been made by the Department of Health and Family Welfare, Government of India in the collaboration of the Indian Space Research Organization by launching several projects in the form of an efficient health delivery system throughout the country in the year 2008, more than 500 telemedicine centers were linked with approximately 50 specialist hospitals [12]. The project is one of the most successful projects by treating approx. 1.2 Lakh patients till December 2017 [11].

Deen Dayal Chalit Aspatal; is another example of mobile units serving the rural population as well to those, who are not able to afford the expensive treatment at the private healthcare system. Vivekananda Girija Kalyana Kendra is working for training of young women to be trained as nurse and midwifery, for efficient running treatment in various hospitals as well to the mobile units, for rural area across the country. Piramal e-Swasthya is one more social welfare scheme initiated by Piramal Healthcare Limited, which a unique telemedicine system is serving to the rural region of Rajasthan State, aimed to address the absence of doctors, inspired by the use of modern technology.

Boat clinic has been started by National Rural Health Mission (NRHM) and the Government of Assam, has been providing basic healthcare services to the islands in the Brahmaputra River through specially designed boats equipped with laboratories and pharmacies since 2005.

Narayana Health and CISCO started work collaboratively in the year 2016 for affordable, real-time assessment of medical device data, audio, high definition two ways video, electro-cardiogram, radiology, other medical reports studied by the help of web-based portal helping the mobile endpoints of patients. The biggest support is the doctors to conduct highly critical diagnostics such as Diacom viewing and detection of thrombolysis in cardiac care units of the distant location [13].

World Health Partners does not have its own network of telemedicine clinics but coordinates a network of 12,000 entrepreneurs having independent clinics located in the States of Bihar and Uttar Pradesh, by the help of a web-based application on laptops and tablets as a platform to integrate commonly available devices to measure blood pressure, pulse temperature, blood sugar, blood count, fetal sounds, and cardiac signals with provision for adding an otoscope for an ear examination and dermoscopy for the skin. The system can work in any digital environment ranging from 2G to 3G, and 4G internet [14].

Sankara Nethralaya, a well-known eye care chain of hospitals, is now offering teleophthalmology services to rural parts of the country, which includes comprehensive eye examination, training school teachers for vision screening programs, organizing diabetic retinopathy screening camps and also performs eye surgeries free of cost at the base hospital.

Sanjay Gandhi Post Graduate Institute of Medical Sciences, Uttar Pradesh, is working for telemedicine-based healthcare, by taking follow-up of patient of various branches primarily of rheumatology, endocrine surgery, nuclear medicine with the help of the Government of India. They had served in extreme locations for disaster management in well-known pilgrimages like Kailash Mansarovar and Kumbh Mela.

2.5 FUTURE POTENTIAL OF TELE-HEALTHCARE SECTOR

As in India, till date, none of the guidance or legislation has been made for practicing telemedicine through video, text, and audio-based applications. The existing legislation under the Indian Medical Council Act (1956), Drugs and Cosmetics Act (1940), and Rules (1945), Clinical Establishment (Registration and Regulation) Act (2010), Information Technology Act (2000), and the IT (Reasonable Security Practices and Procedures and Sensitive Personal Data or Information) Rules (2011), effectively regulates the practice of medicine and the information-sharing aspect. The gap between the existing laws and uncertain future rules of telemedicine is a threat not only to the patient but also to medical practitioners. Although many non-profit organizations are serving the unreached community in-country in a wide variety of forms and for them, practice guidelines will be a key enabler in fostering its growth. For the telemedicine system to be more vibrant, it is important to do a survey in the unreached areas of the country, which can help in tracing the exact need of the particular area. A public–private model can effectively work for the successful execution of a telemedicine system in India. Chances of supply of the inferior type of medicine to the rural could be possible, so surveillance systems should work efficiently to monitor any kind of shortcoming a telemedicine center is facing. In our country already public health sector is divided among various levels, as shown in Figure 2.1, so a possibility is there if all medical colleges should be connected to public health centers and sub-centers on the basis of a single platform of patient health portfolio sharing and for a fixed day, consultant present at the medical center can give consultation through skype or other online services so that unnecessary burden of traveling by the patient to medical college could be saved. The database of disease history, once created, can be saved forever; an outbreak of future disease could be predicted easily. Every aspect can only be successful after the fulfillment of awareness sessions given to the population present in the rural area for the importance of preventive healthcare, encouragement to the community for regular health check-ups, ease of safe drinking water, and knowledge of proper nutrition and sanitation. In a nutshell, IT can work hand in hand with medical services to make the livelihood of mankind.

KEYWORDS

- **e-doctor**
- **healthcare**
- **National Rural Health Mission**
- **telehealthcare**
- **telemedicine**
- **Tello Mobile Clinic**

REFERENCES

1. UNICEF, New York, (2009). *Oxford University for UNICEF, The State of the World's Children, Maternal and Newborn Health Oxford.*
2. UNICEF, New York, (2008). *United Nations Children's Fund*; *2008*. The State of the World's Children Survival.
3. Indian, P. S., Yusuf, S., Pais, P., Afzal, R., Xavier, D., Teo, K., Eikelboom, J., et al., (2009). Effects of a polypill (Polycap) on risk factors in middle-aged individuals without cardiovascular disease (TIPS): A phase II, double-blind, randomized trial, India. *Lancet, 373*(9672), 1341–1351.
4. Lim, S. S., Dandona, L., Hoisington, J. A., James, S. L., Hogan, M. C., & Gakidou, E., (2010). India's Janani Suraksha Yojana, a conditional cash transfer program to increase births in health facilities: An impact evaluation, India. *Lancet, 375*(9730), 2009–2023.
5. John, T. J., Dandona, L., Sharma, V. P., & Kakkar, M., (2011). Continuing challenge of infectious diseases in India. *Lancet, 377*(9761), 252–269.
6. Banerjee, A., Deaton, A., & Duflo, E., (2004). Health, health care, and economic development: Wealth, health, and health services in rural Rajasthan. *Am. Econ. Rev., 94*(2), 326–330.
7. Das, J., & Hammer, J., (2007). Location, location, location: Residence, wealth, and the quality of medical care in Delhi, India. *Health Aff. (Millwood), 26*(3), 338–351.
8. Raj, A., (2011). Gender equity and universal health coverage in India. *Lancet, 377*(9766), 618–619.
9. Reddy, K. S., Patel, V., Jha, P., Paul, V. K., Kumar, A. K., & Dandona, L., (2011). Towards achievement of universal health care in India by 2020: A call to action, India. *Lancet, 377*(9767), 760–768.

10. Sinha, V. D. S., Tiwari, R. N., & Kataria, R., (2012). Telemedicine in neurosurgical emergency: Indian perspective. *Asian J. Neurosurg., 7*, 75–77.
11. Mishra, S. K., Kapoor, L., & Singh, I. P., (2009). Telemedicine in India: Current scenario and the future. *Telemed. J. e-Health, 15*, 568–575.
12. Solberg, K. E., (2006). Telemedicine set to grow in India over the next 5 years. *Lancet, 371*, 17, 18.
13. Nair, P., (2014). ICT based health governance practices: The Indian experience. *J. Health Mang., 16*, 25–40.
14. SAARC, (2005). *Telemedicine Project in India.* Available at: http://www.mea.gov.in/ (accessed on 13 June 2022).
15. Balarajan, Y., Selvaraj, S., & Subramanian, S. V, (2011). Health care and equity in India. *Lancet (London, England), 377*(9764), 505–515.
16. https://healthmarketinnovations.org/programs-list/1296 (accessed on 13 June 2022).

CHAPTER 3

IoT-BASED FRAMEWORK FOR A HEALTHCARE INFORMATION SYSTEM USING CLOUD COMPUTING: OPPORTUNITIES, CHALLENGES, SECURITY, AND FUTURE DIRECTIONS

NIRANJAN LAL[1] and VISHAL SHARMA[2]

[1]*CSE, SET, Mody University, Laxmangarh, Sikar, Rajasthan, India, E-mail: niranjan_verma51@yahoo.com*

[2]*Research Scholar, CSE, SET, Mody University, Laxmangarh, Sikar, Rajasthan, India*

ABSTRACT

The exponential rate at which devices, things, or objects are connected to the internet leads to the development of a newly emerged technology called IoT. This advance that has come up with IoT needs a new network infrastructure. It will bring revolution in various fields smart home systems, domestic systems, healthcare monitoring systems, monitoring of the goods and logistics, sensor device data, vehicle data, research data, and many other related fields.

The main aim of this chapter is to include the use of the latest technologies like cloud computing and the internet of things (IoT) in

IoT and Cloud Computing-Based Healthcare Information Systems. Anand Sharma, PhD, Hiren Kumar Deva Sarma, PhD & S. R. Biradar, PhD (Eds.)

the healthcare information system, which benefits not only patients but the administration staff and hospitals as well. Traditional network infrastructure lacks in implementing the high-level network policies and interfaces and thus becoming a hurdle in IoT-enabled healthcare networks. As we know, IoT is physical objects as a network that connect the various embedded devices to communicate data and information via the internet that can connect the devices to store the huge amount of data on the cloud.

Healthcare is a hot application for various industries and researchers. IoT and cloud computing for healthcare information's system can improve the safety of the patient, staff performance, and enhancement of the efficiency in the medical industry. Overall, the IoT and cloud computing together would allow for the automation of everything around us.

In this chapter, firstly, we have given a framework based on IoT using cloud computing for healthcare information system that will provide a better solution for the medical industry. Secondly, we have discussed various benefits, challenges, opportunities, and various security challenges in healthcare future development with the solution and currently ongoing research along with future directions.

3.1 INTRODUCTION

Nowadays, the internet is used by billion customers worldwide to browse different contents for different purposes like, for e-mails, multimedia, online games, social networking, researcher data, medical data and almost for all types of data, that are available digitally. Nowadays, the internet is only the medium that used to connect the various physical objects or things for everyday life's data and for living things and for the society, even for all the aspects of our lives [12, 13], that becomes the necessity of our lives.

The internet of things (IoT) is the networking of physical devices or things. These physical devices like sensors and networks, which are embedded with software help to collect and exchange the data between different entities. To improve the efficiency and accuracy of physical objects and things, IoT can be controlled network infrastructure remotely using computer-based systems. As the IoT devices ate increasing day-by-day, which are dependent on cloud computing system for computation data and storage for local and real-time data. As the main application of IoT is in the smart homes and healthcare systems, which are popular now a days and becoming popular daily basis to monitor the health industry data of the patient. In healthcare system, IoT integration can improve the quality and effectiveness of service in a healthcare information system. Using IoT devices in the healthcare data can be monitored remotely with emergency notification systems, some examples of monitoring using IoT devices, Blood pressure and heart rate (HR) monitoring, with advanced devices, pacemakers, electronic wristbands, and advanced hearing aids.

In today's era, cloud computing is a good technology and option that help the IoT and healthcare information system storage, as cloud is the repository of database, servers, and networks through the internet. Cloud computing definition so far given by Buyya et al. in 2009 [7, 8]:

> *"Cloud is the parallel and distributed system which consists of the inter-connected and virtualized computers that are dynamically conditions presented as one or more computing resource(s) based on service-level agreements various service provider and consumers."*

Other definition of cloud computing is given by the National Institute of Standards and Technology (NIST):

> *"Cloud computing is a model of ubiquitous on demand network of shared space, which is convenient as per the use of resources (storage, servers, networks and their application and services) and services with minimal effort and cost" [2, 9].*

It is used by almost all organizations for storing and management of big data on the cloud for various business applications (HR, Payroll, ERP, etc.), as shown in Figure 3.1, and architecture level cloud computing shown in Figure 3.2.

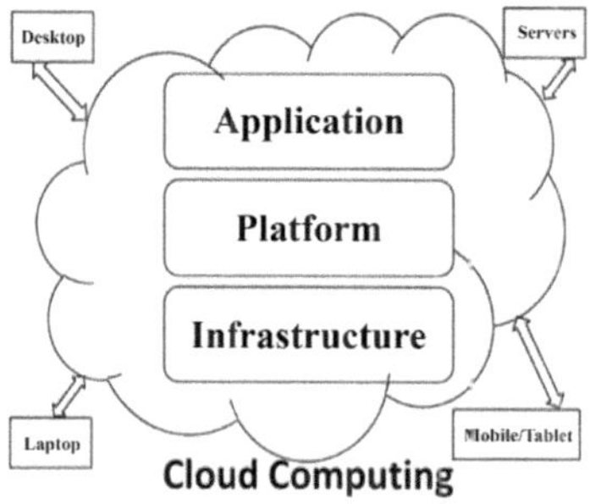

FIGURE 3.1 Cloud computing logical diagram.

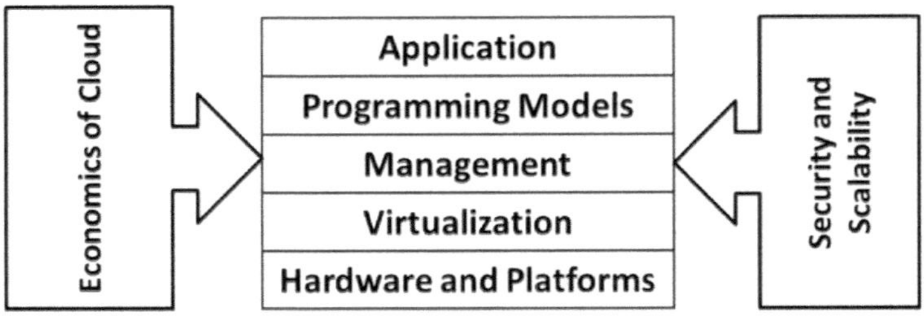

FIGURE 3.2 Architectural level cloud computing.

IoT is the high demand technology in all most all areas that connects the "things" and smart devices with collecting and other information in stimulated time at any location, any time in any environment. It helps the users to live smartly with safe lives. IoT is used in various applications like smart home systems, domestic systems, healthcare monitoring systems, monitoring of the goods and logistics, sensor device data, vehicle data, research data, and many other related fields. In this chapter, we have considered healthcare systems, in which IoT can help for the medical industry to gain quick access to health-related information. IoT is also defined as the "internet of everything," as shown in Figure 3.3.

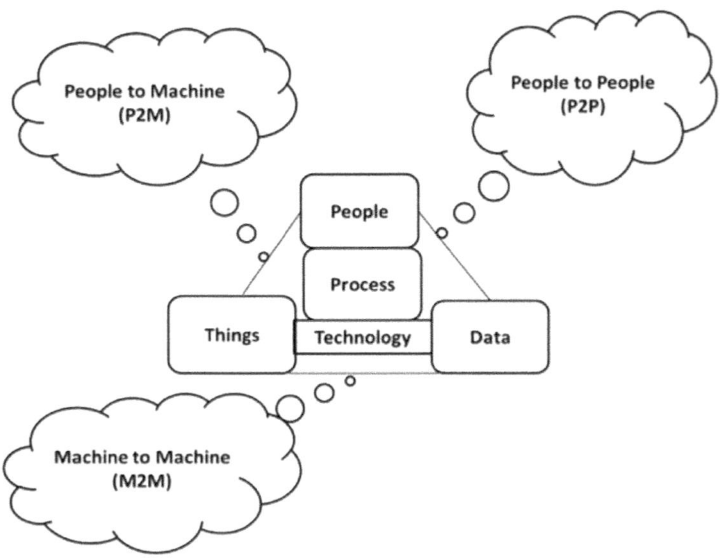

FIGURE 3.3 Internet of everything.

However, the integration of IoT technology with healthcare system may arise many challenges (data storage and management, exchange of data, security, and privacy, etc.). One of the good solutions for these challenges is cloud computing technology.

In this chapter, we have considered cloud computing because: (i) it is of high on demands; (ii) its availability; (iii) it can be used anytime, anywhere for all the users; (iv) it is distributed in nature; (v); it reduces the usage cost as per the requirement; and (vi) it is pay-as-you-go service with minimal use of servers and other resources.

3.1.1 CONTRIBUTIONS OF AUTHORS

In this chapter, we have done a survey on IoT and cloud computing and the application of IoT in healthcare information system. In this chapter, we have also covered the discussion on said technologies, applications, services, standards, and various challenges of the IoT and cloud computing in the healthcare information system. The main contributions points are given below:

- Present a survey on two hot technologies IoT and cloud computing and how both technologies help the society for healthcare system;
- Uses and integration of both the technologies in the healthcare system and issues;
- Discuss various concepts and existing application of said technologies with their advantages and disadvantages;
- Describe industry trends for IoT and cloud computing around the globe;
- Discuss the challenges, opportunities, security issues of both the technologies for healthcare system;
- Various technologies associated with IoT, IoT device features, scenario, and future of IoT in healthcare in industry setting;
- Discuss the future research directions.

This chapter is organized as follows after the introduction section. Section 3.2 covers the related work and background related to our research. Section 3.3 covers how IoT and cloud computing is integrated into the healthcare information sector, which is again divided into many subsections for the discussion related integration, advantages, disadvantages, trends features of IoT, cloud computing, and healthcare systems. Section 3.4 covers the proposed framework for healthcare information systems using IoT and Cloud computing. Section 3.5 discussed the various opportunities and challenges in the healthcare system. In Section 3.6, the main security issues are covered. The second last Section 3.7 mentions some future of said technologies with the healthcare system, and finally, Section 3.8 conclude the chapter.

3.2 RELATED WORK AND BACKGROUND

In this section, we have covered the contents of some researchers who have contributed on cloud computing and IoT in healthcare information systems.

The paper by Islam et al. [16] reviews the various applications and services that can be integrate healthcare system with IoT, and how it can be implemented in medical industry for enhancement in the management. They have also reviewed the various security issues and difficulties that can arise in IoT and healthcare information systems. Mutlag et al. [17] have identified some factors for resource management of healthcare data in the cloud. They have also covered the fog computing in IoT healthcare system with limitations of recent approaches. Kumari et al. [18] include the fog computing description with their challenges and opportunities; they introduce three-layered architecture for real-time data and application of healthcare's information system. García et al. [19] proposed a framework based on fog computing for mobile patients, using their approach response time decreased four times as compared to other approaches. Kraemer et al. [20], written a paper that completed the survey on fog computing requirement for healthcare system with fog computing components and network. Ahmadi et al. [21], also described the IoT architecture for healthcare's information system using cloud computing with some critical issues related to healthcare system and IoT. In a paper given by Baker et al. [22], different elements requirement for IoT in healthcare information have been given like various types of sensors and communication approaches. They have also proposed a framework for IoT healthcare system with cloud computing approach for storing the IoT healthcare data. Farahani et al. [23], introduced a hardware and software e-health ecosystem on recent IoT e-health research. They have also discussed the various challenges, security issues in network and IoT devices with future directions. In a paper written by Hassanalieragh et al. [27], identified various challenges in IoT for healthcare information system with the opportunities for integration of both. Guigang et al. [28] proposed a method, in which we can set some specific rules for the massive IoT medical sensors information to monitor the information of the users and the patients, these rules can also execute rules and for management purposes when some events occur.

In spite of the widespread use of cloud computing, it is still an active area of research, there are many frameworks have been proposed and implemented with IoT in health services Sahi [29]. They have application, security, and efficiency domains of IoT in health services. They have also addressed implementation issues like communication entities and technologies, hardware structure, and data storage flow. A framework was proposed by Zhao et al. [30] for remotely monitored elderly people. Hossain et al. [31] have presented a healthcare industrial IoT for a real-time health monitoring information system, and this proposed system analyzes patients' healthcare data to avoid death situations. Gope et al. [32] presented the body sensor network (BSN) features with IoT developments that can be used for patient data collection and monitoring.

3.3 HOW IOT AND CLOUD COMPUTING HELPS TOGETHER IN HEALTHCARE SECTOR?

The IoT is a hot topic for the researchers, academics, sectors, organizations, and industries. It connects several objects and "things" without involvement of the human into a network and computing resources, it can be used for patient's real-time monitoring using wireless sensor network (WSN) communication [3, 4] for HR, respiration rate (RR), and blood pressure (BP) using this approach easily in a second [5].

IoT enabled various things and the devices across the globe to store the data and process them at a later stage. However, the huge gap between data collection and the ability to process and analyze acts as a major deterrent to realize this potential opportunity. This gap can be filled by creating a framework by helping cloud computing and IoT together, which is the is the latest breakthrough that combines diverse technologies connected via the internet to deliver solutions in varied locations and environments on a real-time basis. Healthcare system can gain the benefit with these emerging technologies with managing anything of medical industry from managing chronic diseases to preventing different health conditions.

3.3.1 CLOUD COMPUTING BENEFITS IN HEALTHCARE SYSTEM

Cloud computing can provide a flexible solution for hospitals. Hospitals can use the store the large volume of data and information related to various stakeholders like employees, staff, doctors, patient data, testing data, and solutions in a secured environment with remote facilities to access the cloud resources and networks. By the BCC research [14], the global healthcare cloud computing market is expected to hit $35 billion by 2022, with 11.6% annual growth rate. As per the survey done in 2018 [14], 69% of respondent's hospital are not planned to store their data on the cloud. In this section, we have given some benefits that can help the medical industry and the hospitals to make the decision for moving their centralized data on the cloud [14]:

- This approach can provide the efficient storage records digitally, with less loss of records;
- Streamline patient data for proper care with less error rate;
- It can decrease the cost of data storage with backup facility and security of patients;
- It can also make use of big data with flexibility and scalability;
- It enhances the patient safety with less treatment time efficiently and accurately;
- It opens and enhance the way for medical researchers;
- It can also work with heterogeneous data and resources.

3.3.2 IOT ADVANTAGES AND DISADVANTAGES IN HEALTHCARE INFORMATION SYSTEM

One of the facilities of IoT for information systems is that it can provide services anywhere, anytime, and on any media [33]. In healthcare, IoT enables the possible benefits for the organizations to exchange the data. Here, we have covered some advantages and disadvantages of IoT in healthcare system [24, 25] that help for better management, convenient, comfort to improve the quality of life. By using cloud-based IoT services, we can transform a complete healthcare system using some other technologies like ZigBee, Wi-Fi, etc. It can be used in several applications, given below:

- Design of database;
- Integration of cloud and hospital information system;
- Real-time sensor for data collection;
- e-storage of heterogeneous and multimedia data (text, images, videos, excel sheets, etc.) [61–66];
- Healthcare data, vehicles, stock market, social media, organization, and industries data.

3.3.2.1 ADVANTAGES

IoT in healthcare system in data centralization carries many significant benefits:

- Easy to monitor remotely patient data with minimal error rates;
- Using IoT-based sensor data occurrence of health problems may be decreased;
- Using IoT-based healthcare doctors, staff, and testing cost can be reduced with good efficiency;
- Using IoT-based healthcare system, data can be access anytime, anywhere with heterogeneous media with mobility facility to the users;
- Automated data collection with using IoT on cloud and/or other storage mediums;
- Reduced the wastage of time of doctors, testing, and other solution for patient treatments;
- Real-time monitoring of data and information with security;
- Continues information to patients for proper treatment with improved healthcare management;
- Enhancements in the chronic disease treatment efficiently;
- All-around technological enhancement with IoT and cloud computing.

3.3.2.2 DISADVANTAGES

Alternatively, there are disadvantages of implementation the IoT in healthcare system that include:

- Restriction due to global healthcare regulations;
- Complexity due to IoT diverse and complex networks;
- Interoperability and compatibility problems due to heterogeneous manufactures and data;
- Unauthorized access to centralization of data and information;
- Generating huge amount health and other data;
- Security and privacy problems is higher side if any personal information is hacked.

3.3.3 IOT DRIVE GROWTH OF HEALTHCARE CLOUD AND CLINICAL APPLICATIONS

As healthcare cloud is expanding in the organizations for clinician applications, IoT data, data storage is flexible and scalable environment. The healthcare uses of cloud computing are expected to grow by 18% through 2023, given in Ref. [15] with uses of various services (SaaS, IaaS) on public, private, and/or hybrid cloud. It will be used for both clinicians and non-clinical applications in the healthcare system. Clinical applications are growing due to an increase in chronic disease and an aging population that increases the patient's data rapidly.

It provides a benefit to organizations in terms of storage, and management of various hardware resources at their end, that will be easily managed by both IoT and cloud computing technologies remotely by various cloud service providers. That scale up or scale down their IT infrastructure (processing power, storage, networking, and users) easily in their environment with modern care facilities.

3.3.4 INTEGRATING CLOUD COMPUTING AND IOT

Integration of IoT, fog computing [10] and cloud computing for healthcare information system is shown in Figure 3.4, using this integration medical industry can access and share the medical data using less infrastructure and resources transparently in pay-as-you-go fashion over the network, and performing operations that meet growing needs [6, 12] and uses of portable devices and other technologies like artificial intelligence (AI) [11].

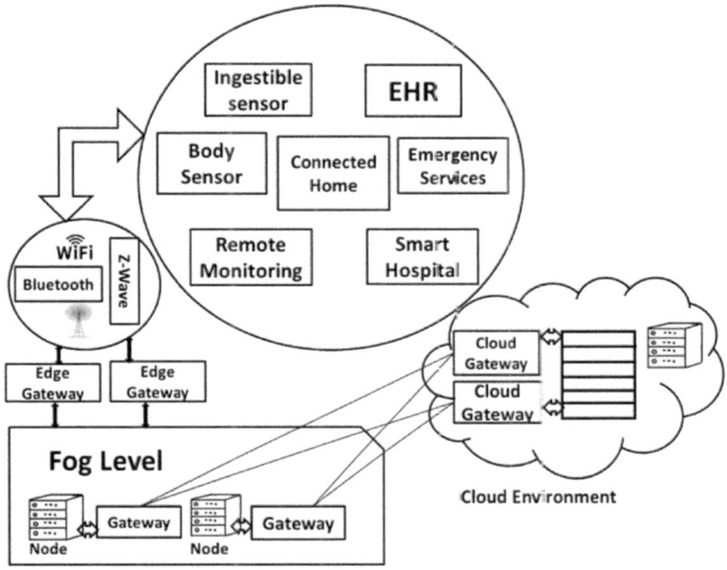

FIGURE 3.4 Layout of integration of IoT and cloud computing with healthcare systems.

3.3.4.1 HEALTHCARE APPLICATIONS AND IOT FEATURES

In IoT and healthcare applications, there are many types of research going on, and it is adopting various other features and innovations to enhance the performance of healthcare information systems. Some features of the IoT devices are [39]: (i) wearability; (ii) long working time; (iii) constancy or stability; (iv) low participation degree of users; (v) possessing data interim storage mechanism; and (vi) IoT scenario in the healthcare industry.

IoT in healthcare information system improve the services in the following aspects [40, 42]: (i) sensor-based electronic flow of information with screening and assessment in-home and other environments to reduce the pressure of hospitals; (ii) proactive model for patients admission and other events; (iii) individual monitoring with improved personalization of healthcare process positive impact on states of patients psychologically;

(iv) improved clinical management of medical data and services; (v) self-care diagnostic processes, diagnoses, and monitoring critical diseases and vital signs using smartphones; (vi) optimized and less of diagnosis with automatic testing and monitoring other parameters related to humans.

Figure 3.5 shows the uses of IoT and cloud computing in hospital environment, how medical situation looks in hospital and medical environment, how various things like sensors, EHR, RFID (for scanning purpose), hospital system, network hubs (connecting device), hospital and doctors, and cloud computing components are connected via internet to store records of labs, health records electronically and prescription histories [34–42].

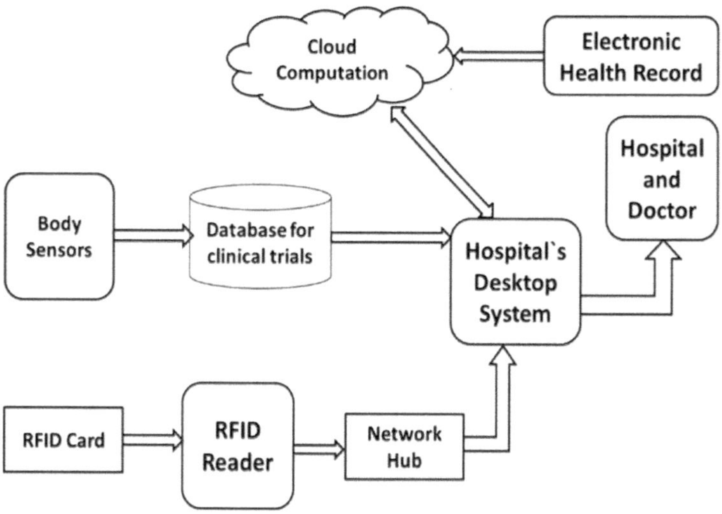

FIGURE 3.5 Layout of IoT and cloud computing with hospital environment.

3.3.4.2 *IOT TRENDS IN HEALTHCARE*

There are many trends that are going nowadays in the development and implementation of startups worldwide: (i) wearables continue to top the market; (ii) surgical robotics become a common reality; (iii) integration of other prominent technologies with the IoT expands the horizon; (iv) internet of medical things (IoMT); (v) mobility using smartphones, etc.

3.3.5 OTHER SUPPORTING TECHNOLOGIES FOR IOT

There are many open challenges that are addressed by new research and investigation, due to heterogeneous manufacturers, complex deployment. Many other technologies are also supporting for IoT, such as RFID, WSN, smartphones, barcodes, cloud computing, etc., are shown in Figure 3.6.

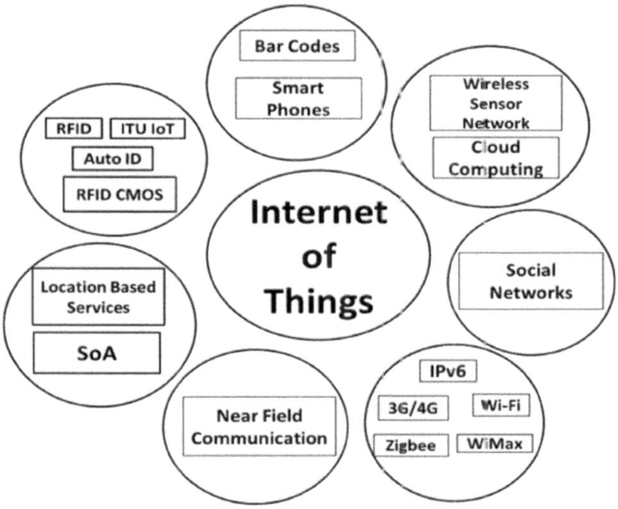

FIGURE 3.6 Supporting technologies for IoT.

3.4 PROPOSED IOT FRAMEWORK FOR HEALTHCARE INFORMATION SYSTEM

In this section, we have given our proposed framework for IoT and cloud computing in healthcare information system. In healthcare information with IoT, we have divided it's in basic components given below which are used for specific purposes separately [56, 57]:

- Topology consists of physical configuration of the things, application, and use cases;
- Structure consists of physical components and various techniques to connects them;
- Platform consists of frameworks, protocols, and various libraries used for IoT-based healthcare information system.

In the increasing demand of the medical industries setting, we have given an IoT-based framework for healthcare information system using cloud computing is shown in Figure 3.7. This framework is based on the cloud services like platform as a service (PaaS) and infrastructure as a service (IaaS), that may help patients to find the best care at the optimal cost in secured storage and shared health information [58].

By using our proposed IoT-based framework with cloud computing in healthcare may offers several advantages:

- Scalability of resources;
- High reliability and efficiency;
- Virtualization;
- Remote accessibility with faster deployment;
- Use of latest technology capability – cloud, IoT, cloud-based radio-frequency identification (RFID), on demand services, backup, etc.;
- Resource sharing facility and reduction in operation cost;
- Proper management and efficient monitoring of medical data;
- Smart health monitoring, information transmission and tracking management;
- One main benefit of this integration, it can reduce the latency and saves the bandwidth.

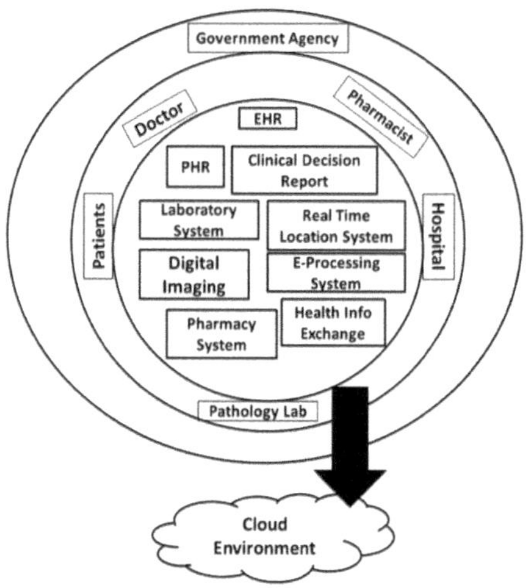

FIGURE 3.7 Proposed IoT-based framework with cloud computing in healthcare information system.

Different layers of our proposed approach in the broader way are shown in Figure 3.8. The main components of both layers are given in diagram with their uses. This is divided in two basic layers: (i) local storage environment – consist of data perception, data aggregation and processing, local security, and access layers, these all provide specific purpose; and (ii) cloud storage environment that is consists of cloud security layer, presentation layer, application, service, and business layers, for computing purpose over the network [48–55].

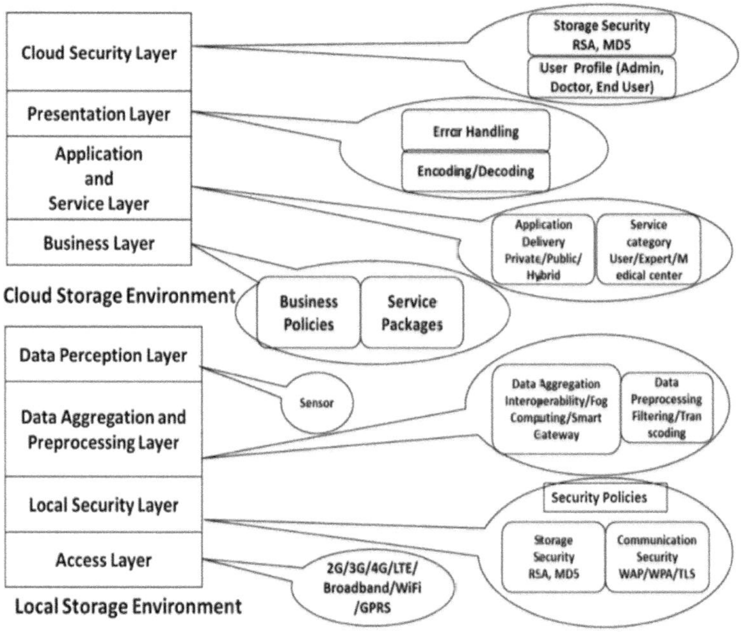

FIGURE 3.8 Platform of IoT framework with cloud computing in healthcare information system.

3.5 OPPORTUNITIES AND CHALLENGES OF INTEGRATING IOT AND CLOUD COMPUTING IN HEALTHCARE INFORMATION SYSTEMS

Due to increasing the population and demands for health services and increasing the diseases like flu, plague disease, corona virus (COVID-19), many challenges may arise for collecting and exchanging the health information, these challenges may stope the success of integration of IoT and cloud computing and other technologies with healthcare information system.

Here we are discussing some challenges that we have find out from various sources and survey that we have done [43–55]:

- Underdeveloped initiatives, integration problems of IoT and cloud computing and healthcare information system.
- How to handle the unified data of patients from healthcare providers?
- How motivate the teamwork of care among healthcare practitioners?
- How to handle the communication deficiency among clinics, departments, staff, employees, healthcare professionals?
- How to verify the patient's information?
- How to handle security, privacy, and risk failure if any healthcare information system has any loopholes?
- Information storage shortage at a single location and patient consent.
- Compatibility and interoperability issue of medical data and technology.
- How to handle heterogeneity problem of manufacture and heterogeneous data using IoT or cloud computing with healthcare information system?
- Geographical access problem, no global clock.
- Different workflow and overlapping of function in the hospital.
- Lack of storage capacity, memory, and technology dependency of hospitals.
- Regular update problem.

In this section, we have found some challenges related to IoT and cloud computing and healthcare information system. There may be more challenges, which can be identified by new researchers and take care these for new development and initiates.

3.6 MAIN RISKS IN IOT HEALTHCARE

Figure 3.9 shows the main risks that may be raised in the integration of IoT with cloud computing in healthcare information system [51–55].

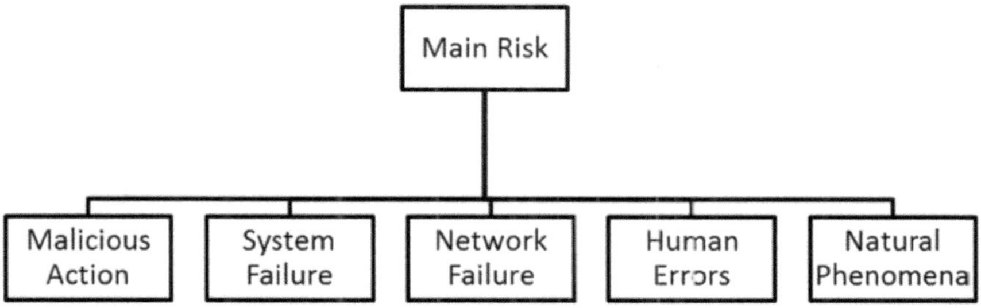

FIGURE 3.9 Main risks in IoT healthcare system.

Other security challenges are: (i) memory constraints; (ii) speed of computation; (iii) power consumption; (iv) scalability; (v) communication channel; and (vi) security updates.

3.7 FUTURE OF IOT AND CLOUD COMPUTING IN HEALTHCARE INFORMATION SYSTEM

There are many big leaders like Apple, Google, and Samsung and many others are involved and investing in the development and improvement of the health services. Figure 3.10 shows the uses of devices in millions at the end of 2015 to 2020 globally [59]:

- A business insider report [59], IoT healthcare technology market will increase to $400 billion by 2022, this is because of increasing the demand, technology improvements and development like 5G connectivity, IoT, AI, machine learning (ML), deep learning in healthcare IT software [59].
- By the end of 2020, many organizations will provide employment only in the healthcare-related development [59].
- Experts said the market value will be increases healthcare cloud computing exponentially by 2020 and beyond. This hits $8.5 in 2018, by 2025, it's expected to be $55 billion [60].
- Healing at home with peace of mind.
- Independent health monitoring.
- Medicines on the right time with well diagnosis.

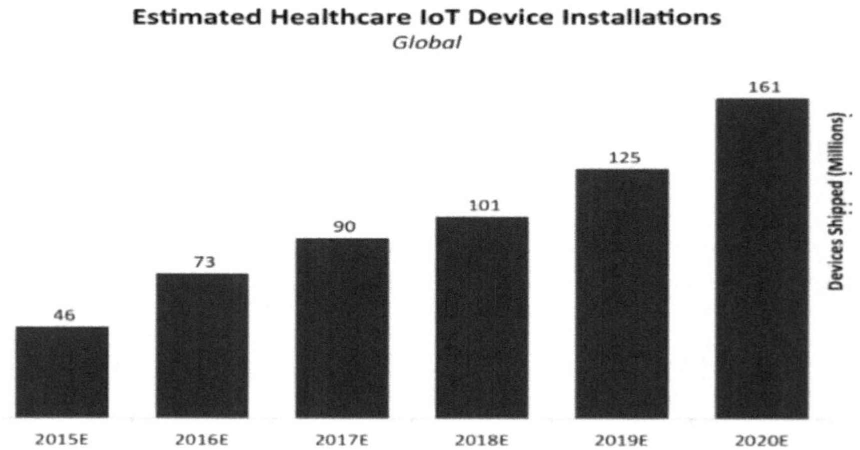

FIGURE 3.10 Increment in healthcare device installation in millions from 2015 to 2020.

3.8 CONCLUSION

As the IoT and cloud computing are growing technologies in healthcare information system. In this chapter, we have studied many research papers related to IoT, cloud computing, fog computing, healthcare information system, various traditional approaches given by many experts of these areas. In this chapter, we have proposed a framework based on IoT and cloud computing in healthcare information system, we have only proposed this framework, using this framework many workload of the medical industry can reduce and improve for health services, our approach can provide various benefits to the medical industry and open the new area of research for IT professionals and medical professionals.

Our integrated system may benefit various stakeholders like patients, administration staff, and hospitals over the traditional network infrastructures. In this chapter, we have also discussed the advantages and disadvantages of IoT and cloud computing in healthcare systems and various trends, features, opportunities, and challenges that open new research areas for new development and innovation. Finally, we have covered some points for the future of the IoT and cloud computing in healthcare information systems.

KEYWORDS

- **artificial intelligence**
- **body sensor network**
- **cloud computing**
- **healthcare**
- **hospital information system**
- **infrastructure as a service**
- **Internet of things**

REFERENCES

1. Johnston, S., (2013). *Seminar on Collaboration as a Service – Cloud Computing.* https://www.cloudcomputing-news.net/news/2013/aug/19/cio-man-behind-Cloud-what-Cloud-solution-will-really-transform-business/ (accessed on 13 June 2022).
2. Lal, N., et al., (2013). Detailed dominant approach cloud computing integration with WSN. In: *9th International Conference on Heterogeneous Networking for Quality, Reliability, Security, and Robustness* (Vol. 115). Published in springer digital library, lecture notes of the institute for computer sciences, social informatics, and telecommunications engineering.
3. Abidi, B., Jilbab, A., & Haziti, M. E., (2017). Wireless sensor networks in biomedical: Wireless body area networks. In: *Europe and MENA Cooperation Advances in Information and Communication Technologies* (pp. 321–329). Springer: Berlin/Heidelberg, Germany.
4. Xu, Q., Ren, P., Song, H., & Du, Q., (2016). Security enhancement for IoT communications exposed to eavesdroppers with uncertain locations. *IEEE Access, 4*, 2840–2853.
5. Scuotto, V., Ferraris, A., & Bresciani, S., (2016). Internet of things: Applications and challenges in smart cities: A case study of IBM smart city projects. *Bus. Process Manag. J., 22*, 357–367.
6. Stergiou, C., Psannis, K. E., Kim, B. G., & Gupta, B., (2018). Secure integration of IoT and cloud computing. *Future Gener. Comput. Syst., 78*, 964–975.
7. Senyo, P., Addae, E., & Boateng, R., (2018). Cloud computing research: A review of research themes, frameworks, methods, and future research directions. *Int. J. Info. Manag., 38*(1), 128–139.
8. Buyya, R., Yeo, C., Venugopal, S., Broberg, J., & Brandic, I., (2009). Cloud computing and emerging IT platforms: Vision, hype, and reality for delivering computing as the 5th utility. *Future Generat. Comput. Syst., 25*, 599–616.

9. Mell, P., & Grance, T., (2011). *The NIST Definition of Cloud Computing.* Special publication 800-145. National Institute of Standards and Technology, U.S. Department of Commerce, USA.
10. Truong, H. L., & Dustdar, S., (2015). Principles for engineering IoT cloud systems. *IEEE Cloud Comput., 2*, 68–76.
11. Minh, D. L., Sadeghi-Niaraki, A., Huy, H. D., Min, K., & Moon, H., (2018). Deep learning approach for short-term stock trends prediction based on two-stream gated recurrent unit network. *IEEE Access, 6*, 55392–55404.
12. Paul, P. V., & Saraswathi, R., (2017). The internet of things: A comprehensive survey. In: *Proceedings of the 2017 International Conference on Computation of Power, Energy Information and Communication (ICCPEIC)* (pp. 421–426). Melmaruvathur, India.
13. Mitchell, S., Villa, N., Stewart-Weeks, M., & Lange, A., (2013). *The Internet of Everything for Cities. Connect. People, Process. Data, Things to Improve 'Livability' of Cities Communities* (pp. 1–21). Cisco.
14. *Healthcare Cloud Computing Market on Track for $35B by 2022.* https://www.healthcaredive.com/news/healthcare-cloud-computing-market-on-track-for-35b-by-2022/516066/ (accessed on 13 June 2022).
15. *Clinical Applications, IoT Drive Growth of Healthcare Cloud.* https://hitinfrastructure.com/news/clinical-applications-iot-drive-growth-of-healthcare-cloud (accessed on 13 June 2022).
16. Islam, S. R., Kwak, D., Kabir, M. H., Hossain, M., & Kwak, K. S., (2015). The internet of things for health care: A comprehensive survey. *IEEE Access, 3*, 678–708.
17. Mutlag, A. A., Ghani, M. K. A., Arunkumar, N., Mohamed, M. A., & Mohd, O., (2019). Enabling technologies for fog computing in healthcare IoT systems. *Future Gener. Comput. Syst., 90*, 62–78.
18. Kumari, A., Tanwar, S., Tyagi, S., & Kumar, N., (2018). Fog computing for healthcare 4.0 environment: Opportunities and challenges. *Comput. Electr. Eng., 72*, 1–13.
19. García-Valls, M., Calva-Urrego, C., & García-Fornes, A., (2020). Accelerating smart e-health services execution at the fog computing infrastructure. *Future Gener. Comput. Syst.* 2018.10.1016/j.future.2018.07.001.
20. Kraemer, F. A., Braten, A. E., Tamkittikhun, N., & Palma, D., (2017). Fog computing in healthcare: A review and discussion. *IEEE Access, 5*, 9206–9222.
21. Ahmadi, H., Arji, G., Shahmoradi, L., Safdari, R., Nilashi, M., & Alizadeh, M., (2018). The application of internet of things in healthcare: A systematic literature review and classification. *Univer. Access Inf. Soc.,* 1–33. 10.1007/s10209-018-0618-4.
22. Baker, S. B., Xiang, W., & Atkinson, I., (2017). Internet of things for smart healthcare: Technologies, challenges, and opportunities. *IEEE Access, 5*, 26521–26544.
23. Farahani, B., Firouzi, F., Chang, V., Badaroglu, M., Constant, N., & Mankodiya, K., (2018). Towards fog-driven IoT e-health: Promises and challenges of IoT in medicine and healthcare. *Future Gener. Comput. Syst., 78*, 659–676.
24. Lim, A. K., & Thuemmler, C., (2015). Opportunities and challenges of internet-based health interventions in the future internet. In: *2015 12th International Conference on IEEE Information Technology-New Generations (ITNG)* (pp. 567–573).

25. Keh, H. C., et al., (2014). Integrating unified communications and internet of m-health things with micro wireless physiological sensors. *Journal of Applied Science and Engineering, 17*(3), 319–328.
26. Nandyala, C. S., & Kim, H. K., (2016). From cloud to fog and IoT-based real-time U-healthcare monitoring for smart homes and hospitals. *Int. J. Smart Home, 10*, 187–196.
27. Hassanalieragh, M., Page, A., Soyata, T., Sharma, G., Aktas, M., Mateos, G., Kantarci, B., & Andreescu, S., (2015). Health monitoring and management using internet of things (IoT) sensing with cloud-based processing: Opportunities and challenges. In: *2015 IEEE International Conference on Services Computing* (pp. 285–292). doi: 10.1109/SCC.2015.47.
28. Guigang, Z., Chao, L., Yong, Z., Chunxiao, X., & Jijiang, Y., (2012). SemanMedical: A kind of semantic medical monitoring system model based on the IoT sensors. *IEEE 14th International Conference e-Health Networking, Applications and Services Healthcom* (pp. 238–243).
29. Sahi, M. A., Abbas, H., Saleem, K., et al., (2017) *A Survey on Privacy Preservation in e-Healthcare Environment.* IEEE.
30. Zhao, W., Wang, C., & Nakahira, Y., (2011). Medical application on the internet of things. In: *Proceedings of IET International Conference on Communication Technology and Application (ICCTA 2011)* (pp. 660–665). Beijing, China.
31. Hossain, M. S., & Muhammad, G., (2016). Cloud-assisted industrial internet of things (IIoT) enabled framework for health monitoring. *Comput. Netw., 101*, 192–202.
32. Gope, P., & Hwang, T., (2016). BSN-care: A secure IoT-based modern healthcare. *IEEE Sens. J., 16*(5), 1368–1376.
33. Ullah, K., Shah, M. A., & Zhang, S., (2016). Effective ways to use internet of things in the field of medical and smart health care. In: *2016 International Conference on Intelligent Systems Engineering (ICISE)* (pp. 372–379). Islamabad, Pakistanpp: IEEE.
34. Serrano, K. J., et al., (2016). Willingness to exchange health information via mobile devices: Findings from a population-based survey. *Annals of Family Medicine*, 34–40.
35. Roy, A., Zalzala, A. M. S., & Kumar, A., (2016). Disruption of things: A model to facilitate adoption of IoT-based innovations by the urban poor. *Procedia Engineering*, pp. 199–209.
36. Sallabi, F., & Shuaib, K., (2016). Internet of things network management system architecture for smart healthcare. In: *2016 Sixth International Conference on Digital Information and Communication Technology and its Applications (DICTAP)* (pp. 165–170).
37. Li, S., Da Xu, L., & Zhao, S., (2015). The internet of things: A survey. *Information Systems Frontiers, 17*(2), 243–259.
38. Dimitrov, D. V., (2016). Medical internet of things and big data in healthcare. *Healthcare Informatics Research, 22*(3), 156–163.
39. Da Xu, L., He, W., & Li, S., (2014). Internet of things in industries: A survey. *IEEE Transactions on Industrial Informatics, 10*(4), 2233–2243.
40. Santos, A., Macedo, J., Costa, A., & Nicolau, M. J., (2014). Internet of things and smart objects for m-health monitoring and control. *Procedia Technology*, 1351–1360.

41. Mohammed, D., & Ahmed, M., (2019). IoT service utilization in healthcare. *Internet of Things (IoT) for Automated and Smart Applications*. doi: http://dx.doi.org/10.5772/intechopen.86014.
42. Al-Fuqaha, A., Guizani, M., Mohammadi, M., Aledhari, M., & Ayyash, M., (2015). Internet of things: A survey on enabling technologies, protocols, and applications. *IEEE Communication Surveys and Tutorials, 17*(4), 2347–2376.
43. Park, H., et al., (2015). Can a health information exchange save healthcare costs? Evidence from a pilot program in South Korea. *International Journal of Medical Informatics, 84*(9), 658–666.
44. Song, Z., et al., (2012). *A Survey of Primary Care Doctors in 10 Countries Shows Progress in Use of Health Information Technology*. Less in Other Areas.
45. Latif, A., Othman, M., Suliman, A., & Daher, A., (2016). Current status, challenges and needs for pilgrim health record management sharing network the case of Malaysia. *International Archives of Medicine, 9*(1), 1–10.
46. Sujansky, W., & Kunz, D., (2015). A standard based model for the sharing of patient generated health information with electronic health records. *Personal and Ubiquitous Computing*, pp. 9–25.
47. Wang, J. Y., Ho, H. Y., Chen, J. D., Chai, S., Tai, C. J., & Chen, Y. F., (2015). Attitudes toward inter-hospital electronic patient record exchange: Discrepancies among physicians, medical record staff, and patients. *BMC Health Services Research.*
48. Hollis, K. F., (2016). To share or not to share: Ethical acquisition and use of medical data. *AMIA Joint Summits on Translational Science Proceedings,* pp. 420–427.
49. Everson, J., et al., (2016). Health information exchange associated with improved emergency department care through faster accessing of patient information from outside organizations. *Journal of the American Medical Informatics Association, 169*(10), 1023–1028.
50. Abomhara, M., & Køien, G. M., (2016). Towards an access control model for collaborative healthcare systems. In: *Proc. 9th Int. Jt. Conf. Biomed. Eng. Syst. Technol. (BIOSTEC 2016)* (Vol. 5, pp. 213–222).
51. Riordan, F., Papoutsi, C., Reed, J. E., Marston, C., Bell, D., & Majeed, A., (2015). Patient and public attitudes towards informed consent models and levels of awareness of electronic health records in the UK. *International Journal of Medical Informatics*, 237–247.
52. Hsieh, P., (2015). 'Physicians' acceptance of electronic medical records exchange: An extension of the decomposed TPB model with institutional trust and perceived risk. *International Journal of Medical Informatics*, 1–14.
53. Mac McCullough, J., et al., (2014). Electronic health information exchange in underserved settings: examining initiatives in small physician practices & community health centers. *BMC Health Services Research.*
54. Swain, M. J., & Kharrazi, H., (2015). Feasibility of 30-day hospital readmission prediction modeling based on health information exchange data. *International Journal of Medical Informatics*, 1048–1056.
55. Zhang, H., Han, B. T., & Tang, Z., (2017). Constructing a nationwide interoperable health information system in China: The case study of Sichuan province. *Health Policy and Technology*, 142–151.

56. Yang, Z., Zhou, Q., Lei, L., Zheng, K., & Xiang, W., (2016). An IoT-cloud based wearable ECG monitoring system for smart healthcare. *J Med. Syst., 40*, 286.
57. Almotiri, S. H., Khan, M. A., & Alghamdi, M. A., (2016). Mobile health (m-health) system in the context of IoT. In: *Proceedings of the IEEE International Conference on Future Internet of Things and Cloud Workshops (FiCloudW)* (pp. 39–42). Vienna, Austria.
58. Tyagi, S., Agarwal, A., & Maheshwari, P., (2016). A conceptual framework for IoT-based healthcare system using cloud computing. In: *2016 6th International Conference – Cloud System and Big Data Engineering (Confluence)* (pp. 503–507).
59. *IoT in Healthcare: Use Cases, Trends, Advantages, and Disadvantages*. https://dzone.com/articles/iot-in-healthcare-use-cases-trends-advantages-and (accessed on 13 June 2022).
60. *Five Trends in Healthcare Cloud Computing for 2020*. https://www.healthitoutcomes.com/doc/trends-in-healthcare-cloud-computing-for-0001 (accessed on 13 June 2022).
61. Lal, N., & Qamar, S., (2015). Comparison of ranking algorithm with dataspace. In: *ICACEA*, (pp. 565–572).
62. Lal, N., Singh, M., & Yadav, S., (2019). Rule-based wrappers for a dataspace system. *IJITEE, 8*(6C), 80–90.
63. Lal, N., Qamar, S., & Shivani, S., (2016). Search ranking for heterogeneous data over dataspace. *Indian Journal of Science and Technology (Scopus Indexed), 9*(36), 1–9.
64. Lal, N., & Kaur, N., (2018). Clustering of social networking data using sparkR in big data. Springer Nature Singapore Pvt. Ltd. *Communications in Computer and Information Science (CCIS), 906*, 217–226.
65. Lal, N., Qamar, S., & Kalra, M., (2017). K-mean clustering algorithm approach for data mining of heterogeneous data. *ICT4SD, LNNS, Springer Proceeding, 10*, 61–70.
66. Lal, N., & Kalara, M., (2016). *Data Mining of Heterogeneous Data with Research Challenges* (pp. 1–6). Presented in CDAN, Published in IEEE Digital Library.
67. Minh, D. L., Md Jalil, P., Dongil, H., Kyungbok, M., & Hyeonjoon, M., (2019). *A Survey on Internet of Things and Cloud Computing for Healthcare, 8*, 768. doi: 10.3390/electronics8070768.

CHAPTER 4

A STUDY ON UNINTERRUPTED SECURITY IN IoT-BASED HEALTHCARE SYSTEMS

ANIRUDHI THANVI,[1] RAGHAV SHARMA,[1] BHANVI MENGHANI,[1] MANISH KUMAR,[2] and SUNIL KUMAR JANGIR[3]

[1]*Department of Information Technology, Jaipur Engineering College and Research Center, Jaipur, Rajasthan, India, E-mail: ani12thanvi@gmail.com (A. Thanvi)*

[2]*Department of Biomedical Engineering, Mody University of Science and Technology, Laxmangarh, Rajasthan, India*

[3]*Department of Computer Science and Engineering, School of Engineering and Technology, Mody University of Science and Technology, Laxmangarh, Rajasthan, India*

ABSTRACT

The internet of things (IoT) is the summation of interconnected smart devices/objects globally through the internet. The swift evolution of IoT and extensive growth of wireless automation open up the recently developed possibilities of extension in many realms, for example, transportation, agriculture, education, and mainly in the medicare area. Initiating the IoT through healthcare implementations brings a lot more advantages,

IoT and Cloud Computing-Based Healthcare Information Systems. Anand Sharma, PhD, Hiren Kumar Deva Sarma, PhD & S. R. Biradar, PhD (Eds.)

inclusive of being cost-efficient through lowered cost of visiting the healthcare centers, healthcare supply charges, conveying charges, human assets costs, and indemnity costs. It conducts to add on the precedence of enhanced grade of care in healthcare. Collaborating healthcare and the latest technologies present in the current scenario leads to the innovation of smart health. The purpose of smart health is to issue medical provision to patients whenever and wherever. The smart health observing method is majorly linked with the wireless network channel which is the utmost endangered for threats. Nevertheless, many attacks are perceived that can jeopardize these health monitoring systems and applications. These attacks are inclusive of timing-based and fingerprint snooping, denial of service (DoS) attack, select, and forwarding attacks, replay attacks, and sensor attack. In this chapter, we will discuss about the end-to-end data security system required for IoT healthcare schemes.

4.1 INTRODUCTION

Modern-day civilization relies on the censorious framework and the amenities they give, here in concern to critical societal services (CSS). They supply us with water, heat, electricity, and various methods to tour, trade, and communicate. Conventionally, these essential structures are kept separately to prevent safety warnings and interference in the presentations. Wellness program implementation is depicting majorly the technologies related to the internet of things (IoT), and it is named as the implementations which are IoT based in wellness programs or healthcare. The civilization leads to development in technologies and wireless networks, and the latest domain has been introduced named IoT [4]. It gives various attributes such as rigorous distant observation of facts or figures, so we can keep a check on the patients on their day-to-day activity by utilizing sensors in adaptable gadgets, for example, mobile phones or portable gadgets. During this, these areas are coming out, they also get new tasks or provocations, chiefly when the attack is on healthcare that itself is a tedious method, requiring compatibility, appropriate, protected, pliable, and power-saving alternative. Medical care and healthcare depict the catchiest implementation fields for the IoT [18].

The internet of things has the capabilities that allow a hike to various healthcare implementations, for example, portable health observation, health initiatives, severe ailments, and care of senior citizens. Compliance with care and medicines at the doorstep and by the suppliers of healthcare is an additional chief possible implementation. Therefore, many of the medical gadgets, imaging gadgets, and diagnostic and sensors can be taken as intelligent gadgets accounting for a very major section of the IoT [33]. These IoT-based healthcare services are anticipated to cut the costing, growth in the standard of living, and enhance the experience of the user. For the providers of the healthcare, the IoT can lower down the gadget downtime with remote provision. Including that the IoT can rightly recognize the best suitable time for refilling contributes to most of the gadgets for their full-fledged functioning. Moreover, the IoT issues the well-organized planning of restricted resources by assuring their perfect utilization and facilities of more patients. Comfort in cost-efficiency relations through secure and seamless connections amongst single patients, healthcare organizations and clinics is a key trend. The latest healthcare connectivity operated by wireless automation is anticipated to bear severe ailments, prior detection, live observation, and medical crisis. Gateways, medical servers, and health databases play a very important role in generating health documentation and giving on-demand health facilities to certified stakeholders [32].

The industry of healthcare is undertaking a shift in paradigm in the way medical staff and patient's converse and function on regular bases. The insurrection of the IoT will take part in a tedious role in relating billions of intelligent objects, wearable devices, tablets, smartphones, and cloud health implementations using many transmission mediums such as wireless sensor lattice, Bluetooth, and RFID. Health IoT implementations extending from patient's scrutiny to channelizing severe ailments will lower the cost of healthcare and make the process of care more prominent. These implementations will operate and transfer the set of data that are convertible alongside the gadgets from various destinations such as clinic, home, ambulance, and hospital.

In this chapter, we review several security challenges and requirements in IoT-based healthcare sector and also about literature review depicting the work that has been done in enhancing IoT-based healthcare security. We also discuss about the IoT architecture in detail where security loop holes are there and a brief outline of future implementation that could be done.

4.2 LITERATURE REVIEW

Basically, the IoT says connectivity of people and things with anything, in any network, from anywhere, at any time wherein anyone can transmit data information. Everything is going global due to the use of the internet. To establish an inter-operable network through IoT, security of data transfer is necessary. This section discusses the various authors' opinions and proposed methods of different researchers regarding security in the IoT-based healthcare system.

Gupta et al., proposed architecture representing the implanted sensors of the equipment instead of via smartphone sensors or wearable sensors for storing basic health-related parameters [6]. Hossain and Muhammad [27] designed an architecture using a cloud-assisted IoT structure to monitor ECG and added healthcare-related information employing smartphone. For security of records to be communicated, the instigators used the watermarking technique.

At e-health systems Zeadelly et al. presented a security threads and challenges, also it discusses about the future issues addressed by designers and developers to face the assaults caused due to wide utilization of new IoT technologies [36].

Rashmani et al. projected a smart e-health gateway. This gateway has the capability of offering various new features, for instance, embedded data mining, local storage, real-time local data processing and many more [23]. Peris-Lopez et al. proposed a grouping code of behavior as it offers the association of medication-prescription-patient to confirmation. It establishes a high-class level of security till the PIN is in the limit entropy and it is easy to implement [19].

Wu et al. [34] proposed their work implementing self-directed wireless body area network using healthcare application connected to IoT. A research methodology expressing a smart healthcare framework supported by IoT application was modeled by Bhatia et al. [2] to offer everywhere healthcare to human being throughout his/her workout sessions. Data acquired architecture for wearable devices were proposed to provide an efficient diagnosis [22]. Muhammad explained a model that allows doctors and caretakers to persistently monitor patients' stances remotely and accordingly take suitable action through facial recognition system [17]. Khan designed a health supervising system with (RFID) radio-frequency recognition [7]. For elderly people, an IoT-based healthcare system was proposed named we-care by Pinto and their team [21]. Similarly, many more inventions or technologies have been developed in the healthcare sector using IoT where security plays a major role in data authentication and verification.

The above-referred research methodologies empower automatic patient supervising and give the likely nature of the social insurance without trading off with the patient's relief. The essential focal point of every one of these undertakings is to accomplish an advanced level of proficiency, unwavering quality, and cost-viability of their frameworks Albeit a portion of these editorials referenced the security concerns with electronic clinical proceedings and wearable sensors, none of them installed security arrangements with their telehealth frameworks.

4.3 IOT ARCHITECTURE FOR HEALTHCARE

Healthcare IoT frameworks are particular in which they are worked to serve a person, which inalienably elevates the prerequisites of wellbeing, dependability, and security. In addition, they need to give constant notifications and reactions with respect to the patient's status. In an ordinary human care IoT framework, to observe patients' exercises and crucial signs, the framework needs to guarantee the security of patients. Furthermore, doctors, patients, and different caretakers' figures request a trustworthy framework wherein the outcomes are exact and convenient, and the administration is dependable and secure.

To ensure these prerequisites, the keen parts in the framework require an anticipated inertness and dependable correspondence with the upper figuring layer. The ordinary or traditional cloud-based methodologies can't guarantee the prerequisites of IoT healthcare frameworks, as the association with the cloud is the least dependent and might acquire extra inertness. Right now, use a novel framework design as a reasonable world-view to address the previously mentioned necessities.

The IoT healthcare network architecture alludes to a diagram for the specification of the IoT healthcare network physical components, their useful association, and their standards of working and methods. To begin, the essential reference design, Figure 4.1, is introduced for the telehealth and surrounding helped living systems prescribed by Continual Health Alliance. The major problems have been rectified for this architecture [37] – the invulnerability of the gateway of IoT and the wireless local area network (WLAN)/wireless personal area network (WPAN), secure, and mixed media spilling interchanges between IoT doors and caregivers. Numerous investigations [3, 5, 9, 11, 13, 14, 20, 26, 31] have justified that the IPv6-based 6LoWPAN is the premise of the IoT healthcare network.

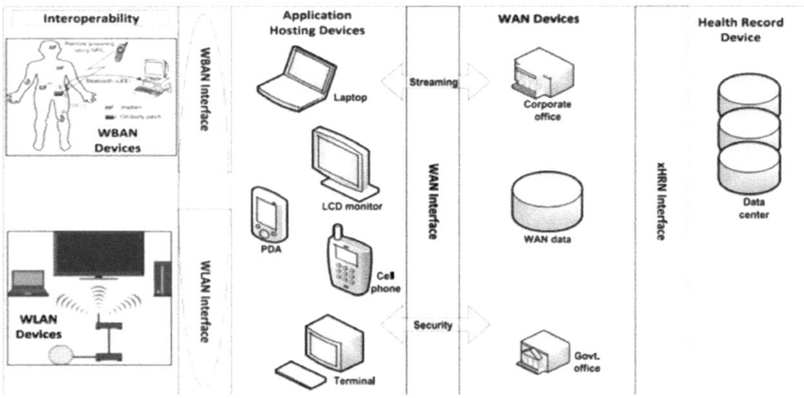

FIGURE 4.1 Simplified reference architecture: Continua Health Alliance.
Source: Reprinted with permission from Ref. [8]. Open access.

As planned in Ref. [28], Figure 4.2 shows the construction of the 6LoWLAN layer. As per the IoT healthcare network idea, wearable, and sensors use IPv6 and 6LoWPAN frameworks for circulation of the information over the 802.15.4 convention. Data sent is then responded back by sensor hubs with the intervention of the client datagram convention (UDP). To acquaint portability arrangement with the 6LoWPAN, a convention for marketing messages between versatile base systems, patient hubs, and visited systems is proposed in Ref. [26]. To address versatility, four elective strategies are considered in Ref. [3], including requesting switches, sitting tight for another coordinated non-cyclic diagram (DAG), data object (DIO), connecting to other accessible parent hubs, and sending DAG data sales (DIS) messages.

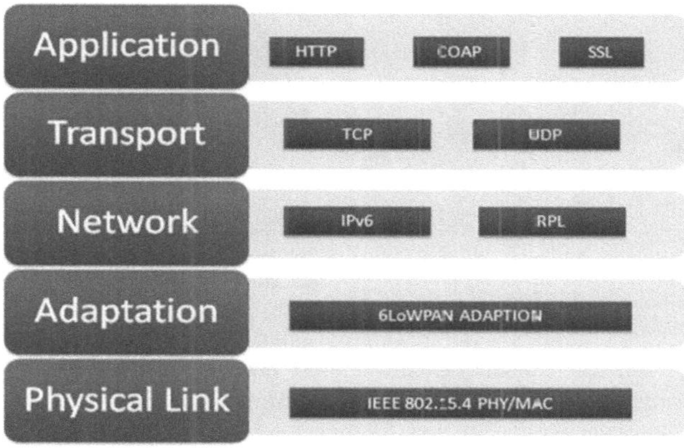

FIGURE 4.2 Protocol stack of 6LoWPAN.

Among these, requesting transition and sending DIS messages speak to the quickest techniques since they are started by the versatile hub itself. A regular passage convention stack for network clinical administrations is portrayed in Ref. [35]. This stack expressly portrays how occasional congestion, irregular congestion, and question-driven congestion can be overseen inside the health network. A complex e-health administration conveyance strategy comprising of three stages that has been projected in Ref. [30], which includes organization, signalization, and information transmission. Signalization conventions assist primarily as the premise of complex help structure, nature of administration (QoS) exchange, and asset assignment methods in the IoT health network.

In a run-of-the-mill medicinal services IoT framework, to screen patients' crucial signs and exercises, the framework needs to guarantee the security and protection of patients. Doctors and different parental figures request a trustworthy framework wherein the outcomes are precise, opportune, and the administration is solid and secure [16]. To ensure these necessities, the shrewd parts in the framework require an anticipated idleness, dependable, and strong correspondence with different segments of social insurance IoT frameworks. The triple-layered framework design of our intended social insurance IoT framework on which the arrangements of security can be implemented appears in shown Figure 4.3.

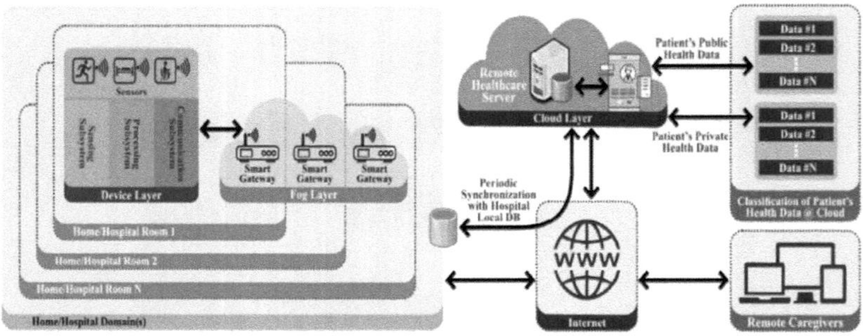

FIGURE 4.3 The secure uninterrupted end-to-end architecture of healthcare IoT framework. *Source*: Reprinted with permission from Ref. [16]; © 2018 The Author(s). Published by Elsevier B.V. https://creativecommons.org/licenses/by-nc-nd/4.0/

In this type of framework, data related to a patient's wellbeing is stored by implantable or wearable clinical sensor hubs with which the patient is prepared for individual observing of different constraints [1]. The usefulness of every layer is as per the following:

1. **Device Layer:** The most minimal layer comprising of a few physical gadgets including wearable or implantable clinical sensor hubs that are coordinated into a little remote module to gather relevant and clinical information.
2. **Fog Layer:** The center layer comprises of a system of interrelated brilliant portals. A shrewd entryway gets information from various sub-systems, executes convention transformation, and gives other more elevated level administrations [12]. It goes about as a storehouse (neighborhood database) to incidentally store sensors' and clients' data, and gives knowledge at the systems edge.
3. **Cloud Layer:** This layer incorporates transmitting, information warehousing and large information examination servers, and clinic neighborhood record that intermittently executes information synchronizing with the mobile medicinal services database server in the cloud.

4.4 IOT HEALTHCARE SECURITY

It has been well said, "An activity cannot be managed well if it cannot be measured." A very controlled collaboration and information sharing is required as at any time the healthcare providers can change as people travel a lot so data can be lost. Similarly, support for adaptiveness is also crucial. Security and privacy risks changes dynamically, a level of security and privacy should be maintained during the changes [25]. There is an extensive acceptance of IoT and new e-health devices are being made to use these days. These devices and their applications transact with a vital private data such as delicate information of a person related to health. Therefore, a new target of attackers could be IoT healthcare domains, so for full acceptance of IoT healthcare it is necessary to recognize and scrutinize the features of discrete features of IoT privacy and security from the healthcare perspective (Figure 4.4) [8, 15].

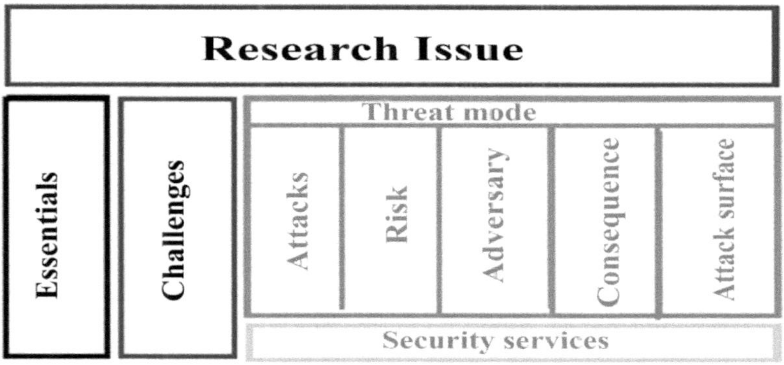

FIGURE 4.4 IoT-based healthcare security issues.

4.4.1 SECURITY REQUIREMENTS

IoT healthcare-based solutions in terms of security requirements are alike to those of typical communication scenarios. To get the security services in IoT systems, then there is a need to consider some security requirements:

1. **Data Confidentiality:** The privacy protection means the inaccessibility of medical information for users that are not permitted. Also, these messages refuse to accept in revealing their substance to eavesdroppers.
2. **Data Integrity:** Integrity guarantees that any antagonist should not alter the medical information received in transit. Besides, it should not compromise stored data and content.

3. **Data Authentication and Authorization:** Authentication empowers an IoT well-being gadget to guarantee the uniqueness of the friend with which it is exchanging the data and information.
4. **Availability of Data:** Data information availability ensures the survivability of IoT medical-based administrations (either neighborhood or worldwide administrations through the cloud) to approve gatherings when required even below the denial of service (DoS) assaults.
5. **Freshness of Message:** This ensures the data receiving is new and recent; no attacker replays the old messages. This network gives a time-varying measurement technique.
6. **Fault Tolerance:** At the time of any faults in devices or networks, the security scheme should continue to provide particular security.
7. **Mobility Support:** Mobility is solitary the most significant difficulties in IoT healthcare frameworks which expands the pertinence of these innovations. Besides, mobility permits the patient to shift from his/her supported MSN to different spaces for clinical tests without trailing the persistent checking.
8. **Uninterrupted Security:** It is one of the significant necessities in medicinal service-based IoT frameworks. This element empowers the end-purposes of an IoT healthcare framework, which is parental figures and clinical sensors, to safely converse with one another past the autonomous system.

4.4.2 SECURITY CHALLENGES

All these IoT security necessities are not ensured by safety skills, and these are required to be addressed as new challenges of IoT framework [29]. Challenges and difficulties for secure IoT healthcare framework incorporates are: computational limitation (low-speed processor with less of security performance), memory limitations (not enough memory to carry out complex security protocol), energy limits (devices have inadequate battery power), mobility (devices are not stagnant but portable so proper availability of connection to network), scalability (global connection of devices are increasing so maintaining scale as well as security is a difficult task), multiplicity, and simplicity of device, vibrant network topology, regularized security updates, and tamper-resistant packages [24].

4.5 CONCLUSION

Researchers globally have explored various technologies regarding the security in IoT healthcare framework. This chapter overviews various parts of IoT-based healthcare advances and presents different IoT architecture and also it analyzes the security requirements and their challenges. Security objectives of e-health IoT scenarios are specified and there is a need to share information with a very high privacy regulation. In this approach, security is a big challenge in medical and its usability is the next challenge. The examined literature certainly leaves no doubt that security should be a significant part of the future deployment of IoT in basic administrations. In the current event of threats/dangers not paid attention to may lead to trouble in the future, like an interwoven of numerous innovations with such a large number of gaps.

4.6 FUTURE SCOPE

We live in a world of dynamic technological rebellion. It's very much difficult to keep track of the various new innovations that are intensely influencing our lives in unparalleled traditions. The IoT is one such drastic innovation that looks as if it has grabbed everyone's interest in recent times.

The current outcome has been executed in a confined cloned atmosphere where all sensors for e-health and their interfaces are not taken into consideration. The authentication of optimization for multi-objective through ACO isn't introduced. The evaluation of administration has just been investigated. Further onwards, the energy and the cost efficiency of sensor gadgets can also be taken into consideration as parts of the efforts of development. The feature of optimization ants could be situated in a future outcome as here the segments of determining the strength of the pheromones, which are assessed in accordance with the data of the medically interrupted sensing path of IoT gadgets. The incorporation of the colony and the significantly related libraries of mediators can take part relevantly to observe the security intimidation between parallel programming. The standards of optimization could also be contented, and consequently, the non-polynomial issues of traversing and searching the tedious graph can be mediated computationally.

KEYWORDS

- **healthcare system**
- **Internet of Things (IoT)**
- **privacy**
- **security**
- **smart health**
- **wireless local area network**
- **wireless personal area network**

REFERENCES

1. Aski, V., Gupta, S., Conference, & B. S. I. G., & (2019). An authentication-centric multi-layered security model for data security in IoT-enabled biomedical applications. *IEEE 8th Global Conference on Consumer Electronics (GCCE)* (pp. 957–960). Osaka, Japan. Ieeexplore.Ieee.Org. Retrieved from: https://ieeexplore.ieee.org/abstract/document/9015217/ (accessed on 13 June 2022).
2. Bhatia, M., Sood, S., & Sood, S. K., (2018). *Article in Computers in Industry.* Elsevier. https://doi.org/10.1016/j.compind.2017.06.009.
3. Bui, N., Bressan, N., M. Z.-E. W., (2012). *Interconnection of Body Area Networks to a Communications Infrastructure: An Architectural Study*. Ieeexplore.Ieee.Org. Retrieved from: https://ieeexplore.ieee.org/abstract/document/6216833/ (accessed on 13 June 2022).
4. Butt, S. A., Luis, D. J., Jamal, T., Ali, A., & Shoaib, M., (2019). IoT smart health security threats. In: *2019 19th International Conference on Computational Science and its Applications (ICCSA)* (pp. 26–31). https://doi.org/10.1109/ICCSA.2019.000-8.
5. Doukas, C., & International, I. M. S., (2012). *Bringing IoT and Cloud Computing Towards Pervasive Healthcare.* Ieeexplore.Ieee.Org. Retrieved from: https://ieeexplore.ieee.org/abstract/document/6296978/ (accessed on 13 June 2022).
6. Gupta, P. K., Maharaj, B. T. J., Malekian, R., Maharaj, B. T. J., & Malekian, R., (n.d.). *A Novel and Secure IoT Based Cloud-Centric Architecture to Perform Predictive Analysis of Users Activities in Sustainable Health Centers*. In: Springer. Retrieved from: https://link.springer.com/article/10.1007/s11042-016-4050-6 (accessed on 13 June 2022).
7. Industrial, S. K. I. C., (2017). *Health Care Monitoring System in Internet of Things (IoT) by Using RFID.* Ieeexplore.Ieee.Org. Retrieved from: https://ieeexplore.ieee.org/abstract/document/7917920/ (accessed on 13 June 2022).
8. Islam, S. M. R., Kwak, D., Kabir, M. H., Hossain, M., & Kwak, K. S., (2015). The internet of things for health care: A comprehensive survey. *IEEE Access, 3*, 678–708. https://doi.org/10.1109/ACCESS.2015.2437951.

9. Istepanian, R., Hu, S., & N. P. C., (2011). *The Potential of Internet of m-Health Things "m-IoT" for Non-Invasive Glucose Level Sensing*. Ieeexplore.Ieee.Org. Retrieved from: https://ieeexplore.ieee.org/abstract/document/6091302/ (accessed on 13 June 2022).
10. Jara, A., & M. Z. I. I. J., (2013). *Interconnection Framework for m-Health and Remote Monitoring Based on the Internet of Things*. Ieeexplore.Ieee.Org. Retrieved from: https://ieeexplore.ieee.org/abstract/document/6585881/ (accessed on 13 June 2022).
11. Jara, A. J., Zamora-Izquierdo, M. A., Skarmeta, A., Jara, A. J., Alcolea, A. F., Zamora, M. A., & Alsaedy, M., (2011). Drugs interaction checker based on IoT internet of things and future application-level security mechanism view project selected papers from the 2nd Global IoT Summit: IoT technologies and applications for the benefit of society view project. *Drugs Interaction Checker Based on IoT*. Ieeexplore.Ieee.Org. https://doi.org/10.1109/IOT.2010.5678458.
12. Jia, X., He, D., Kumar, N., & Choo, K. K. R., (2019). Authenticated key agreement scheme for fog-driven IoT healthcare system. *Wireless Networks, 25*(8), 4737–4750. https://doi.org/10.1007/s11276-018-1759-3.
13. López, P., Fernández, D., & A. J. I. N., (2013). *Survey of Internet of Things Technologies for Clinical Environments*. Ieeexplore.Ieee.Org. Retrieved from: https://ieeexplore.ieee.org/abstract/document/6550583/ (accessed on 13 June 2022).
14. Mohd, W., Muzaaliff, N., Musa, W., Touati, F., Khriji, L., Al-Busaidi, A., & Mnaouer, A. B., (2014). Embedded gateway services for internet of things applications in ubiquitous healthcare wireless ECG patch view project water pipeline monitoring based on WSN view project. *Embedded Gateway Services for Internet of Things Applications in Ubiquitous Healthcare*. Ieeexplore.Ieee.Org. https://doi.org/10.1109/ICoICT.2014.6914055.
15. Moosavi, S. R., Gia, T. N., Rahmani, A., Virtanen, S., Tenhunen, H., & Isoaho, J., (2016). End-to-end security scheme for mobility enabled healthcare internet of things. *Future Generation Computer Systems*. https://doi.org/10.1016/j.future.2016.02.020.
16. Moosavi, S. R., Seppo, I., Levorato, M., & Levorato, M., (2018). Science direct end-to-end security schemes in performance analysis of schemes in healthcare IoT security performance analysis of security schemes in performance analysis of security schemes in healthcare IoT healthcare IoT healthcare. *Procedia Computer Science, 130*, 432–439. https://doi.org/10.1016/j.procs.2018.04.064.
17. Muhammad, G., Alsulaiman, M., & Access, S. A., (2017). *A Facial-Expression Monitoring System for Improved Healthcare in Smart Cities*. Ieeexplore.Ieee.Org. Retrieved from: https://ieeexplore.ieee.org/abstract/document/7941992/ (accessed on 13 June 2022).
18. Pang, Z., (2013). *Technologies and Architectures of the Internet-of-Things (IoT) for Health and Well-being*. Retrieved from: http://www.diva-portal.org/smash/record.jsf?pid=diva2:621384 (accessed on 13 June 2022).
19. Peris-Lopez, P., & Orfila, A., A. M., (2011). *A Comprehensive RFID Solution to Enhance Inpatient Medication Safety*. Elsevier. Retrieved from: https://www.sciencedirect.com/science/article/pii/S1386505610001796 (accessed on 13 June 2022).
20. Petrescu, A., Imadali, S., Karanasiou, A., Petrescu, A., Sifniadis, I., & Angelidis, P., (2013). e-Health service support in future IPv6 vehicular networks Véronique vèque

école supérieure d'electricité e-health service support. In: *IPv6 Vehicular Networks*. Ieeexplore.Ieee.Org. https://doi.org/10.1109/WiMOB.2012.6379134.
21. Pinto, S., Cabral, J., Gomes, T., Pinto, S., Cabral, J., Gomes, T., & Algoritmi, C., (n.d.). *We-Care: An IoT-based Health Care system for Elderly People*. Ieeexplore. Ieee.Org. https://doi.org/10.1109/ICIT.2017.7915565.
22. Lomotey, R. K., Pry, J., Sriramoju, S., Kaku, K., & Ralph, D., (2017). Wearable IoT data architecture. *IEEE World Congress on Services (SERVICES)*, 44–50.
23. Rahmani, A. M., Nguyen, G. T., Negash, B., Anzanpour, A., Azimi, I., Jiang, M., & Liljeberg, P., (2017). Exploiting smart e-health gateways at the edge of healthcare internet-of-things: A fog computing approach. *Future Generation Computer Systems*. https://doi.org/10.1016/j.future.2017.02.014.
24. Robinson, Y., Krishnan, R., & Data, S. R. I., (2020). *A Comprehensive Study for Security Mechanisms in Healthcare Information Systems Using Internet of Things* (Vol. 180). Springer. Retrieved from: https://link.springer.com/chapter/10.1007/978-3-030-39119-5_15 (accessed on 13 June 2022).
25. Savola, R. M., Abie, H., & Sihvonen, M., (n.d.). *Towards Metrics-Driven Adaptive Security Management in e-Health IoT Applications*. In: asset.nr.no. Retrieved from: http://asset.nr.no/images/5/5a/SeTTIT2012_Savola_Abie_Sihvonen.pdf (accessed on 13 June 2022).
26. Shahamabadi, M., & B. A., (2013). *A Network Mobility Solution Based on 6LoWPAN Hospital Wireless Sensor Network (NEMO-HWSN)*. Ieeexplore.Ieee.Org. Retrieved from: https://ieeexplore.ieee.org/abstract/document/6603711/ (accessed on 13 June 2022).
27. Shamim, H. M., & Muhammad, G., (2016). *Cloud-Assisted Industrial Internet of Things (IIoT)-Enabled Framework for Health Monitoring* (Vol. 19, pp. 1–11). Elsevier https://doi.org/10.1016/j.comnet.2016.01.009.
28. Shelby, Z., & Bormann, C., (2011). *6LoWPAN: The Wireless Embedded Internet*. Retrieved from: https://books.google.com/books?hl=en&lr=&id=3Nm7ZCxscMQC&oi=fnd&pg=PT9&dq=+The+Wireless+Embedded+Internet&ots=xqdpP8XCES&sig=JAriTnb8HDfBt5G_DGpRE64b4r4 (accessed on 13 June 2022).
29. Srivastava, G., Parizi, R. M., & Dehghantanha, A., (2020). The future of blockchain technology in healthcare internet of things security. In: Choo, K. K., Dehghantanha, A., & Parizi, R., (eds.), *Blockchain Cybersecurity, Trust, and Privacy. Advances in Information Security* (Vol. 79, pp. 161–184). https://doi.org/10.1007/978-3-030-38181-3_9.
30. Świątek, P., & A. R.-I. C., (2013). *IoT as a Service System for e-Health*. Ieeexplore. Ieee.Org. Retrieved from: https://ieeexplore.ieee.org/abstract/document/6720643/ (accessed on 13 June 2022).
31. Tabish, R., Ghaleb, A., & R. H. M. E., (2014). *A 3G/Wi-Fi-Enabled 6LoWPAN-Based U-Healthcare System for Ubiquitous Real-Time Monitoring and Data Logging*. Ieeexplore.Ieee.Org. Retrieved from: https://ieeexplore.ieee.org/abstract/document/6783258/ (accessed on 13 June 2022).
32. Vasanth, K., Ti, & J. S.-T. I., (2016). *Creating Solutions for Health Through Technology Innovation*. In: ti.com.cn. Retrieved from: http://www.ti.com.cn/cn/lit/wp/sszy006/sszy006.pdf (accessed on 13 June 2022).

33. Vyas, A., & Jangir, S. K., (2019). Advances in approach for object detection and classification. *National Conference on Information Technology & Security Applications*, (978), 1–3.
34. Wu, T., Wu, F., Redoute, J., & Access, M. Y. I., (2017). *An Autonomous Wireless Body Area Network Implementation Towards IoT Connected Healthcare Applications* Ieeexplore.Ieee.Org. Retrieved from: https://ieeexplore.ieee.org/abstract/document/7950903/ (accessed on 13 June 2022).
35. You, L., Liu, C., & Congress, S. T., (2011). *Community Medical Network (CMN): Architecture and Implementation.* Ieeexplore.Ieee.Org. Retrieved from: https://ieeexplore.ieee.org/abstract/document/6103930/ (accessed on 13 June 2022).
36. Zeadally, S., Isaac, J. T., & Baig, Z., (2016). Security attacks and solutions in electronic health (e-health) systems. *Journal of Medical Systems, 40*(12). https://doi.org/10.1007/s10916-016-0597-z.
37. Zhang, X., (2011). *An Open, Secure and Flexible Platform Based on Internet of Things and Cloud Computing for Ambient Aiding Living and Telemedicine*. Ieeexplore.Ieee.Org. Retrieved from: https://ieeexplore.ieee.org/abstract/document/5778905/ (accessed on 13 June 2022).

CHAPTER 5

IoHT: HEALTHCARE WITH THE INTERNET OF THINGS

EKTA SONI and KHYATI CHOPRA

Department of Electronics and Communication Engineering, G.D. Goenka University, Gurgaon, Haryana, India, E-mails: ekta.soni@gdgoenka.ac.in (E. Soni); khyati.chopra@gdgoenka.ac.in (K. Chopra)

ABSTRACT

Revolution in information technology (IT) is being well utilized by many fields. Internet connectivity and cloud computing further make the exchange of data more convenient. The exchange of data initially happened between a host device and the cloud through the internet. Gradually more than one host device has been connected to share the data collected with the cloud, and that is known as the internet of things or 'IoT.' Connecting healthcare with IT is already facilitating people. This kind of system is also proved a miracle for remote and rural area patients, etc. The need for IoHT is also projected due to the negligence towards health in urban areas because of the busy life of individuals and which is eventually be paid off by paying huge hospital bills and high health risks towards diseases. The high amount charging hospitals and the long queues are also some big issues to be resolved. In the shadow of these above issues and the advantages provided by IT, a regular and home-based portable design of the health signal monitoring system can be realized.

IoT and Cloud Computing-Based Healthcare Information Systems. Anand Sharma, PhD, Hiren Kumar Deva Sarma, PhD & S. R. Biradar, PhD (Eds.)

The IoHT sometimes interchangeably used with telemedicine. Telemedicine yet a deeper concept as it includes not only sharing the body signals with physicians then also on-line monitoring, video consultation, etc. So, telemedicine and IoHT become synonyms.

The technology is ever-changing and improving, so its applications and the benefits. The medical field does not remain limited. Interdisciplinary inventions are facilitating it by making it more autonomous and error-free. In IoHT the medical field meets with the IoT technology, signal processing, etc. The IoHT is expanding by reducing human intervention in it by including machine learning (ML) and artificial intelligence (AI). ML and AI help to keep the network congestion free. While sending an abandon of data, every AI can train the system with the known data set in the way that it can only send the signal with some distortion than the normal. So, it can reduce the amount of the sent data. Further to reduce more bandwidth, the compression of the signals is the technique added to release the burden from the communication networks before sending it to the physician's end.

5.1 INTRODUCTION

Currently, the things or devices connected are exceeding the total population of the world. In this kind of scenario, the utilization of IoT by fields like transportation, home automation, healthcare, industrial automation, city management, etc., is increasing rapidly. It enables different physical objects to join together and utilize their diversity to make intelligent decisions [1]. These objects connected in the network are not computers but can be some devices or sensors connected through the internet. In a very useful example, all the appliances of a home can be connected to the internet and controlled by a remote smartphone or computer. These appliances have the capability of internet connectivity through IP or Zigbee and have software to control them.

Healthcare is utilizing IoT by shifting its focus from the hospitals to the patient's home. It makes possible the cross-boundary integration of in-home medical devices and the far monitoring end. It can also be utilized in hospital healthcare by connecting all the devices at rural healthcare to urban setups using the internet, mobile, and satellite. Hence the IoT in healthcare can also be termed as internet of health things or IoHT [2].

The IoHT infrastructure includes the acquisition of medical data, storage, processing, and then transmission to a distant end using the internet [2–4]. Thus, it is removing the physical and geographical barriers to help people and proved beneficial for both the hospital and the patient. Its aim is to make the lifestyle and daily activities healthier. The existing sensors for healthcare signals like heart rate (HR), respiration, blood pressure, weighing, hyper, and hypotension [5], body temperature sensor, human capacitance measurer, fall detection, ECG sensors, hand gesture recognition, swallowing monitoring, and gait analysis, etc., [6] can be work in pair. These sensors are then connected with a development board containing microcontrollers like Arduino and Raspberry pi.

In the subsequent paragraphs, there are some of the important aspects of IoHT has been discussed and that will be followed by the detailed architecture and working of IoHT.

5.2 IMPORTANT ASPECTS OF IOHT

5.2.1 IOHT IN INDIA

India is a developing country where the ratio of literacy is still low. Two-thirds of the population of India resides in villages that are deprived of even basic amenities. The ratio of doctor to the citizen is 1:1500 means only one doctor is available over 1,500 citizens. The authorized criterion by The World Health Organization (WHO) recommends 1 doctor per 1,000 residents. The scenario of the remote locations is even poorer. These areas rely on government hospitals only. The common sight of doctor to citizen ratio in this area is even going to 1:10,000. This is really a matter of dwell upon. In that case, if any disaster happens to like the pandemic of COVID-19, the spread of deadly coronavirus, the situation becomes even worsen and unmanageable [7].

To insert IoHT in India is also a challenge from both the perspectives, i.e., financial and mental. People are not ready to adopt the change due to unawareness and ignorance. Besides that, also "According to the IoT India Congress (2018), the Indian IoT market is expected to grow from $1.3 billion in 2016 to $9 billion by 2020 across sectors such as telecom, health, vehicles, and homes, among others. According to accenture estimates, the value of IoHT will top US $163 billion by 2020" [8].

Yet it is projected that in the upcoming years, the healthcare sector will reach at the top of industries using IoT [8]. The Indian healthcare system of big hospitals has started taking steps towards inheriting IoT in the culture. This will not only make the life of the patient easier but also reduce pressure from the hospitals and the doctors. Most of the consultations and monitoring are done through the internet only. This is opening new ways for centralizing healthcare and make it to access for each and every person. Inventions are being done to make the system affordable to even poorer people.

5.2.2 LIFESTYLE DISEASES AND IOHT

As discussed earlier also that IoHT becomes the way of maintaining a healthy lifestyle as well as it can be applied in the tracking of chronic diseases. The lifestyle dependent diseases like blood pressure and diabetes that are generally ignored in our life are the real reason behind many kinds of other chronic illnesses. Thus, timely management of these small IR-regulations of the body can help to regulate chronic diseases of the future. In the virtue of a regular monitoring of the signals may increase the burden over the hospitals and will make the situation chaotic if one goes every day for the checkup. This scenario can be replaced by a home-based measurement system. The home-based system is a wide idea that includes not only monitoring at home while at any place whether during traveling, at the workplace, athletes, in the remote areas or in the war zone also where it's a way impossible to track one's health.

For example, to monitor diabetes level handheld conventional invasive devices are available in the market that can be used in home. But this conventional invasive technique is nowadays get replaced by a non-invasive technique based on Arduino, implemented to calculate the sugar level in the human body through the dedicated VOC sensor, that can measure ketone levels in the body [9]. Similarly, for obesity BMI (body mass index) can be calculated. In the case of blood pressure measurement there are both handheld and Arduino based system can be used. There are shields available to calculate the blood pressure in the body.

In this way if these small body signals can be measured and regulated every day, they can save one from any major illness in the future such as dysfunctional eyes, kidney failure, etc., are the long-term effect of diabetes that can be controlled by if diabetes would have ruled out at the initial stage. In the same manner lever related problems, cholesterol, etc., can be intimated by obesity level and blood pressure fluctuations.

5.2.3 BRIDGING THE GAP (DOCTOR AND PATIENT)

IoHT is designed to fill the gap between the patient and the doctor which is formed due to the location and the availability of the patient. Remotely located patient or a rural patient or elderly patients with reduced mobility would not be at immediate accessibility to the physician. IoHT is only the way to bridge the gap between both the ends. The hospital visits are also reduced and so the cost of healthcare [10]. IoHT can be designed for both hospital and patient's end. In hospitals where the ratio of doctor to the patient generally remains low and where there is a need for continuous monitoring of patients in such scenarios, IoHT works like wonder. If the patients at their respective beds are connected through IoT and send real-time signals to the caregivers, then wherever the caregivers are, they can monitor them and can do the requisite. That proves IoHT a win-win situation for both the ends, i.e., hospitals, and patients. Hospitals and doctors can monitor many patients at the same time and treat according to the seriousness of the disease. Healthcare consumers are now demanding higher quality and convenience. That can only be realized through telemedicine or IoHT. The scenario of the traditional health center is changing rapidly and getting replaced by health monitoring at the ease of patient. It has also reduced the mortality rate and complications related to life-threatening diseases like heart diseases, cancer, etc. [10].

5.2.4 PRIVACY THREAT IN IOHT

The IoHT network must contain some essential features such as geographic coverage, transparency, scalability, and security. Where geographic coverage is the area covered by the IoHT network, scalability is the ability to add or delete the number of devices from the network, transparency means no hidden node in the network and the security is keeping the network safe from any privacy breaching network attack.

The network is prone to many hostile attacks. Sometimes its main advantage of providing mobility to its user becomes its limitation. Because during mobility network changes and so the security configurations which makes them vulnerable to confidentiality attacks such as "information interference, attacks based on host properties and attacks based on network properties." If the devices are uniquely identifiable, then the location of them can also be traced easily.

Most of the health sensors and the networks are made cheaper in order to facilitate IoHT to the poor people also. The cheaper IoHT system has limited memory, less durability and a low level of security while using public networks for sending the health signals along with patient's personal information. The public networks are openly accessible or weekly encrypted hence vulnerable to attacks and leakage of personal information. Literature has suggested some techniques to make the system robust for cyber-attacks are network segmentation, robust authentication, etc. [10, 11]. Game theory with Stackelberg security equilibrium (GTSSE) [13] is also a method mentioned in the literature towards solving the problem of security of networks.

Security threat is coming out as a major obstacle in the path of success of IoHT. Hackers are easily attacking the personal information of the users saved in the cloud network and try to misuse that. So, this is a challenge to save the patient's information from any unauthorized person. With the technology improvement, there are more chances to make the system more secure.

5.2.5 PROMINENT HURDLES AND POTENTIAL BARRIERS IN MAKING IOHT A HABIT

Other than the security and safety of the networks there are some more hurdles in the way of realization of IoHT in the real environment. The road to success is not as easy as it seems. The theory changes itself when a concept coming to get practically implemented. Mobile phones and the internet have become fashionable and necessary all over the world. People are using them for their entertainment. But they hesitate to use the technology for their own benefit. The big telecom companies should also take decisions in the way of encouraging their consumers to implement IoHT through their networks. The lack of awareness towards their health becomes the true hindrance in the way of implementation. Similarly, fear of the unknown and not adopting the change are some key challenges to work upon. People should get educated about the dos and don'ts towards their health. Other challenges like availability of service, authentication of devices, fault tolerance, device malfunctioning information, etc., also make implementation difficult. The heterogeneity of devices is one more challenge to consider while designing an IoHT based system. All the devices connected in a network differ in computational and communication capabilities [11]. This can be solved by choosing the best-suited protocols and architecture according to the designed system, network requirements and application. Data management and self-configuration are also things to be considered.

5.2.6 ARTIFICIAL INTELLIGENCE (AI), PREDICTIVE ANALYSIS, AND MACHINE LEARNING (ML) IN IOHT

To make the system automated, it is required to take the decisions itself and reduce human interventions, and the system is needed to get adapted 'by' technology instead of we or system adapt 'to' technology. To resolve these artificial intelligence (AI) and machine learning (ML) are need to be considered. According to John McCarthy (1956), "AI involves machines that can perform tasks that are characteristic of human intelligence." In 1959, Arthur Samuel defined it as "the ability to learn without being explicitly programmed." AI is something related to making the machine intelligent enough to take its own decisions by training it with language, pictures, audios, problem-solving, etc. On the other side, ML is the way of achieving AI. AI cannot be achieved without using ML as without ML the coding would be complex. ML trains the algorithm to learn how things are actually happening by feeding it by huge amounts of data so that algorithms would improve itself after every iteration. Basically, the ML is the way of training the device to work like the human brain. Later take its decision according to the information fed to it. ML has many approaches such as inductive logic programming, reinforcement learning, Bayesian networks, deep learning, clustering, etc. Artificial neural networks (ANNs) are algorithms of deep learning work like the function of the interconnecting neurons in the brain. The sensor data works like the human body and AI as the human brain gets data from the different sensors to train itself. The combination of AI, ML, and IoT is useful in three areas viz. "remote patient monitoring (RPM), wellness, and prevention and operations" [11].

The AI system is not supposed to be placed randomly in the system architecture, but it should be located according to the availability of data. After collecting data from the devices or sensors, it is stored and fed to the AI system. The process is related to selecting a particular set of information to decide the method of AI. For example, heart sensor data is fed to the network of a random number of people and according to the trend of data AI system can fix the range of heartbeat for a particular age can easily trace any change from trained values in the new incoming data [12]. The reply from AI should be properly interpreted. The AI gives an answer that includes digits that make sense with only proper context. In this way, the new incoming data is linked with the knowledge located in the system in order to conclude the response to a particular problem. In this way, the system can properly react, so make the decision. AI methods have high processing power, so they need to be placed on external servers this is also beneficial for using multiple devices at the same time [11].

5.2.7 COMPRESSION FOR IOHT

IoHT, where at one place helpful for regular real-time monitoring of health signals but at another place responsible for increasing required bandwidth to send signals, storage space and congestion due to abandoning the amount of data sent every day. For example, if we consider only a single type of health signal like ECG signal. The useful bandwidth of an ECG signal ranges from 0.5 to 50 Hz. This can be further extended up to 1 kHz for intensive care applications (pacemaker detection) [14]. A single physician may require 4 megabits per second (Mbps) of speed. The 4 Mbps includes browsing, non-real-time image downloading and remote monitoring [15]. The average speed of the internet in India is 2.5 Mbps [16]. It makes the storage and transmission of this signal difficult. The available bandwidth is nowhere matching the required bandwidth for transmitting the signals in real-time. This is only about one body signal, if we talk about the composite bandwidth required for all the body signals the situation becomes even worst. This huge difference in bandwidth requirements and available bandwidth will induce the need for real-time compression of medical data before sending them to a remote location [17]. The compression will be based on utilizing the redundancy of the signal elements without loss in the diagnostic details. At the transmission end, the signal gets compressed and sent to the receiving end where the signal gets decompressed in order to fetch the important diagnostic information.

5.2.8 FUTURE HEALTH MARKET AND STRATEGIES

Every nation is working towards realizing better health services for its citizens, whether it's developing or developed. For this telemedicine is adopted by every country such as u-Japan health policy, National strategy for health in Sweden, object-naming service (ONS) of France in IoHT network, Industry 4.0 strategic initiative of Germany, e-health development strategy of China, etc. Even countries like India, Pakistan, and Arabia all are investing in IoHT services. The WHO is also making efforts to promote m-health and e-health [10].

These efforts make the future of IoHT very bright around the globe. Both hardware and software innovations due to new technologies and enhanced capabilities are the factors behind the development of IoHT. The lower cost of technology also attracts users [10].

5.3 ARCHITECTURE OF IOHT

The architecture for working of IoHT is shown in Figure 5.1. The architecture is depicted in layers in which the first is the perception layer that includes sensors and hardware platforms, the second is the network layer that includes the internet and cloud, and the third is the application layer that includes the far monitoring end. Other than these layers, two more layers are included in the architecture of IoHT in Ref. [11]. These two additional layers are gateway layer and middleware layer and are added between the existing layers, i.e., between perception and the network layer and between network and application layer, respectively [11]. The gateway layer used for communication with the network layer and the middleware layer communicates to the application layer to transfer the data. The gateway layer also communicates the data between the intelligent objects.

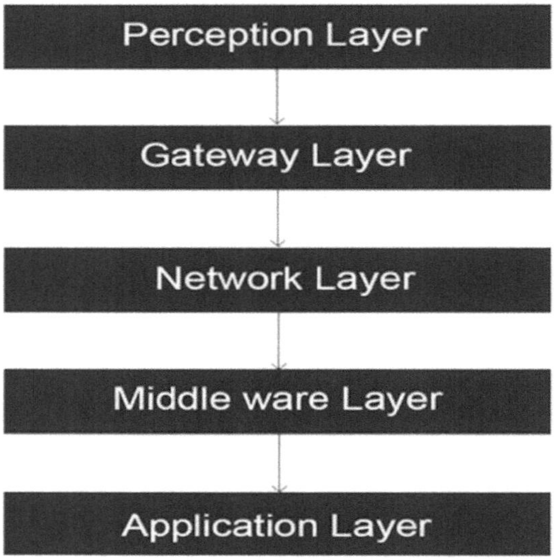

FIGURE 5.1 Architecture of IoHT [11].

5.4 METHODOLOGY

This is depicted previously also that the methodology of IoHT includes the acquisition of vital body signals then it is shared with the cloud, and in the end, they are monitored from the far end. The whole process includes well-programmed system hardware in order to accomplish the goal. To understand the working of the system more deeply here, the whole process is explained in parts in subsections.

5.4.1 SENSORS

The sensor is the device used to gather the information of its surroundings and fed to a processor to use the information. The healthcare sensors are used to sense the vital body signals that can be monitored for a long time in order to track the health of a person. There are many kinds of health sensors are available for different parts of the body such as sensors for the heartbeat, for electro cardiogram signal (trace any inadequacy of the heart), for brain signals, i.e., electro encephalogram signals, for respiration, for blood pressure, for weighing, for hyper and hypo-tension [5], for body temperature signals, for human capacitance measurer, for fall detection, for hand gesture recognition, for swallowing monitoring, for gait analysis, etc. [6]. These sensors are sometimes supported by other environmental sensors like temperature sensors, humidity sensors, distance sensors, etc., in order to make an intelligent system of IoHT. IoT makes all these sensors to work together as it can reduce the cost of sending data and also the time consumed. The combined sensor data goes to the processing hardware, cloud, and to all the subsequent parts of the system which will be discussed in the later sections.

5.4.2 PROCESSING HARDWARE

All the physical sensors are connected to common hardware to process the data received from them. That hardware platform must enable the received analog signal to change into digital as it must contain an onboard transducer for the purpose. Then the signal will be gone through noise cancelation; for further cleaning, it uses the onboard filters. To enable these features, here an Arduino or raspberry pi based developing boards have been suggested [20]. These boards contain a microcontroller IC on them in addition to the above-mentioned required circuit components. After processing the sensor data, the data is required to be transferred to far monitoring end through the cloud. This will require internet connectivity to send real-time data. For this purpose, both the developing boards contain an ethernet port on them. To get detailed knowledge about these boards they are discussed hereunder.

5.4.2.1 ARDUINO

Arduino is a small developing board that is primarily used by the beginners of IoT. It has almost all the features present which is required for an IoT system. The microcontroller used is an Atmel 8-bit AVR microcontroller ATmega 'X.' A linear regulator of 5V, a 16 MHz crystal oscillator or ceramic resonator to provide clock frequency to the circuit. Arduino *Uno* is the most used among all available versions of Arduino. It has 14 digital I/O pins including six for pulse width modulation. Other than these, six analog inputs pins that can be used as digital I/O pins. A USB connection to connect with a host computer or a laptop and a power jack to get power along with an ICSP header and a reset button is accompanied on the board. The software used is an integrated development environment (IDE) written in Java. The program is written is called sketch and saved as text files with the file extension .ino [21].

5.4.2.2 RASPBERRY PI

The Raspberry Pi is a small computer, used for the purpose of IoT. Like Arduino, it also has a series of versions. It is better than Arduino in terms of its ARM-compatible central processing unit (CPU) and on-chip graphics processing unit (GPU). The processor speed varies from 700 MHz to 1.5 GHz of the latest version, i.e., Pi4 with 4GB RAM. It has a secure digital (SD) card slot to store the operating system and program memory. In addition to these, the boards also have five USB ports. It supports video output, HDMI, and composite video and audio output. It has GPIO pins also for the lower levels of output. Onboard Wi-Fi 802.11n and Bluetooth are available for networking. The software used is Raspbian, a Debian-based (32-bit) Linux distribution. Other than these Ubuntu, Windows 10 IoT Core, RISC OS is also supporting software available for the same [22].

Arduino is a microcontroller while Raspberry pi is a mini-computer. It can run multiple programs at a time, unlike Arduino which can run only a single program. Interfacing sensors is not as easy as with the Arduino. The clock speed of Raspberry pi is 40 times faster than Arduino, but the workability of Arduino can be expanded by using shields for different purposes, which is not the case with Raspberry pi. Arduino has 32 KB onboard storage while raspberry pi needs an SD card to store the data. Thus, from the features discussed above, it has been concluded that Arduino is good at doing a simple task, but Raspberry pi is used for more complex, less repetitive, and multiple tasks together, for example, in robots.

Same with the case of healthcare, when we need to monitor only one signal at a time than it is a repetitive kind of simple operation that requires Arduino as a controller but if more than one health signal is being monitored at a time then Raspberry pi will be the choice for the parallel operation.

5.4.3 CLOUD

The signals after processing go to Cloud, and cloud computing is a collective term used for both the services delivered using the internet and the hardware used to deliver them. The analysis of data sent to the cloud is done by software services. The cloud is categorized into two types, i.e., public, and private. It is public when anyone can use it by paying a decent amount for it. Public clouds are used for small devices, by hobbyists or technical personnel. While private clouds are usually made for big organizations to use them solely. This kind of cloud is beyond the reach of the general public [23]. The cloud is the medium of transferring data, and the destination of data would be the monitoring end.

5.4.4 MONITORING END

The monitoring end is the last destination of the physical data where they get analyzed. This could be a hospital, a physician, or a health center. Hospitals and the health centers are having many physicians are at work. So, it is easier to analyze the health data even in real-time. After analysis, the findings may be sent back to the patient with the recommendations and treatment requirements. Sometimes the relatives of the patient are also informed about the condition of the health of a patient. This is normally the case of chronic illness or life-threatening disease where rapid action is must be required.

5.4.5 THE IOHT STRUCTURE AND BLOCK DIAGRAM

The block diagram of IoHT has been shown in Figure 5.2. Figure 5.2 depicts the main building blocks and the overall architecture adopted for the IoHT system. This is a combined picture of all the parts discussed previously. According to this, the first step involves health data acquisition through sensors, and then it's further processing using any development board. In this, the host PC will work as a display unit connected with the microcontroller device.

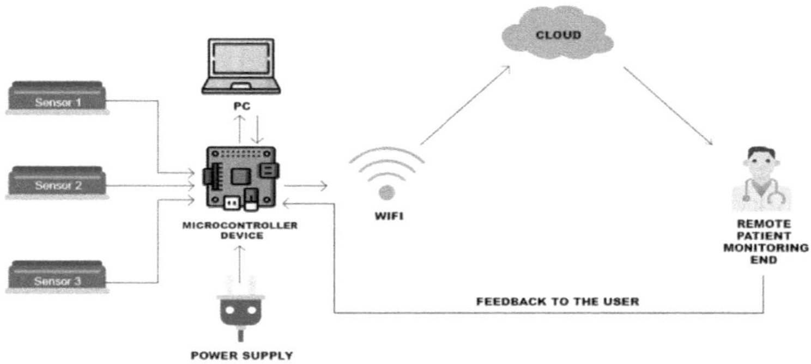

FIGURE 5.2 IoHT structure.

The collected physical signals are then transmitted to the cloud. From the cloud, the data will be transmitted to the remote end for further monitoring by a health practitioner. Health feedback and findings can be sent to the patient end back by the practitioner.

5.4.6 FLOW DIAGRAM

The flow of data in the network is as follows: physical signals accessed by the sensors, raw data fed to the processing board for filtering and compression, it is displayed on the computer attached to it, then the Wi-Fi shield joined with the developing board make the data transfer to the cloud, from the cloud the physician will get the data almost in real-time (Figure 5.3).

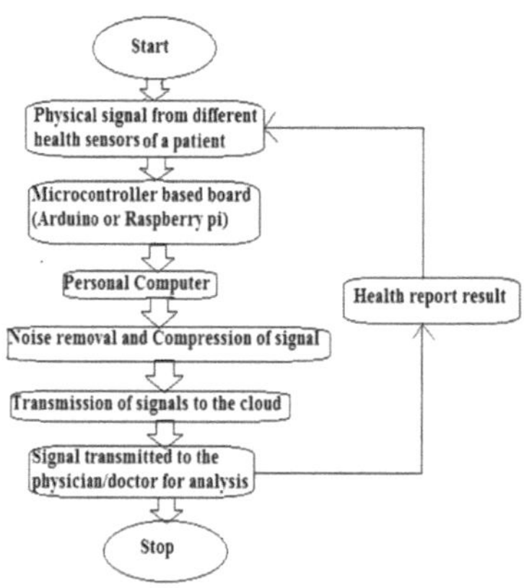

FIGURE 5.3 Flow diagram of IoHT.

The result will be fed back to the consumer or the patient. The system is flexible enough to add ML algorithms and AI while the data is getting compressed in the personal computer. So that a preliminary idea about the distortion in the set values of the signals and the reason behind them can be interpreted at the patient end only before sending. The data sent to the physician end may take some time, but the authenticity of the result will be proved after the report is analyzed by the physician only. So, ML and AI are useful for a 'rough real-time data' interpretation.

5.5 CONCLUSION

IoHT is the technology for healthcare. Its area of application is not limited to the chronic patients but also to the patients facing geographical barriers and hit by any natural calamity like earthquake or tsunami. The after-disaster management health services can only be provided by tele-medicine. The whole world is facing its all-time biggest disaster this time due to the spread of COVID-19 virus. Big developed countries like the USA is also not able to get over to this pandemic. In the present scenario when the hospital beds are full of corona patients, and there is a danger of unnecessary exposure to the disease if someone physically goes to the hospitals. It is better to avoid going out by using these IoHT devices at their homes and get instructed by the respective physician through any of the multimedia services.

Its low cost makes it a must-have. In addition, it also has the capability of self-care, ML, high performance, and flexibility to add extra sensors to it [19, 24]. It's proved to be a very beneficial platform for both home-based as well as hospital-based systems. The design solves the purpose of the remote monitoring of various health systems for a healthy life. The capability of Arduino and Raspberry pi has boosted the operability of the given system in the way of accomplishing simultaneous tasks. In the less complex system, it is to be suggested to use Arduino, which is a cheaper solution too and can support many shields. Raspberry pi is suggested to use when the design uses repetitive task and the system is of complex type. Other than this an SMS feedback service can be included to make to inform guardians and patients about alarming health signals. Other areas that are not touched till now are like stroke rehabilitation, mental disorder tracking, weight control, etc., are to be worked in the future [18]. IoHT can also be utilized for children with any mental or physical health problems.

The security aspect of the IoT devices is not commonly taken into due consideration that makes the system vulnerable to attacks. The attackers may misuse the health data of the patients. So, it is necessary to apply the required security to the whole network. Compression of the data acquired without sending them to the other end is also an important feature to be considered by IoHT.

KEYWORDS

- **Arduino**
- **artificial intelligence**
- **health sensors**
- **home-healthcare**
- **information technology**
- **raspberry-pi**
- **telemedicine**

REFERENCES

1. Babu, B. S., Srikanth, K., Ramanjaneyulu, T., & Narayana, I. L., (2016). IoT for healthcare. *International Journal of Science and Research, 5*(2), 322–326.
2. Wilson, L. S., & Maeder, A. J., (2015). Recent directions in telemedicine: Review of trends in research and practice. *Healthcare Informatics Research, 21*(4), 213–222.
3. Bui, N., & Zorzi, M., (2011). Health care applications: A solution based on the internet of things. In: *Proceedings of the 4th International Symposium on Applied Sciences in Biomedical and Communication Technologies* (p. 131). ACM.
4. Ukil, A., Bandyoapdhyay, S., Puri, C., & Pal, A., (2016). IoT healthcare analytics: The importance of anomaly detection. In: *2016 IEEE 30th International Conference on Advanced Information Networking and Applications (AINA)* (pp. 994–997). IEEE.
5. Fanucci, L., Saponara, S., Bacchillone, T., Donati, M., Barba, P., Sánchez-Tato, I., & Carmona, C., (2012). Sensing devices and sensor signal processing for remote monitoring of vital signs in CHF patients. *IEEE Transactions on Instrumentation and Measurement, 62*(3), 553–569.
6. Mukhopadhyay, S. C., (2014). Wearable sensors for human activity monitoring: A review. *IEEE Sensors Journal, 15*(3), 1321–1330.
7. Kumar, R., & Pal, R., (2018). India achieves WHO recommended doctor population ratio: A call for paradigm shift in public health discourse! *Journal of Family Medicine and Primary Care, 7*(5), 841.

8. Available online at: https://www.dqindia.com/reinventing-healthcare-internet-things-iot-john-samuel-accenture/ (accessed on 13 June 2022).
9. Rydosz, A., (2018). Sensors for enhanced detection of acetone as a potential tool for non-invasive diabetes monitoring. *Sensors, 18*(7), 2298.
10. Albesher, A. A., (2019). IoT in healthcare: Recent advances in the development of smart cyber-physical ubiquitous environments. *International Journal of Computer Science and Network Security, 19*(2), 181–186.
11. Poniszewska-Maranda, A., & Kaczmarek, D., (2015). Selected methods of artificial intelligence for internet of things conception. In: *2015 Federated Conference on Computer Science and Information Systems (FedCSIS)* (pp. 1343–1348). IEEE.
12. Available online at: https://www.iotforall.com/the-difference-between-artificial-intelligence-machine-learning-and-deep-learning/ (accessed on 13 June 2022).
13. Somasundaram, M., & Sivakumar, R., (2015). Game theory-based security in wireless body area network with Stackelberg security equilibrium. *The Scientific World Journal, 2015*.
14. Hu, F., Xie, D., & Shen, S., (2013). On the application of the internet of things in the field of medical and health care. In: *2013 IEEE International Conference on Green Computing and Communications and IEEE Internet of Things and IEEE Cyber, Physical and Social Computing* (pp. 2053–2058). IEEE.
15. Available online at: https://www.healthit.gov/topic/about-onc/health-it-strategic-planning (accessed on 13 June 2022).
16. Available online at: http://gadgets.ndtv.com/internet/features/indias-fastest-broadband-internet-service-providers-810697 (accessed on 13 June 2022).
17. Yakut, O., Solak, S., & Bolat, E. D., (2014). Measuring ECG signal using e-health sensor platform. In: *International Conference on Chemistry, Biomedical and Environment Engineering, Antalya* (pp. 71–75).
18. Santos, M. A., Munoz, R., Olivares, R., Rebouças, F. P. P., Del Ser, J., & De Albuquerque, V. H. C., (2020). Online heart monitoring systems on the internet of health things environments: A survey, a reference model, and an outlook. *Information Fusion, 53*, 222–239.
19. Nguyen, H. H., Mirza, F., Naeem, M. A., & Nguyen, M., (2017). A review on IoT healthcare monitoring applications and a vision for transforming sensor data into real-time clinical feedback. In: *2017 IEEE 21st International Conference on Computer Supported Cooperative Work in Design (CSCWD)* (pp. 257–262). IEEE.
20. Ghosh, A. M., Halder, D., & Hossain, S. A., (2016). Remote health monitoring system through IoT. In: *2016 5th International Conference on Informatics, Electronics and Vision (ICIEV)* (pp. 921–926). IEEE.
21. Available online at: https://en.wikipedia.org/wiki/Arduino (accessed on 13 June 2022).
22. Available online at: https://en.wikipedia.org/wiki/Raspberry_Pi (accessed on 13 June 2022).
23. Suen, C. H., Kirchberg, M., & Lee, B. S., (2011). Efficient migration of virtual machines between public and private cloud. In: *2011 IEEE Third International Conference on Cloud Computing Technology and Science* (pp. 549–553). IEEE.

24. Haripriya, K., Aravind, C. M., Karthigayen, V., & Ganesh, P., (2016). Patient health monitoring system using IoT and cloud-based processing. *Indian Journal of Science and Technology, 9*.

CHAPTER 6

CLOUD COMPUTING IN HEALTHCARE

SHIVANI MONGA and KAVITA

Department of CS and IT, Faculty of Engineering and Technology, Jayoti Vidyapeeth Women's University, Jaipur, Rajasthan, India, E-mail: Shivanimonga385@gmail.com (S. Monga)

ABSTRACT

The development of cloud computing guides us to new and creative advancements for various application domains. With the headway in innovation, healthcare is evolving both in its technicality and organization. Today, storing patient data is of utmost concern because it needs to be handy for the doctor to acquire the previous history of the patient at the hour of emergency. This can be especially right for healthcare with tremendous significance in the present society, thus making it worth to explore the appropriate perspectives. Cloud computing in healthcare is defined as the services provided by hardware and software within the data centers and services provided over the internet. The important characteristics of the healthcare system are – in order to get the patients' medical history; data should be available for the doctors. Medical informatics should be available even when the patient is unconscious and updating the data should be easy and natural. All this data should be stored in a centralized pool or storage. The constant improvement in innovation develops new and creative circumstance that must be dissected utilizing complete and integrative exploration.

IoT and Cloud Computing-Based Healthcare Information Systems. Anand Sharma, PhD, Hiren Kumar Deva Sarma, PhD & S. R. Biradar, PhD (Eds.)

6.1 INTRODUCTION

Over the last 50 years, technology and advancements have become a must for human beings in many ways. Cloud computing is a self-service, internet structure that encourages the client to utilize processing assets anyplace and at whenever. Cloud computing is one of the speediest creating innovation, and numerous associations are currently introducing a gigantic assortment of cloud services.

It is assuming a critical part in the medical care area. The internet-based processing innovation utilizes a secured organization of online facilitated distant workers to keep, oversee, and handle information that can be effortlessly gotten to from anyplace in the world.

Cloud computing in the healthcare system can be a productive procedure to interface and synchronize the entire medical care framework. Utilizing this patient, emergency clinics, facilities, dispensaries, research centers, laboratories, specialists, drug specialists, medical consultants, and clinical advisors would all be able to be made a portion of a framework to control the work process.

The use of cloud computing in overseeing healthcare can improve the nature of administrations yet can likewise be a help for patients who remain to profit because of adaptability and accommodation that the framework offers. Cloud computing provides trustworthy and excellent service to users on a scalable and flexible infrastructure. It very well may be a bunch of heterogeneous processing units composed together yet it works like a homogeneous single machine.

To convey high caliber and solid administrations medical services needs composed and logical innovations, so that system can work in a cost effective and efficient way.

Technology platform comprises modules directly from arrangements, line the board, e-wallet or money cards with payment gateway and status, clinical records the executives, e-prescription conveyance, and request the executives and continuum of care.

The organization gives continuous announcement online, patient record sees, access, and income contributions to specialists from their cell phone anyplace whenever.

Nowadays, this service is one of the most important research topics in healthcare and information system therefore getting higher consideration.

6.2 WHAT IS A CLOUD?

Cloud can be described as providing data to connected devices and allocating computing resources on demand. The main three benefits of the cloud for healthcare domain are: economic, operational, and functional.

- Economic benefit – it reduces the IT cost as heavy capital expenses, because IT resources are taken on stipulate as desirable and paid for as a running cost;
- It offers scalability and flexibility to meet demand;
- To protect against both types of threats (outsider and insider), cloud service provides data centers which are very secure and protected;
- Cloud service models can be chosen according to the need and requirements of user and healthcare domains;
- Opening cost, hiring period, age of resources and maintenance cost, all affect the pricing of the cloud model.

6.2.1 TYPES OF CLOUD

To deploy cloud computing mainly three types of cloud models are considered:

1. **Private Cloud:** Cloud which works individually for a particular organization; managed and hosted internally or externally.
2. **Public Cloud:** A cloud where services are delivered over the network and available for public use. These services and facilities are rendered for without any cost.
3. **Hybrid Cloud:** Combining of two or more clouds that remain a distinctive entity but are tied collectively and provides the advantages of various models.

Cloud computing includes three types of models according to their service point of view (Table 6.1):

i. SaaS;
ii. PaaS; and
iii. IaaS.

TABLE 6.1 Types of Cloud

SL. No.	Feature	SaaS	PaaS	IaaS
1.	Usage and permissions	Software application is installed in cloud framework and this partial service is given to the users.	It is used when an infrastructure platform is required by the user to run the services or applications.	More permissions and liberty are given to the user.
2.	Control	It permits the users to use the company application from a distant (isolated) application.	Clients are given more control over the applications and custom applications created exclusively for the organization.	Users are provided with the maximum control over the cloud infrastructure.
3.	Applicable	A SaaS cloud could be suitable for a physician with less practice and with a smaller nonexistent IT department.	A PaaS cloud might subsist for medium-sized clinical practices with a good-sized IT department or specialist that could benefit from custom application.	IaaS cloud could be fit for bigger institutions such as health systems, hospitals, and medical groups and institutions with a huge number of staff.

6.2.2 SECURITY AND PRIVACY REQUIREMENTS

1. **Privacy:** It means keeping the information top secret and hidden from unauthorized use. In the healthcare system, patients' information is stored which includes useful and crucial data. To guarantee the privacy issues information requires to be encrypted and the key for decryption should be only with authorized users.
2. **Integrity:** Authorized users are provided with a verification key to check the authorized data.
3. **Trust:** A trust to doctors and patients that their information is kept at accurate place and recovered without making any changes.

6.2.3 BENEFITS OF CLOUD-BASED HEALTHCARE SERVICES

With the use of cloud computing in healthcare services, the problems of doctors, research scholars, patients, hospitals, and pharmacies can be solved out. Doctors can get the patients details whenever they require and can start the treatment of a patient at the earliest. On the part of researchers, they can collect the data from a single place without any efforts. With electronic health records, patients are able to view the prescriptions and information about the doctors, hospital, and can choose the best option which they want.

1. **Better Patient Care:** The overall data about patient's records and treatment provided to them is available to doctors every time.
2. **Reduced Treatment Cost:** Before investing in primary setup and functional cost health department can simply acquire the latest techniques and treatment for any diagnosis.
3. **Resource Scarcity Resolved:** with the assistance of cloud computing issue of shortage of it resources are resolved as remote medical services are being for patient treatment. In case of emergency, a specialist can work remotely which will save time and cost.
4. **Improved Quality:** Healthcare organizations, doctors, patients, and researchers play a role of user and avail the information which is stored on the cloud and helps in improving the facilities and safety of patients.
5. **Help to Researchers:** In cloud computing healthcare services, a huge measure of information is put away, which incorporates patient's set of experiences, their disease, and most recent therapies which are around the world open. With the assistance of this, specialist can develop a creative and improved version with insignificant time and speculation (Figure 6.1).

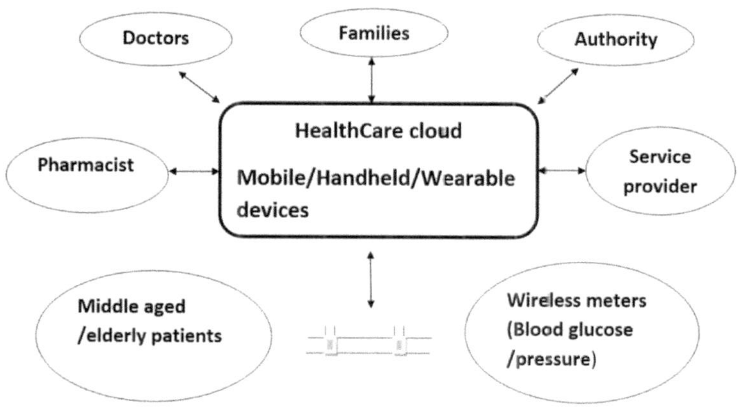

FIGURE 6.1 Healthcare cloud.

An analysis is done on the different technologies and methodologies that work in the healthcare system and their pros and cons that need to be addressed in the future for better services (Table 6.2).

TABLE 6.2 Comparisons of Methodology Used in Healthcare Systems

SL. No.	Techniques Used	Pros	Cons
1.	Monitoring patients through Raspberry Pi	Cost effective technique and 24 hours observation Suitable for village healthcare	It is not easy to set up wireless sensor network nodes as compared to wired networks.
2.	Patient's health parameters through electronic sensors	Ease for people where public transportation is an issue.	The system does not provide direct interaction between patient and doctor.
3.	Electronic pharmacy in Dubai hospitals	System alerts the doctor to any pharmacological interventions. Systems empower specialists to compose the remedy of enlisted patients electronically.	People of the city do not rely on the technology, so they do not use it.
4.	ADAMA medicine website	Good speed and accuracy in completing orders. Save time, effort, and money.	Focuses more on making income than on providing good services.
5.	Fouda pharmacy	Message is sent to the customer if there is a change in the price of medicine.	Prices of medicines changes very frequently and disappoint customers.
6.	Technology model	Easily accessible and highly recognized technology is used.	Adoption of new technology difficult for elders to equip with new technology

6.3 WHERE ARE WE LAGGING BEHIND?

1. **Infrastructure:** It contains gaps like transportation, accessibility of framework including cooling, power flexibly or continuous force gracefully. The framework issues can be addressed by assimilating investigative procedures, developing streamlined health IT

systems, building clinics in villages, and improving effectiveness and efficiency.

2. **Second Sort of Gap:** It is a requirement for information and skilled laborers in the medical services area, particularly in the primary care and to an enormous degree in the secondary framework. We have a lack of specialists and attendants who are either not prepared or prepared enough to have the option to adapt up to cutting edge innovation or not profoundly prepared to deal with various sorts of hardware measures. Confronting this, patients can't get reliable treatment.

6.3.1 CHALLENGES IN UP-GRADATION FOR HEALTHCARE DOMAIN

1. **Technology:** Healthcare is far behind in implementing new advanced technologies like cloud computing, mobile computing, and big data analytics. Headway in innovation needs heaps of venture and human resources. Most of the best hospitals are equipped with the latest technology, yet the medical clinics in country territories come up short on every one of these offices, so customary innovation requires total framework and staff to be refreshed and prepared by new innovation.
2. **Security and Confidentiality:** Confidentiality is a big issue in cloud computing. Storage and management of these kinds of medical applications needs central storage infrastructure which works in distributed architecture.
3. **Legal Issues:** Contract law, data jurisdiction, privacy, and intellectual property rights are various legal issues in cloud computing.

6.4 CONCLUSION

Cloud computing appliance in healthcare renovates the system from capital-intensive to pay-per-usage model. It helps in maintaining a centralized medical history record of patients, which helps the doctor to know the complete medical history and the treatment provided. Rural hospitals lack basic infrastructure, and availability of doctors, and many employees are not equipped to technology due to lack of funds. Uniform healthcare technology adoption can only be done by the sustained efforts from both the government and private sector. Cloud technology with IT in hospitals can cut down expenditure cost and deploying expensive technology.

KEYWORDS

- **cloud computing**
- **cloud technology**
- **healthcare**
- **healthcare services**
- **homogeneous**
- **hospital information system**

REFERENCES

1. Al-Shibli, A., & Al-Jaradi, S., (2017). Electronic pharmacy system (EPS): Case study in Oman. *International Journal of Computation and Applied Sciences IJOCAAS* (pp. 284–290).
2. Chintan, M. B., & Peddoju, S. K., (2016). *Cloud Computing Systems & Applications in Healthcare: A Volume in the Advances in Healthcare Information Systems & Administration (AHISA) Book Series.*
3. Kevin, C., & Teseng, C. C., (2014). An expert fitness diagnosis system based on elastic cloud computing. *The Scientific World Journal*, 10.
4. Jafar, S. A. M., Jayakumar, K., & Lokeshkumar, R., (2019). Patient health informatics system using cloud computing and IoT. *International Journal of Innovative Technology and Exploring Engineering (IJITEE)*, 2162–2165.
5. Prabal, C. P. A., (n.d.). Online pharmacy in India: A study on digital marketing perspective. *International Journal of Research in Engineering, IT and Social Sciences*, 232–242.
6. Rajvardhini, K. B. K., (2013). Survey of health monitoring management using the internet of things (IoT). *International Journal of Science and Research (IJSR)*, 1144–1147.
7. Repu, D. M. M., (2016). Cloud computing for medical applications & healthcare delivery: Technology, application, security, and swot analysis. *ACEIT Conference Proceedings*. Lucknow, UP, India: School of telemedicine & biomedical informatics, Sanjay Gandhi Post Graduate Institute of Medical Sciences.

8. Sasippriya, S. K. G., (2017). A survey on health care monitoring system using IoT. *International Journal of Pure and Applied Mathematics, 117*, 249–253.
9. Shweta, K. C. G., (2019). *Trust, Privacy, Issues in Cloud-Based Healthcare Services*. Chapter 75: IGI Global.
10. Vladimir, S., & Ricardo, C.-P., (2014). Cloud computing-based systems. *The Scientific World Journal*.
11. Yogesh, P. P., & Shubhangi, B., (2017). A survey on patient's health monitoring system in real-time using raspberry pi. *International Journal of Advanced Research in Electrical, Electronics and Instrumentation Engineering*, 4451–4454.

CHAPTER 7

IMPACT OF DELIBERATE RESOURCES (CLOUD COMPUTING) TO SUSTAIN A SMART AND PREVENTIVE HEALTH ECOSYSTEM

RAHUL SHARMA

Department of Computer Science and Engineering, Chandigarh University, Mohali, Punjab, India, E-mail: prof.rahuls@gmail.com

ABSTRACT

Current cloud services are created and deployed on very much provisioned and midway-controlled frameworks. Be that as it may, there are a few classes of services for which the current cloud model may not fit well; some don't require solid execution ensures, the evaluation might be excessively costly for a few; and some might be obliged by the information development expenses to the cloud. To fulfil the prerequisites of such services, some remotely utilized voluntary resources is proposed here, those given by end-user hosts to shape clouds, more dispersed and less managed clouds. Initially, the necessities of cloud services and the difficulties in meeting these prerequisites in such intractable clouds are examined. At that point, some potential answers for these difficulties are presented, and furthermore, this chapter talks about open doors for additional upgrades to make clouds a suitable cloud model.

IoT and Cloud Computing-Based Healthcare Information Systems. Anand Sharma, PhD, Hiren Kumar Deva Sarma, PhD & S. R. Biradar, PhD (Eds.)

7.1 INTRODUCTION

The hidden basic equipment needed for a business or society to operate is generally claimed and overseen by the cloud service providers (e.g., Amazon, IBM, Google, Microsoft, and so forth), while the client addresses a specific cost for their utilization of the helpful services and important supplies. There is also the idea of valuable supply and performance guarantees that something will occur or that something will function as depicted in between the cloud supplier and the client that makes sure about and sees the exhibition they hope to see. Computer services by different organizations accomplish over the Internet in general fall into more than two, however, not a great deal of classes. Long haul state and information stockpiling, one-shot eruption of calculation [16], and intuitive end client situated administrations [15].

7.2 EXPERIMENTAL CLOUD SERVICES

These are services that at the end may send out and used on a production framework which itself can be a business cloud. In any case before the real use, the service developers might need to do a "test drive" to prepare it production ready after debugging its functional ability and another company does for you over the internet to measure gauge user popularity with demand. To complete such military service, they may require sustained access to a large-scale "test cloud," which can give a realistic use of military service and surrounding conditions without the costs and strength and health of a production setting (Figure 7.1).

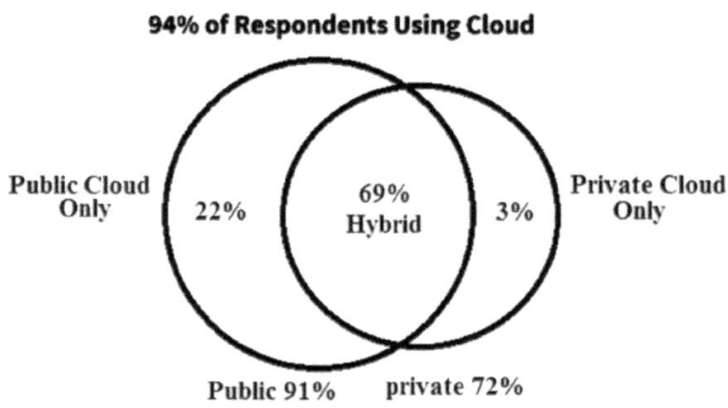

FIGURE 7.1 Respondents using cloud.

7.3 DISPERSED DATA-INTENSIVE SERVICES

These are services which depend on large amounts of broken up and moved away data, and where transferring data to a cloud (operated by one central place) can be way, way too expensive and inefficient. In this case, it would be better than move the math-based valuable supplies closer to the data while providing good enough computer-based ability. For example, a bunch of scientists want to give a service that would carefully study a large number of remotely user shared online writing pages containing text, sound, and video content to find interesting social popular ways.

7.4 SHARED SERVICES

These services would be given by clients, users or associations that want to freely share their own private computer programs with others as a "public service," but require military service and valuable supplies e.g. network radio frequency. In any case, since these services may not be business oriented and it conveys and clients might not have any desire to pay the expense for running the services. Simultaneously, these services may require arbitrary scale-up/downsize dependent on client interest.

For example, a user has created a personalized "tour" of his recent trip to any place that includes images, maps, video, explanation/statement of opinions, etc. This trip is too framework alert; specified user number that describe a location, position, and in order explode up. As this inspect with its data enormous in measurement, it would require a major amount of net radio recurrence or capacity to give out the agreeable to included customers.

A lot of the above services may have frail recital and strength and health needed things, so that paying for strict needed things of high availability, class of being very close to the fact or right digit, and presentation, as given by numerous present cloud provider may be pointless and unwanted.

To congregation such services, I suggest the idea of clouds: additional broke up and moved away, less oversaw clouds, constructed utilizing something you decide to do is not required. Those contribute by the end user host and sometimes may symbolize a change from a single thing to an additional pathway. Volunteer uses equipment for precious calculation, but not a lot of reasons. Volunteer useful equipment or precious materials are attractive for more than two, but not a lot of reasons:

1. **Scalability:** Many existing volunteer raised, flat supporting surfaces consist of millions of hosts and users, provided that many useful things valuable supply ability to hold or do something and the ability to be made bigger or smaller.
2. **Dispersion:** Volunteer nodes are likely to be related, where the detailed calculation need to figure out.
3. **Small Cost of Operation:** Unpaid assistant useful things or valuable supplies are fundamentally available for without any charge or at incredibly less charge. These are simply not operating and working now but able to access valuable supplies previously in the organization. They do not force on people some added and more hardware, preservation, or force costs, away from what they are previously with.
4. **Irritated Module Communications:** Nearly all on hand residence system are calculated for pathetically analogous computation anywhere present is no communication amid the dissimilar figure out or calculate household tasks. Though for organization running on a cloud as well as total of everything or everyone performance goals, needing, ordering careful setting apart and distributing of only occurrence or accessible in single tiny position nodes for their implementation.
5. **Locality and Context Awareness:** As accessible at house and P2P system perform not to tell the disparity amid diverse nodes in the system for giving out, figure out or calculate odd jobs and statistics in a cloud, especially for broke up and moved away data exhaustive and common services, the data calculation place, as well as the facts of the customer higher perspective their place, machine capacity to hold or accomplish something and so on would be basic in making accommodating item or significant flexibly separating and hand out outcome.
6. **Dynamic State Maintenance:** Many computer services other companies do for you over the Internet. Rather than house application anyplace calculations be generally stateless and can be re-executed effectively, clouds should keep up tenuously common position that can be simply retrieved and worn by a repair (Figure 7.2).

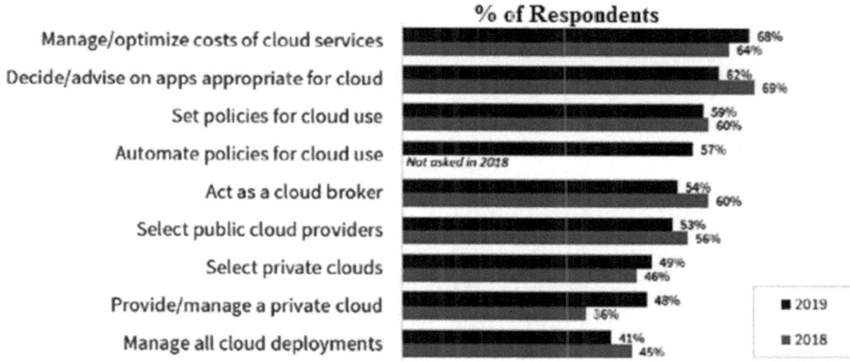

FIGURE 7.2 Role of enterprise central IT in cloud.

7.5 NECESSITIES WITH CHALLENGE

In this segment, a number of needed things are drawn to choose but are not required. Fundamental tools desirable for a trade to function must work pleased by meeting a need or reaching a goal to be acceptable as a doable possible cloud raised, flat supporting surface and needed things.

7.5.1 REQUIREMENT 1: SUPPLY CHECK CENTRIC ACT DEMARCATION

In the direction use many services on a nebula and to hold numerous customer requirements for an examine. The raised, flat supporting surface must provide using different things and service clearly stated for particular performance numbers that measure things, such as response time, throughput, etc.

Whereas this form is suitable for single attempt busty, math based or paper forms or computer based online system that ask for a job, money, admission, etc., a hosted computer service another company does for you over the Internet would be seen as part needs life form submit by end-user, and these desires would have to be run at the same time or together in the cloud. The cloud would then entail machines, methods, or ways to tell or to show the difference between tasks going along with matching up to different requests and organize in the correct order and their outcome disjointedly.

7.5.2 *CHALLENGE*

Conference overhaul centric presentation needed things is taxing because of the group of different things mixed together and time changing or different behavior of something you choose to do, but is not required on nodes. As an illustration, I sent out and used a simple computer service another company does for you over the Internet as of the field of bioinformatics called BLAST (basic local alignment search tool) [3] on a common cloud with testing lab. A far above the ground degree of mixed up nature was watched or followed, both in terms of the math based or computer based ability to hold or do something and communication radio frequency or ability of the contributing knots (Figure 7.3).

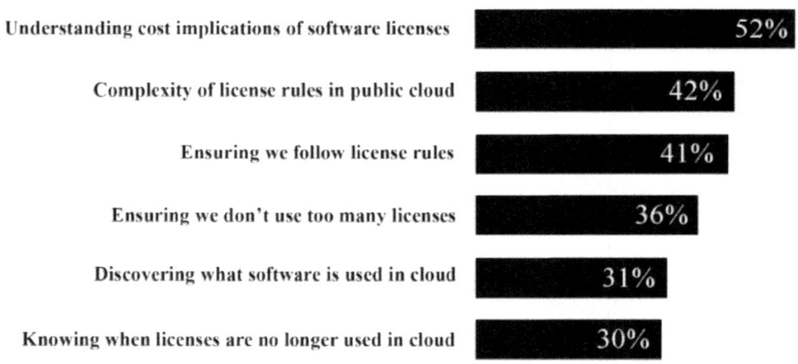

FIGURE 7.3 Challenges of software in the cloud.

7.6 STRUCTURE CLOUDS: PROBABLE SOLUTIONS

Some of the approaches are currently sketched that can be worn to defeat confront organized and listed below.

7.6.1 *MANAGING HETEROGENEITY*

Many different kinds of people or things of unpaid assistant nodes have to be captured and controlled in a service clearly stated or particular way. Here, a mixed-up nature is focused as it hits and affects performance.

First of all, large-scale useful things, or valuable supply discovery ways of doing things [5, 18, 19] could be employed to select a good set of used services. These useful things or valuable supplies would be selected based on their abilities and their long-term firm and steady nature or lasting nature and strength.

Further, service performance numbers that measure things would govern how mixed-up nature of selected useful things/valuable supplies is to be handled, and one such model is presented here. Numerous services pulled in to clouds would be those that need enormous calculations, for example, large scale picture investigation or logical sorting out/ascertaining.

Such services are agreeable to working together processing each service request would be rotten into separate undertakings and run on various volunteers. The reaction time for each service solicitation can be diminished under basic equipment needed for a business to operate mixed-up nature capacities to hold something for load balancing. For example, as the finishing point of the request is de-suspended on the slowest node, the tasks should be set apart and given out according to individual node abilities (e.g., by allocating bigger errands to quicker nodes with quicker correspondence ways). Thus, errands might be estimated in relation to the hub capacities (to hold or accomplish something) for load balancing, and may also be rotten into smaller fixed sizes to account for performance unsteadiness [18]. Almost the same ways of doing things can be used for fully using for profit mixed-up nature in a nebula for giving service oriented performance.

7.6.2 HANDLING DATA COMPUTE DEPENDENCE

Selecting something you decide to do, however, isn't needed nodes for work separating and distributing have to take into version the site of desirable facts. The primary confront is to position statistics assuming its spot isn't known a prior. A loaded organized things exist for finding descriptive data by name, picture, GPS location, etc. but is not required in P2P networks [7]. When the statistics of area are realized the organization space from conceivable unpaid assistant nodes should be measured about believed to assemble act goal (Figure 7.4).

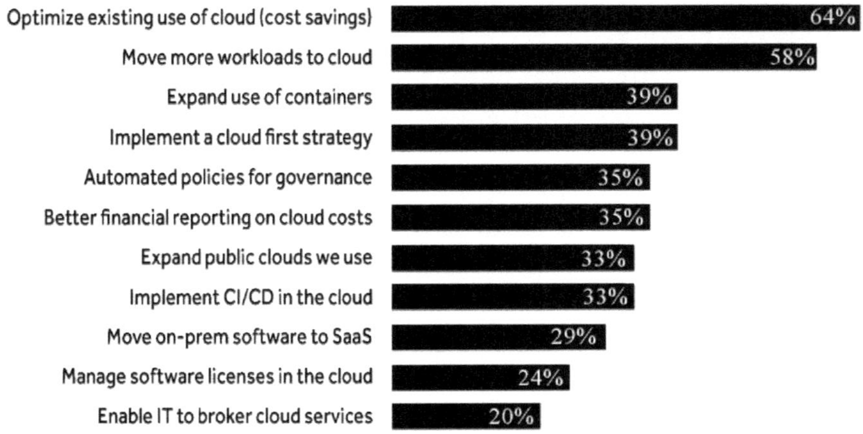

FIGURE 7.4 Top cloud initiatives in 2019.

7.7 CONCLUSION

This chapter offers the idea to create cloud by basic tools required for an industry. These clouds are geared towards hosting computer and services to do over the Internet. Clouds can exist as matching, basic equipment needed for a business or society to operate, and can even serve as a change from one node to another node for a lot of inspection that would ultimately be deployed on clouds.

KEYWORDS

- **business cloud**
- **cloud computing**
- **computer services**
- **deliberate resources**
- **health ecosystem**
- **scalability**
- **smart and preventive**

REFERENCES

1. Azure Services Platform. http://www.microsoft.com/azure/default.mspx (accessed on 13 June 2022).
2. *The Basic Local Alignment Search Tool (BLAST)*. http://www.ncbi.nlm.nih.gov/blast (accessed on 13 June 2022).
3. BOINC Stats. http://boincstats.com (accessed on 13 June 2022).
4. Castro, M., & Liskov, B., (2019). *Practical Byzantine Fault Tolerance*. In OSDI.
5. Amazon Elastic Compute Cloud (Amazon EC2). http://aws.amazon.com/ec2 (accessed on 13 June 2022).
6. Folding@home distributing computing project. https://folding.stanford.edu (accessed on 13 June 2022).
7. Foster, I., & Kesselman, C., (2007). Globus: A meta computing infrastructure toolkit. *International Journal of Supercomputer Applications, 11*(2), 115–128.
8. Google App Engine. http://code.google.com/appengine (accessed on 13 June 2022).
9. Google Maps. http://maps.google.com (accessed on 13 June 2022).
10. Gottfrid, D. (2007). *Self-service, Prorated Super Computing Fun*! http://open.blogs.nytimes.com/2007/11/01/self-service-prorated-super-computing-fun (accessed on 13 June 2022).
11. *IBM Cloud Computing*. http://www.ibm.com/ibm/cloud (accessed on 13 June 2022).
12. Kim, J., Chandra, A., & Weissman, J., (2018). *OPEN: Passive Network Performance Estimation for Data-intensive Applications*. Technical Report 08-041, Dept. of CSE, Univ. of Minnesota.
13. Network Weather Service. https://nws.cs.ucsb.edu (accessed on 13 June 2022).
14. Oppenheimer, D., Albrecht, J., Patterson, D., & Vahdat, A., (2014). Distributed resource discovery on PlanetLab with SWORD. In: *First Workshop on Real, Large Remotely Systems (WORLDS '04)*.
15. Public Data Sets on AWS. http://aws.amazon.com/publicdatasets (accessed on 13 June 2022).
16. Saroiu, S., Gummadi, K. P., Dunn, R. J., Gribble, S. D., & Levy, H. M., (2012). *An Analysis of Internet Content Delivery Systems*. In OSDI.
17. Stoica, I., Morris, R., Karger, D., Kaashoek, M. F., & Balakrishnan, H., (2011). Chord: A scalable peer-to-peer lookup service for internet applications. In: *Proceedings of SIGCOMM*.
18. Trivedi, R., Chandra, A., & Weissman, J., (2006). Heterogeneity-aware workload distribution in donation-based grids. *International Journal of High-Performance Computing Applications, 20*(4), 455–466.

CHAPTER 8

MEDICAL IMAGE AUTHENTICATION USING A WATERMARKING TECHNIQUE IN CLOUD COMPUTING

RAJESH YADAV and ANAND SHARMA

School of Engineering and Technology, Mody University of Science and Technology, Laxmangarh, Rajasthan, India,
E-mail: yadav.rajesh27@gmail.com (R. Yadav)

ABSTRACT

In modern healthcare technology, innovative software for medical image processing has increased great interest. It also provides an improved medical information and expand the diagnosis and treatment. This field still requires a more implementations in software and hardware. But its cause increases the medical cost and required the improved infrastructure. The cloud computing techniques in medical tried to mitigate this problem. The cloud computing, specially software-as-a-service (SaaS) and platform-as-a-service (PaaS) are very helpful in the healthcare industry. Through improved software healthcare can easily diagnose the patients from anywhere and check their medical history which is store in cloud platform. If required to discuss with another healthcare professional, it's very easy and fast.

Interestingly, the cloud computing techniques reduce the cost of medical functionality because their cost is based on the utilization of

IoT and Cloud Computing-Based Healthcare Information Systems. Anand Sharma, PhD, Hiren Kumar Deva Sarma, PhD & S. R. Biradar, PhD (Eds.)

resources and software. Also, it offers an improved quality of service (QoS), elasticity, fast request and response time, security assurance, etc., irrespective of cost benefits in the healthcare industry, the cloud computing rise to security and privacy issues. A lot of security mechanisms and methods are suggested to reduce these problems and make trust in cloud computing. In this respect, many cryptographic techniques are used in digital medical images. But these methods can reduce the performance of cloud services. In medical, most of the information is in textual and images form, but we are required to prevent the images data. This can be happened through convert the images into pixels and after that encrypting the pixels. Then add the patient's information with encrypted images. Patients' information can be authenticated through id and password in the cloud. That two-way authentication provides more security on the cloud. For encryption, we use the full watermarking techniques.

8.1 INTRODUCTION

Cloud computing is a technique that uses the resources and services which is placed centrally through the internet. Cloud computing permits consumers and organizations to utilize the software without installation and access information in any device on-demand basis [1]. Cloud computing provides the architecture for the organizations. It frequently provides the services through internet in the form of platform-as-a-service (PaaS), infrastructure-as-a-service (IaaS), and software-as-a-service (SaaS) [2]. This provides fast, manageable, and minimum maintenance infrastructure for the organizations that fulfill all business requirements [3]. The user point of view, the cloud provides remote data storage is more beneficial like it can access from anywhere, no maintenance, no need to bother about hardware and software maintenance, etc.

With many advantages of cloud computing, there are a number of disadvantages in it. Data security and stopping unauthentic access is the main disadvantage in cloud. That issue is faced by both the cloud providers and their users. In respect of security a lot of security algorithms are proposed [4]. There encryption technique is one of the most important technique to protecting the text and medical images.

8.1.1 CLOUD ARCHITECTURE

The cloud computing architecture is having two sections, front-end, and back-end. The front-end is the client's machines their applications are accessed and performed the procedures. In cloud computing having different user interfaces, through client can access the applications (Figure 8.1).

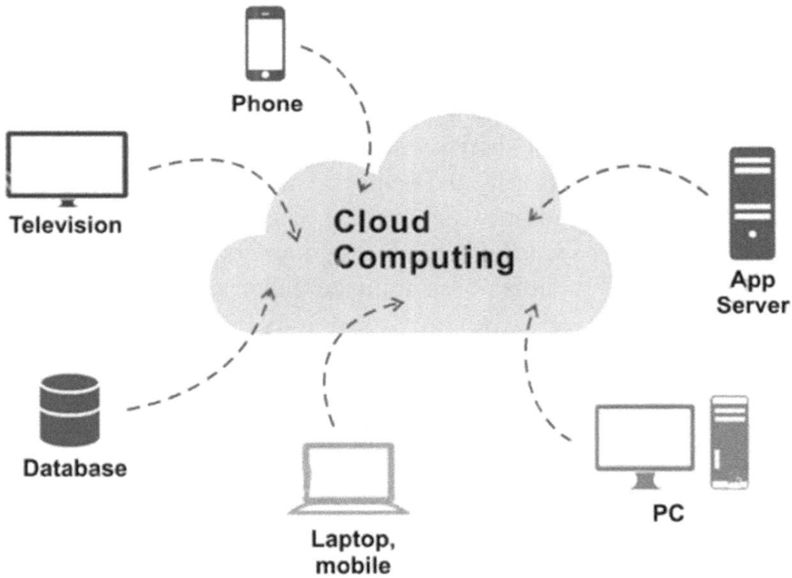

FIGURE 8.1 Cloud architecture.

The back-end is the centric place (Servers, Data Storage system) where data is stored and accessed on authorized client machine on demand. The admin centrally monitors the traffic and handles all servers so functionalities are working smoothly. In between client and server, a middleware is there, its handles all communications between authorized users [5]. Cloud computing use the concept called virtualization, which reduced the physical machines by maximum uses of server capacity.

8.1.2 TYPES OF CLOUD DEPLOYMENT MODELS

1. **Public Cloud:** The public cloud resources are used by public organizations free of cost or pay-per-usage bases. A public cloud service provider creates information technology (IT) resources like applications, storage places available to any user. In this deployment model, user can use services on-demand or pay per bases [6]. For example, AppEngine, Windows Azure, Amazon Elastic compute cloud, etc. The drawback of public cloud is there having no control over the resources, security of data and network performance.
2. **Private Cloud:** This cloud is just opposite to the public cloud, there infrastructures are operating individually by each organization, and it's not shared with other organizations. It provides the high level of security and control. The private cloud is the best for those organizations which want to whole control of the infrastructure and its security. It's delivered more consistent processes, but it's partial in terms of scalability and their size [7].
3. **Community Cloud:** This cloud is shared the infrastructure in between many organizations for common computing. The main purpose of this cloud is to have contributing organizations profits like public cloud but an additional level of security and privacy like the private cloud [8].
4. **Hybrid Cloud:** The hybrid means a combination of more than two things; same as hybrid cloud is a combination of public and private cloud. Normally organizations compute the resources using private cloud, but in high demand or peak load also use the public cloud [5]. On the demand bases automatically transfer the cloud from private to public and handled the requirement graciously.

8.1.3 CLOUD SERVICE

1. **Infrastructure-as-a-Service (IaaS):** It provides all things through virtualization concepts, like virtual machine, infrastructure, storage, and hardware resources that use by users [1]. The service provider can handle the entire infrastructure, while the user only responsible for deployment processes.

2. **Platform-as-a-Service (PaaS):** In this cloud service providers manage the virtual machine, OS, applications, and deploy frameworks [3]. The user can deploy the application or use the applications which are already available on the platform. Service providers maintain or handle all the application; users don't need to worry about that. They only concern about the installation and management of the application.
3. **Software-as-a-Service (SaaS):** This is the top layer of the cloud computing, and it's also directly used by end-user [9]. This service provides the interface where clients can use the different types of software and services. It's also minimizing the need of infrastructure because user can handle that remotely and all things are updated automatically.

8.2 CLOUD COMPUTING IN HEALTHCARE ORGANIZATION

These days a healthcare sector is rapidly growing, and new things are introduced constantly. In this regard it's required to heavy investment for infrastructure and facilities. In terms of introducing new technology in healthcare sectors, the organizations can reduce the cost, time, and improve the performance through cloud computing. Using a cloud computing store, the patient's complete medical history and that can share with many healthcare professionals. e-Health record can manage and share with insurance companies, doctors, and other healthcare professionals. All healthcare organizations want to handle the more demands with already available resources. For improving the quality of services (QoS) it's required computation skills because the patient's data are increasing rapidly. Cloud computing meet the healthcare sector requirements, because it's having capability to store huge amount of patients' data and easily, fast, and secure processed whenever its required. With these features one more benefit that healthcare industry rapidly moves on cloud that is there no geographical barriers for providing services to patients. Through cloud many doctors which are seated on different places can access patient's health record can discuss and gives better treatments.

8.2.1 E-HEALTH BENEFITS

There are lots of benefits using cloud in e-healthcare:

1. **Enriched Patient Attention:** At a time, many doctors who are placed in different places can take care of and gives treatment according to better discussions between them.
2. **Reducing Cost:** Healthcare organization no need to setup expensive s/w and h/, also no need to spend money for their maintenance.
3. **Save Energy:** Because there no large setup is required, so that their energy bill is also decrease.
4. **Disaster Retrieval:** Any emergency, cloud service can protect organization data and if lost then easily recover them.
5. **Exploration:** There central data depository so anyone can use the data for new inventions.
6. **Fast Deployment:** In any type of new requirements solution can be done immediately.
7. **Information Availability:** Patients data is all time available for all healthcare providers [10].

8.2.2 E-HEALTH SECURITY RISK

Security, data confidentially is the main risk of cloud computing. In medical organizations also the patient's data is more confidential. So that in cloud we required to maintain that confidentiality. For that applied many encryption standards for securing the sensitive information. But in cloud that maintenance is very difficult because their huge amount of data is stored and their possibility to leak or exchange the data between users, also there possible to change or delete the data by unauthorized person intestinally.

A healthcare organization specially contains the images files like X-ray, CT scans, radiology, etc., their records are called electronic healthcare records (EHR) [11]. The cloud can contain all EHRs and manage them and that can be accessed by patients and doctors at anywhere and at any time. Therefore, the patient's personal and health information are distributed throughout the networks and there is more probability to misuse by anyone. In healthcare data, the image is more sensitive data, if in decryption time it's not properly done then that records can be useless, or doctors can't give proper treatments. The pharmacy company can misuse the patient's information for hiking the cost of medicines and all. The insurance company can increase the insurance cost according to patient's health data.

8.2.3 E-HEALTH SECURITY ISSUES

The International Medical Information Association (IMIA) concern of data safety and security in e-health networks system [12]. The U.S. Department of health and human services (HHS) published about personal health records (PHRs), that patients, healthcare providers could access using the internet, not necessary to patients is seeking medical care [12]. The security and privacy are not only concerns to deal with abiding by availability, confidentiality, and reliability (ACI) model. The security threats in cloud data like spoofing through attacker imagining to be a legal user, interfering with the data through malicious changes and modification of the information, and denial of the service [13]. For creating the trust in cloud computing applications satisfied the many security requirements. Some of them are:

1. **Confidentiality:** That means patients data is not accessible to any unauthorized person. That create more trust on e-health system and patients are ready to share more and accurate information to their doctors. That confidentiality can get by encryption techniques.
2. **Integrity:** It means the health data is accurate and consistent. It's totally the same as it provided by patients and healthcare providers [14]. The e-health cloud services and information must be errorless. The erroneous data create serious concern on patient's health. There must be some restrictions before using the data by anyone.
3. **Availability:** The information must be available whenever it's required. If the data is not available when it's required to its useless and in e-health, it create more trouble to patients. The data availability can be breach by hardware failure, any upgrade or denial of service (DoS) attack, etc.
4. **Possession and Privacy (PP) of Information:** Ownership is very important to protect against unauthorized access or any misuse of medical data [13]. It can be done through authorization via encryption and other techniques. The user can allow or deny sharing our information to any healthcare professionals.

5. **Authenticity:** In healthcare, is very important to know that the provided information is authentic or not. It can be carriage new problem, like man-in-the-middle attacks, and eased with username and password. Many cryptography protocols make authentication.
6. **Nonrepudiation:** In healthcare, the patients and doctors can't be denying their signature authenticity after misusing the data.
7. **Access Control:** It decides that a particular data is used by which person. With this every one can only access that information which is related to that. The Role-based access control and Attribute-based access control is very famous in healthcare applications [15].
8. **Data Updating:** In healthcare required patients' data should be up to date. It's very dangerous to delay in storage or inconsistency, especially in emergency situation.

8.2.4 HEALTHCARE IMAGE AUTHENTICATION METHOD

This section explains the secret share creation and watermark construction algorithm used for securing the medical images.

- **Algorithm 1: Secret Share Creation:**
  - **S 1:** Use H to produce a **v** × **v** LF sub-band.
  - **S 2:** Complete l × l block dividing on the LF sub-band to generate v/l × v/l non-overlap blocks.
  - **S 3:** Use Arnold transform on W to produce watermark SW.
  - **S 4:** Repeat S 4-S 9 for every bit W_{ij} of watermark.
  - **S 5:** Use Arnold transform (k_i, k_j) to choose a block for Mshare formation, and increment by 1.
  - **S 6:** Use SVD to particular block to generate M, N, and O matrices.
  - **S 7:** Compute the Hu's invariant moment.
  - **S 8:** Generate a 3-bit Mshare out of the sign bit.
  - **S 9:** Encode Mshare and SW with calculation to produce Sshare of size m × m.
- **Algorithm 2: Watermark:**
  - **S 1:** Use contourlet transform on H and generate v × v sub-band.
  - **S 2:** Perform a l × l block dividing on LF sub-band to generate v/l × v/l overlying blocks of S 3.

- **S 3:** Perform S 4 to S 9 element of Sshare.
- **S 4:** Use Arnold transform on (k_i, k_j) to select the block of Mshare creation and increment by 1.
- **S 5:** Use SVD to certain block to produce M, N, O matrices.
- **S 6:** Calculate Hu's invariant moment.
- **S 7:** Generate a 3-bit Mshare out of the sign bits.
- **S 8:** Compute Y from Sshare with equation.
- **S 9:** Subtract Mshare from Y to get SW.
- **S 10:** Use Arnold convert to decode SW to develop W.

8.3 REVIEW LITERATURE

Luis et al. [16] proposed architecture there use the picture archiving and communication system (PACS) that maintain more than one cloud suppliers. There two key components are used in the public cloud. First is DICOM and second is the Data Storage system. For security divides the images into chunks and encrypt by AES algorithm and then store into cloud.

Arkaa and Chellappana [17] proposed a secure shared platform in cloud computing. There medical images are shared between healthcare professional by mobile device. The author proposed architecture there uses the four blocks, picture creation device, image viewer, database, and server. Compression algorithm and cryptography are used for image security.

Yang et al. [18] used cryptography and statistical analysis technique for securing the images. There medical data is divided into many categories. The patient's information is encrypting symmetric encryption and other data saved with plaintext.

Pan et al. [19] used the reversible watermarking techniques for medical image authentication and its integrity. For that use, the advanced encryption standard (AES). There one more technique is used for tracing the unauthorized access that is called OrBAC (organization-based access control).

Fabian et al. [20] introduced the Ciphertext Policy Attribute-Based Encryption for cloud security. There uses the DSA signature for protecting the ownership uses the SHA1 function. After encryption store the medical image into different cloud provider, so its escapes the unauthorized disclosure of important part of the image.

Brindha and Jeyanthi [21] used the visual cryptography technique to secure the storage. There use the Apache POI applications to convert file into text format. It's improved the confidentiality and integrity of file in cloud computing.

Kaur and Khemchandani [22] for image security used a visual cryptography with RSA algorithm. There first divide the image into multiple pieces and then encrypt all images.

Nelmiawati and Ibrahim [23] proposed the security framework there use the Pixel based dispersal scheme. In this regard use the Shamir's Secret Scheme and Robin's Information Dispersal Algorithm for securing patient's information.

Ansari [24] used the SVD approach for semi-fragile watermarking. They put the watermark in the medical image through SVD calculation and then quantizing the value in each image block.

Syifak et al. [25] used the watermarking approach for achieving numbering pattern for precise detection of image recovery.

8.4 PROPOSED METHOD

As above, we explain a lot of techniques that have been used by many authors for securing the medical images, but as we know that the medical images are very sensitive. If in decryption time any small changes can done, that's not exactly similar to the original image, then that is totally useless for medical service providers or can give wrong treatment to patients. So, in this chapter proposed the framework that maintained the originality of image after decryption and also provides the strong security through authentication in cloud computing.

The proposed framework having four sections: data, user, cloud, and authority. The data is encrypted by watermarking algorithm and merge with patient information like patient Id, patient name, etc., before merging the text data is also secure by MAC cipher text. Then that merged data is stored in the cloud. At cloud, the encrypted data is partially decrypts because that reduce the owner computational cost. Figure 8.2 explains the encryption of the original image and again decrypting the data by the user end. After data encryption, their owner can upload on the cloud. The symmetric key (k2) is used for the encryption process and another encryption key (k1) is used for itself. After encrypting the image send on cloud there, this encrypted data is again authenticated by user id and password. So, with this technique we secure the data by two-way authentication on different places.

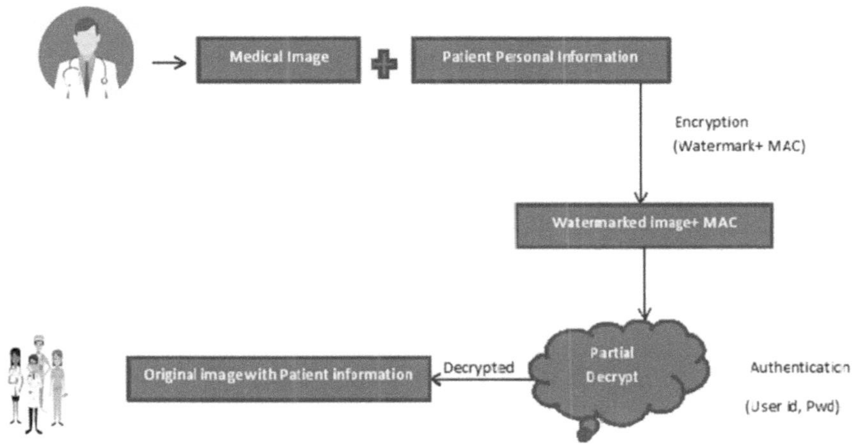

FIGURE 8.2 Framework of overall authentication process.

Authentication Process: The authentication process follows the following steps:

- Read the image sent by radiologist;
- Radiologist accesses the image for study;
- It's got contact to secret share from e-health record server;
- Radiologist shares the image with attached secret share (Algorithm 1) to build watermark (Algorithm 2);
- Radiologist decrypts the Watermark and contact the file;
- Radiologist gets access e-health record of the patient.

8.5 EXPERIMENTAL RESULTS

For experiment use the MATLAB. The algorithm applied on many medical images of different methods like CT, MRA, Ultrasound, PET, X-ray with size 512 × 512. In starting the image is breakdown to produce an LF band of size 256 × 256. It's distributed 128 × 128 non-overlapping blocks of size 2 × 2. For Master Share (Mshare) in starting assumed $k_i = 32$ and

TABLE 8.1 NC Values under MATLAB Attacks

Attack	Modality						
	CT	**Mammogram**	**MRA**	**Nuclear**	**PET**	**Ultrasound**	**X-Ray**
JPEG compression quality factor: 50%	0.9999	0.9855	0.9999	1	0.9997	1	0.9992
Average window size: [9 × 9]	0.9999	0.9892	0.9999	1	0.9997	1	0.9994
Median window size: [9 × 9]	0.9999	0.9885	0.9998	1	0.9999	1	0.9993
Blur window size: [9 × 9]	0.9999	0.9885	0.9998	1	0.9999	1	0.9995
Sharpening + 50% sharpness	0.9999	0.9876	0.9999	1	0.9998	1	0.9992
Gaussian noise: 30%	0.9999	0.9755	0.9998	1	0.9997	1	0.9987
Contrast sharpness: +50%	0.9999	0.9905	0.9999	1	0.9997	1	0.9988
Gamma correction (Gamma value: 0.6)	0.9999	0.9842	0.9999	1	0.9999	1	0.9995
Histogram equalization	0.9999	0.9826	0.9999	1	0.9996	1	0.9988
Resizing scale factor: 0.5	0.9999	0.9806	0.9999	1	0.9996	1	0.9986
Rotation angle: 30	0.9999	0.9853	0.9999	1	0.9996	1	0.9987
Distortion warp factor: 3	0.9999	0.9833	0.9998	1	0.9997	1	0.999

k_j.= 32 there i = 5. The Mshare is attached with watermark to generate the Sshare. At another end it's combined with Sshare to construct the watermark. Compared the structure with proposed by Hsu and Hou [26]; Wanf and Chen [27]; and Rawat and Raman [28]. There we run the attack with parameter identified in Rawat and Raman [28] with MATLAB. The evaluation is based on NC values to set of attacks. Table 8.1 result shows that the proposed structure is better robust as compared to the rest of the structures (Figure 8.3).

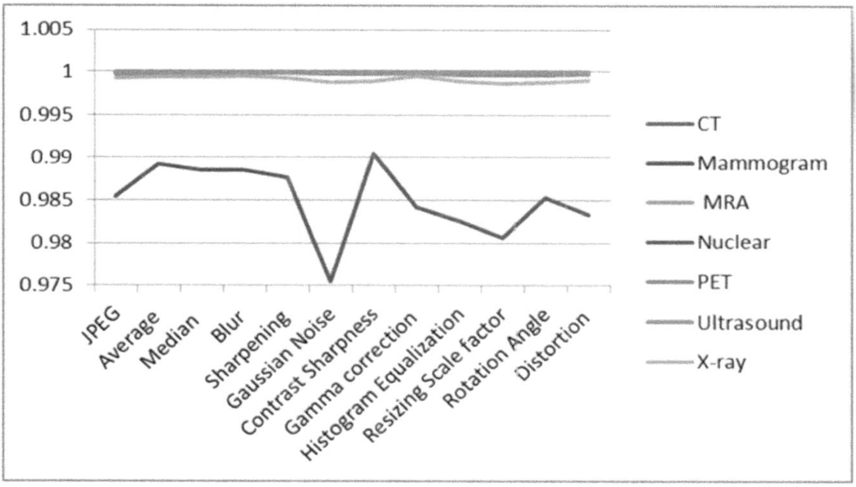

FIGURE 8.3 Comparison with existing watermarking schemes.

8.6 CONCLUSION AND FUTURE SCOPE

The proposed technique is based on watermarking for authentication of patient data on the cloud. And the comparison with the same data shows that the proposed technique is better than the previous techniques, and it reduces the attack probability. Future work tries to improve the performance of data decryption and reduce the time delay. There is also scope of using more techniques to improve the security of patient's data on cloud computing.

KEYWORDS

- **cloud computing**
- **electronic healthcare records**
- **healthcare**
- **infrastructure-as-a-service**
- **quality of service**
- **security**
- **watermarking**

REFERENCES

1. Nishitha, R., & Sreerekha, B., (2015). Enhancing security of personal health records in cloud computing by encryption. *International Journal of Science and Research (IJSR)* (Vol. 4, No. 4, pp. 298–302). ISSN 2319-7064.
2. Gunasekaran, S., & Lavanya, M. P., (2015). A review on enhancing data security in cloud computing using RSA And AES algorithms. *IJAER* (Vol. 9, No. 4). ISSN 2231-5152.
3. Rashmi, S. G., & Deepali, M. K., (2017). Architecture for data security in multicloud using AES-256 encryption algorithm. *International Journal on Recent and Innovation Trends in Computing and Communication (IJRITCC)* (Vol. 3, No. 5). ISSN: 2321-8169.
4. Rizwana, K. M. S., Somasekhar, T., DivyaShree, K. B., & Pooja, G., (2016). Design and implementation of security for healthcare billing system using cloud computing. *International Journal of Electrical, Electronics and Computer Systems (IJEECS)* (Vol. 4, No. 7). ISSN (Online), 2347-2820.
5. Vinoth, K. B., Ramaswami, M., & Swathika, P., (2017). Data security on patient monitoring for future healthcare application. *International Journal of Computer Applications(IJCA), 163*(6).
6. Abha, S., & Mohit, B., (2013). Enhancing cloud computing security using AES algorithm. *International Journal of Computer Applications (IJCA)* (Vol. 67, No. 9). ISSN 0975 – 8887.
7. Divya, R., & Smita, J., (2016). Cloud based information security and privacy in healthcare. *International Journal of Computer Applications (IJCA)* (Vol. 150, No. 4, pp. 11–15). ISSN 0975 – 8887.
8. Sri Varsha, B., & Suryateja, P. S., (2014). Using advanced encryption standard for secure and scalable sharing of personal health records in the cloud. *International Journal of Computer Science and Information Technologies(IJCSIT)* (Vol. 5, No. 6). ISSN 0975-9646.

9. Namita, N. P., & Meghana, N., (2015). Enhanced security for multi cloud storage using AES algorithm. *International Journal of Computer Science and Information Technologies(IJCSIT)* (Vol. 6, No. 6). ISSN 0975-9646.
10. Dong, N., Jonker, H., & Pang, J., (2011). Challenges in e-health: From enabling to enforcing privacy. In: Liu, Z., &. Wassyng, A., (eds.), *Foundations of Health Informatics Engineering and Systems-FHIES 2011: Lecture Notes in Computer Science* (pp. 195–206). Springer.
11. Abbas, A., & Khan, S. U., (2014). A review on the state-of-the-art privacy-preserving approaches in the e-health clouds. *IEEE Journal of Biomedical and Health Informatics, 18*(4), 1431–1441.
12. US Department of Health & Human Services (HHS), (2005). *Health Information Privacy*. US Department of Health & Human Services (HHS), Washington, DC, USA.
13. Metri, P., & Sarote, G., (2011). Privacy issues and challenges in cloud computing. *International Journal of Advanced Engineering and Technology, 5*(1), 5, 6.
14. Xiao, Z., & Xiao, Y., (2013). Security and privacy in cloud computing. *IEEE Communications Surveys & Tutorials, 15*(2), 843–859.
15. Hagner, M.,(2007). Security infrastructure and national patent summary. In *Proceedings of the Tromso Telemedicine and e-Health Conference*. Tromsø, Norway, June.
16. Luis, A., Bastiao, S., Carlos, C., & Oliveira, J. L., (2012). A PACS archive architecture supported on cloud services. *Int. J. CARS, 7*(3), 349–358. Springer.
17. Arkaa, I. H., & Chellappana, K., (2014). Collaborative compressed I-cloud medical image storage with decompress viewer. In: *Proceedings of the International Conference on Robot PRIDE, Procedia Computer Science* (pp. 114–121). Elsevier
18. Yang, C. T., Chen, L. T., Chou, W. L., & Wang, K. C., (2010). Implementation of a medical image file accessing system on cloud computing. In: *Proceedings of the International Conference in Computational Science and Engineering (CSE)* (pp. 321–326). IEEE.
19. Pan, W., Coatrieux, G., Bouslimi, D., & Prigent, N., (2015). Secure public cloud platform for medical images sharing. *Stud. Health Technol. Inf., 210*, 251–255.
20. Fabian, B., Ermakova, T., & Junghanns, P., (2015). Collaborative and secure sharing of healthcare data in multi-clouds. *Inf. Syst., 48*, 132–150. Elsevier.
21. Brindha, K., & Jeyanthi, N., (2015). Secured document sharing using visual cryptography in cloud data storage. *Cybern. Inf. Technol., 15*(4), 111–123.
22. Kaur, K., & Khemchandani, V., (2013). Securing visual cryptographic shares using public-key encryption. In: *Proceedings of the International Conference on Advance Computing Conference, IACC* (pp. 1108–1113).
23. Nelmiawati, N., Salleh, M., & Ibrahim, S., (2015). Medical image dispersal using enhanced secret sharing threshold scheme. In: *Proceedings of the International Conference on Health Informatics and Medical Systems, HIMS 2015* (pp. 132–138).
24. Ansari, I. A., Pant, A., & Ahn, C. W., (2016). Robust and false-positive free watermarking in IWT domain using SVD and ABC. *Eng. Appl. Artif. Intell., 49*, 114–125.

25. Syifak, I. H., Afifah, N. M., Gran, B., Nasrul, H. J., & Jasni, M. Z., (2017). Numbering with spiral pattern to prove authenticity and integrity in medical images. *Pattern Anal. Applic.*
26. Hsu, C. S., & Hou, Y. C., (2005). Copyright protection scheme for digital images using visual cryptography and sampling methods. *Optical Engineering, 44*(7), 1–10. Article ID 077003.
27. Wang, M. S., & Chen, W. C., (2009). A hybrid DWT-SVD copyright protection scheme based on k-means clustering and visual cryptography. *Computer Standards and Interfaces, 31*(4), 757–762.
28. Rawat, S., & Raman, B., (2012). A blind watermarking algorithm based on fractional Fourier transform and visual cryptography. *Signal Processing, 92*(6), 1480–1491.

CHAPTER 9

A LOW POWER BLUETOOTH-BASED PULSE-OXY TRACKER

RITIKA UPADHYAY and BISWAJEET CHAMPATY

School of Engineering, Ajeenkya DY Patil University, Pune, Maharashtra – 412105, India,
E-mail: biswajeet.champaty@adypu.edu.in (B. Champaty)

ABSTRACT

Oxygen is vital to human life, so determining oxygen saturation and its monitoring can detect the concerning symptom and abnormalities at a very early stage so as to save lives, especially for old aged, low immune patients having chronic or infectious diseases. This can be applied in professional diagnostic centers or normal home care. Patients with heart medical procedures are more in danger of poor surrounding perfusion, and capillary oxygen saturation (SpO_2) estimation is customary consideration for examination of blood oxygen saturation in these patients continuously. To display the detection of abnormality and other measurements, a mobile application is proposed.

9.1 INTRODUCTION

The concentration of blood oxygen present in the blood is termed as "blood oxygen saturation" and are subsequently some of the physiological and standard parameters when respiratory and circulatory diagnosis

IoT and Cloud Computing-Based Healthcare Information Systems. Anand Sharma, PhD, Hiren Kumar Deva Sarma, PhD & S. R. Biradar, PhD (Eds.)

comes into play. Various symptoms like dizziness, memory loss, anxiety, inattention, and others combined with the above can be depicted as "Hypoxia," myocardial hypoxia can lead to some serious problems such as ventricular fibrillation and cardiac arrest, some major issues such as myocardial failure, blood pressure and blood circulation failure can come into framework while sever or long-term hypoxia, above all, it can damage cerebral cortex leading to brain tissue degeneration and necrosis. There are many people who have high pressure due to the working culture followed in today's society; people don't give importance to their regular health checkups, so to improve blood oxygen saturation level, the proposed study can be helpful.

Oxygen is firmly managed inside the body on the grounds that hypoxemia can prompt numerous intense unfavorable impacts on individual organ systems. It includes brain, heart, and kidneys. Oxygen saturation can be explained as a proportion of the amount of hemoglobin is at present bound to find oxygen contrasted with unbound hemoglobin present. Considering molecular level, hemoglobin consists majorly of four protein subunits. In which, each subunit is further associated with heme group. Each hemoglobin molecule is subsequently having four binding sites that are available for the oxygen bind. During the flow of oxygen in blood, it is observed that the hemoglobin can carry oxygen molecules but is limited to four. Because of the critical nature of the issue regarding the consumption of oxygen in the human body, it becomes essential to monitor the current oxygen saturation [1]. A pulse oximeter can be utilized to estimate oxygen saturation. A noninvasive system which is set on the patient's finger is then quantifies the wavelength of light to determine the degrees of oxygenated hemoglobin in proportion to deoxygenated hemoglobin present. It is viewed as a fifth fundamental sign as well as it is one of the basic requirements for clinicians to understand the activities and limitations of pulse oximeter. Therefore, they are used to have fundamental information on oxygen saturation.

The MAX30100 is a well-defined heart rate (HR) and pulse oximetry sensing method frequently used for monitoring purpose [2]. It consists of a photodetector, two LEDs, optimized optics, and a low-noise signal processing unit for analog signals for the detection of required signals [3]. The two light emitting diodes in which one is made to transmit red light having a wavelength of 650 nm whereas other provide infrared (IR) radiation having wavelength of about 950 nm. By adopting the basic principle of non-contact type of oxygen saturation measurement that when arterial pulse changes, light absorption in the arterial blood takes place and change in the amount of light absorbed gives the state of pulsation of pulse wave. According to the Beer-Lambert law, when both path transmission and absorption of light into arterial blood changes the arterial pulsation due to change in the volume, then the change in the intensity is observed by the amount of light received by the diode [4].

9.2 REQUIREMENTS

MAX30100 Sensor Module, REES52 Bluetooth Transceiver Module and Arduino UNO. The above specified sensors and elements are used in the proposed work. Laptop specification for the proposed work is given as – Intel Core i5–3320M 2.6GH.

9.3 METHODOLOGY

The Pulse-Oxy Tracker system uses MAX30100 and Arduino UNO for its designing, working as micro-controller for the work. The MAX30100 chip, which consists of two LEDs, i.e., red, and IR, a photodetector with a low-noise signal processing for the analog signals for the detection of the two signals, i.e., pulse oximetry and HR [4]. A first in first out (FIFO) is used to store the absorption data. The data has a buffer of about 64 bytes for both IR and red light. This has majorly two operating modes described below.

9.3.1 THE HEART RATE (HR) MODE

In the pulse or HR mode, just the IR LED will be turned ON, but in double mode, both LEDs, i.e., IR, and red LEDs will glow. A 60 Hz low-pass filter has been incorporated additionally. Filtration will be done through power line noise despite everything it will not represent environmental noise and other fluctuations present while taking readings. When the heart pumps blood because of having more blood, an expansion in oxygenated blood will occur. As soon as, the heart unwinds the amount of oxygenated blood diminishes, and the pulse rate is resolved.

9.3.2 OXYGEN SATURATION MODE

In the oxygen saturation mode, unlike heart mode Red LEDs were switched ON. It is based on the principle that the more IR light is absorbed in oxygenated blood, the redder lights are passed. On the other hand, red light is absorbed by the deoxygenated blood and passes IR light accordingly. MAX30100 provide its output by reading the level of absorption by both the sources which is then stored in buffer so as to read them through I2C.

In this chapter, since we had done the oximetry and HR monitoring by using MAX30100, therefore detection of both the parameters HR and oxygen saturation can be done simultaneously. The light transmitted by both LEDs passes through the finger of the patient and then by the photodetector, which is fabricated within the chip, will sense the absorption of light for the two different wavelengths.

9.3.3 FUNCTIONING

9.3.3.1 INTERFACING MAX30100 WITH ARDUINO UNO AND HC-05 BLUETOOTH MODULE

Firstly, the libraries were downloaded for MAX30100. It works on I2C Communication Protocol, and therefore, the serial data line (SDA) and serial clock line (SCL) are connected to the I2C pin of Arduino, i.e., A4 and A5. This Bluetooth is an UART module and will be connected to the TX and RX pins of Arduino.

All pinouts of MAX30100 were connected using wires, in which the female part of a jumper was connected with sensor while the male part kept open so as to interface Arduino with it. All the wiring is shown in Figure 9.1. At first MAX30100 is connected, afterward connection of HC-05 to Arduino UNO needs to be done. The data received by Arduino is sent to Bluetooth device via serial communication. Range of the described Bluetooth device needs to be 10 meters minimum. For the connection of other devices with our system we use HC-05 as a slave.

After the proper connection of MAX30100 with Arduino UNO and HC-05, this system was connected to the laptop. A Red LED glows continuously in MAX30100 as well as HC-05 signaling that the system is powered correctly. The baud rate of uploaded code will be taken as 9600.

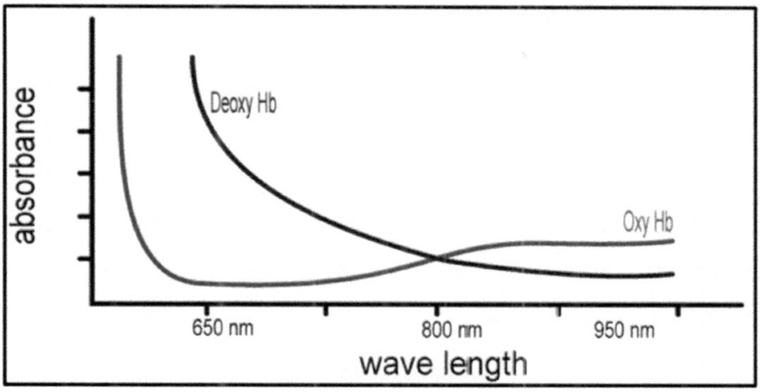

FIGURE 9.1 Absorbance graph of oxy-Hb and deoxy-Hb.

For making the Bluetooth application, MIT App Inventor 2 was used. The designing and coding of the application was done under designer and blocks window .apk file will be saved to the application available on Android phone and then installed in phone. The next step is to turn 'ON' the Bluetooth connection. The mobile is connected to HC-05 to get the data on the mobile application. On placing the fingertip on the sensor, the parameters BPM and Oxygen Saturation was available on Bluetooth application pulse oxy-tracker (Figures 9.2–9.4; Tables 9.1 and 9.2).

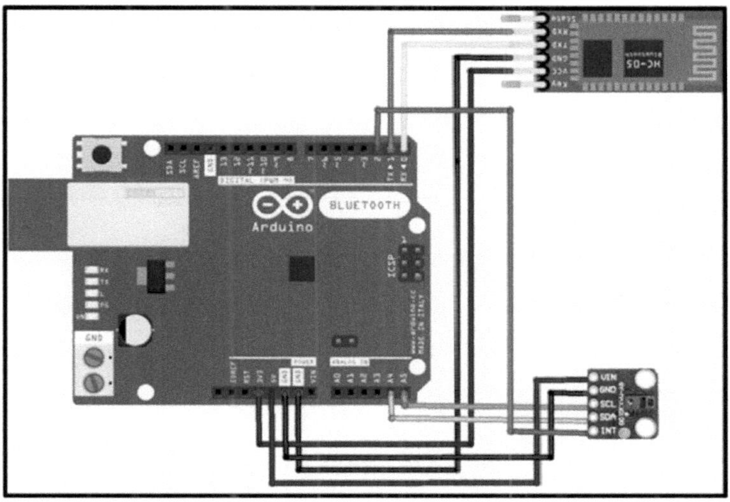

FIGURE 9.2 Connections of MAX30100 with Arduino UNO and HC-05 Bluetooth modules.

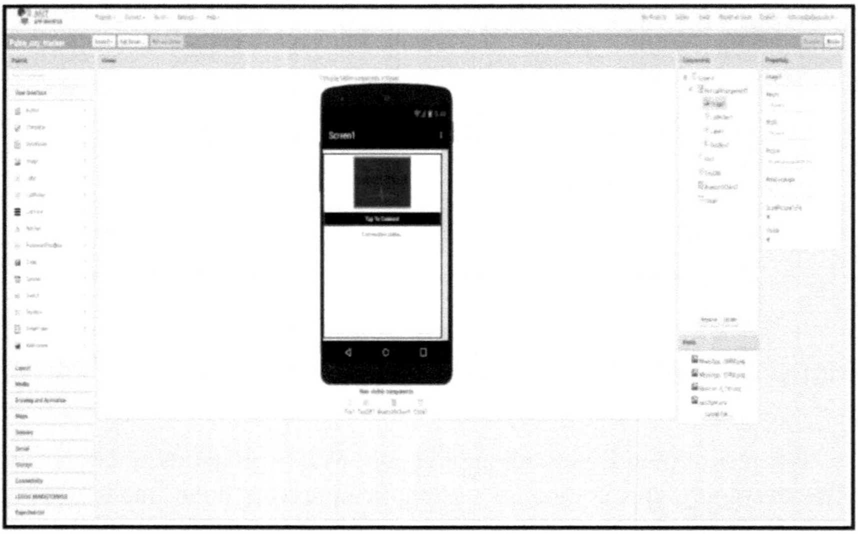

FIGURE 9.3 Bluetooth applications on MIT inventory app.

TABLE 9.1 Pin Connection of Arduino UNO with MAX30100

Pin: MAX30100	Pin: Arduino UNO
GND	GND
VIN	5V
INT	D2
SCL	A5
SDA	A4

TABLE 9.2 Pin Connection of Arduino UNO with HC-05 Bluetooth Module

Pin: HC-05 Bluetooth	Pin: Arduino UNO
VCC	3.3 V
GND	GND
TXD	RXD
RXD	TXD

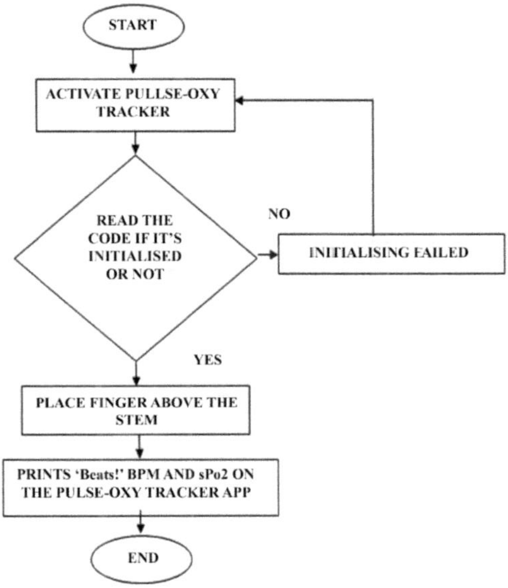

FIGURE 9.4 Flow chart of working model.

9.4 RESULTS

This section will show the results (Figures 9.5–9.7).

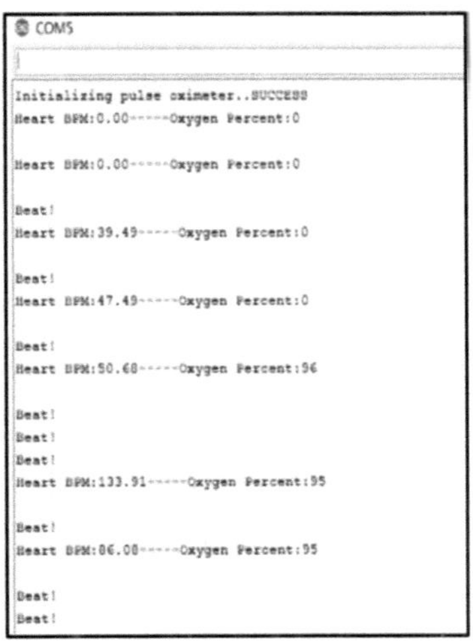

FIGURE 9.5 Readings of heart rate and SpO_2 on the serial monitor after placing a finger over the system.

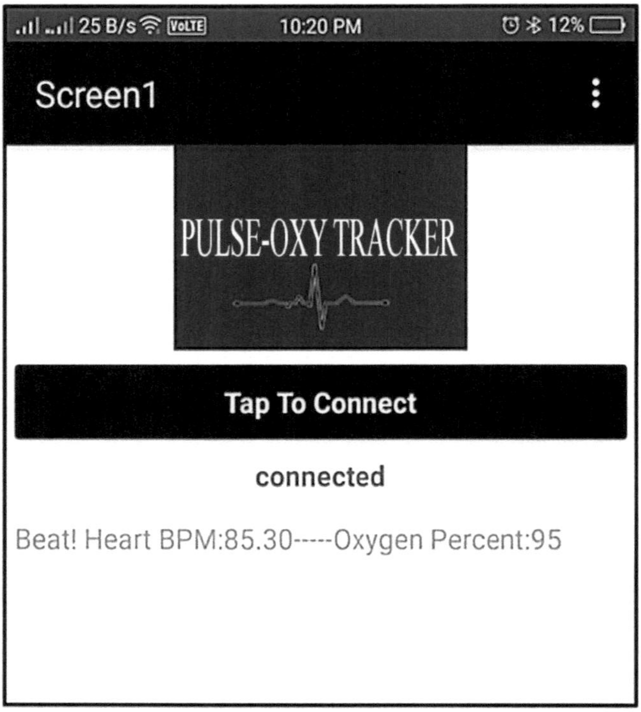

FIGURE 9.6 Heart rate and SpO_2 readings after placing a finger over the system – Example 1.

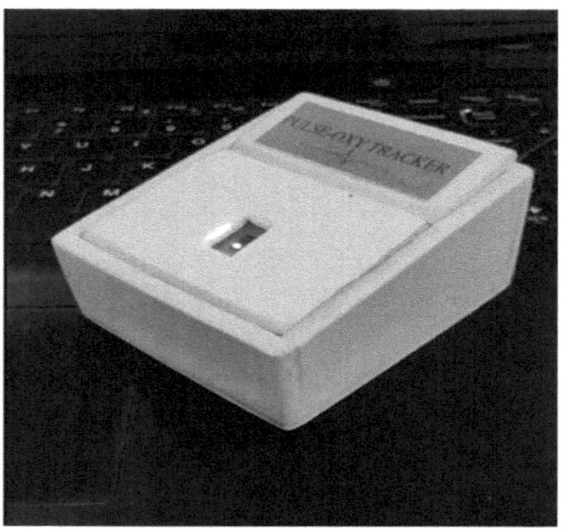

FIGURE 9.7 Heart rate and SpO_2 readings after placing a finger over the system – Example 2.

9.5 CONCLUSION AND DISCUSSION

The Bluetooth-based Pulse-Oxy Tracker using a mobile application has been a relatively successful device compared to general Pulse Oximetry and Pulse-Rate devices that are used in hospitals. Very low power is used by the system, which makes it preferable to even operate using the battery, which was the foremost intention of the proposed module. Its operational voltage range can be given as 1.8 to 3.3 V. Thus, our aim to make the system accessible and portable has been proven and tested thoroughly. With this device, patients, as well as doctors, can get acquired results on their mobile.

KEYWORDS

- **Bluetooth**
- **low power**
- **myocardial hypoxia**
- **pulse oximeter**
- **serial clock line**
- **serial data line**
- **SpO2**

REFERENCES

1. Hafen, B. B., & Sharma, S., (2018). *Oxygen Saturation*. StatPearls [Internet]: StatPearls Publishing.
2. Dyaneshwar, S., Monica, K., Jaiyashri, G., & Amutha, R., (2018). Cloud assisted recovery scheme for compressively sensed medical sensor data. *IEEE International Conference on System, Computation, Automation and Networking (ICSCA)* (pp. 1–6). IEEE.
3. Banet, M., Morris, B., & Visser, H., (2006). *Vital Sign-Monitoring System with Multiple Optical Modules*. Ed: Google Patents.
4. Yossef, H. O., et al., (2018). Pulse oximetry with two infrared wavelengths without calibration in extracted arterial blood. *Sensors, 18*(10), 3457.
5. Lakshmi, P. N. R., & Venkatesan, P., (2018). Smart watch for healthcare monitoring. *International Journal of Engineering Technology Science and Research, 5*(3), 1107–1111.

CHAPTER 10

DEVELOPMENT OF A LOCATION TRACKER APP FOR A PATIENT TRACKING SYSTEM

S. R. JAYASIMHA and J. USHA

Department of Master of Computer Applications, RV College of Engineering, Bangalore, Karnataka, India, E-mail: jayasimhasr@rvce.edu.in (S. R. Jayasimha)

ABSTRACT

The combination of cloud computing with healthcare has the potential to improve several healthcare-related activities, such as telemedicine, post-hospitalization care plans, and virtual medication adherence. It also improves access to healthcare services through telehealth. Today's healthcare organizations must focus on a lot more than the health of their patients. The infrastructure it takes to support clinical care delivery continues to expand, with cloud computing being one of the most significant contributors to that growth.

In this chapter, we discuss cloud computing technology, challenges in healthcare technology, and AWS applications in healthcare. Initially, a patient is required to register in the mobile application. The patient should provide the history and symptoms. These details are then relayed as notifications to a nearby specialty doctor who is also registered for the application. All the data is stored in the cloud. The doctor communicates with the patient through this application immediately. The application will

IoT and Cloud Computing-Based Healthcare Information Systems. Anand Sharma, PhD, Hiren Kumar Deva Sarma, PhD & S. R. Biradar, PhD (Eds.)

notify the location information of the patient through the GPS connections and sends information to the administrator. The doctor can get the location of the patient and the path direction from the doctor's location to the patient location. Doctors can prescribe the necessary treatment protocol to the patient and monitor the patient remotely. If the patient is afflicted with a contagious disease, measures can be taken to avoid the spread of the disease in the community. Once the patient consults the doctor about their disease, the doctor can also track the patient's earlier movements by looking at the history.

10.1 INTRODUCTION

Cloud computing is a delivery model delivery based on-demand computing services over the internet on a pay-as-you-go basis rather than managing files on a local storage device. This is also called anytime anywhere with any device existing for any services. It has universal access, data storage in the cloud is with the help of servers' which are scalable, and services are available in the cloud on pay as you go model. In cloud computing, the user will pay for what he uses, if he must scale up, he will have to pay more, if he wants to scale down, he will have to pay less. There is no need to invest in servers as cloud computing provides infrastructure on demand. Also, no experts are required for hardware and software maintenance. It provides better data security; security standards are high. Mechanisms for disaster recovery, high flexibility, automatic updates of software, teams can collaborate from widespread locations. Data can be tracked and shared anywhere over the Internet. Initially, days before the cloud exists, peoples were using a number of servers to store the data. The users had to invest on servers or buy from the service providers [1]. During the maintenance of web portals, the problem faced was the huge network traffic. The server monitoring and maintenance is easy. The troubleshooting was a big issue faced by managing with the client. The important thing is data handling data through these servers is difficult. Nowadays, everything is online, e.g., shopping, bill payment, reading, listening, watching movies, and reading books. Since everything is online transaction, data handling requires huge memory. The maintenance of the data requires a separate space that is called cloud. Cloud service providers do the maintenance activities such as billing, traffic maintenance, and storage.

Figure 10.1 shows the space available in the cloud, and it provides a huge space to store your data and run applications based on the needs of the user. Cloud is nothing but a collection of data centers. The cloud data centers take care of functions, applications; manage resources by combining the space available in the cloud. The adoption of cloud in healthcare is particularly important to track the information of a patient. It helps to store the diseases/ailments of the patient and his personal information, and the application sends the patient location to the administrator or to the concerned person or the doctor. Through this application, the administrator can track the patient activity and the movement [2]. The application helps the administrator to restrict the patient movement by sending notifications. This can avoid the spread from one patient to another. This application is deployed through the public platform in the cloud. The cloud healthcare application deployment is a dynamic process and easy to use. It is simplified to track the patient easily. The cloud usage in the healthcare industry will not cause much infrastructure problem as everything goes on online. The patient location can be tracked using GPS tracker implemented in the AWS EC2 instances and tested. Once the patient is registered through his mobile to the healthcare application, the application can track the patient and information through the mobile number and the internet protocol address is mapped to the server the server will track the patient location details and movement. Confidentiality of the data will be maintained to prevent misuse.

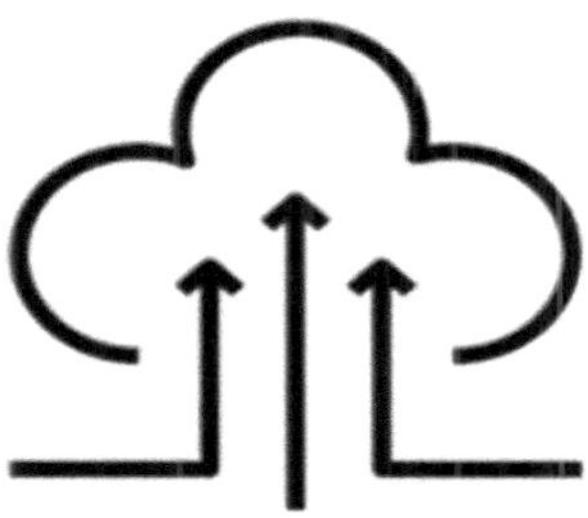

FIGURE 10.1 Structure of cloud.

10.2 DEPLOYMENT MODELS/TYPES OF CLOUD COMPUTING

In the cloud computing, the cloud service provider provides an appropriate type of service model for the user to work on. Figure 10.2 shows the types of data storage in the various organizations can be stored through any one of these models [3].

10.2.1 PUBLIC CLOUD

In this cloud, cloud infrastructure is made available to the general public over the internet and is owned by cloud provider, the cost is less, and the user will pay only for recourses they use. Public service is a type of service provided to the public. The internet is the main source of communication between the user and the server. The third-party service providers provide the services. Public cloud is available to everyone. The service provider makes the resources available to everyone through the world wide web such as AWS, SUN CLOUD, MICROSOFT AZURE.

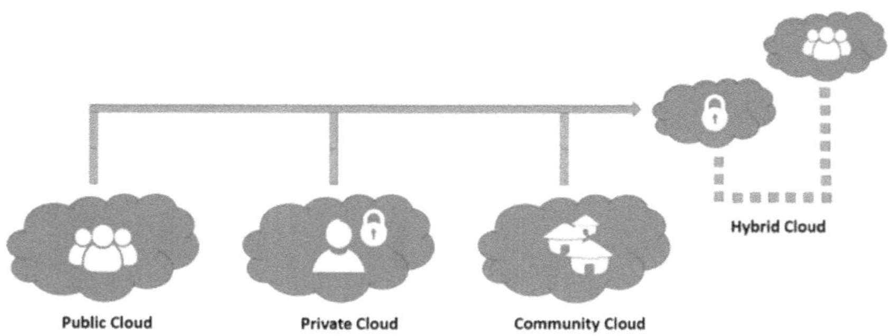

FIGURE 10.2 Models of cloud computing.

10.2.2 PRIVATE CLOUD

In this cloud, the cloud infrastructure is exclusively operated by a single organization. The cost is huge and can be managed by a third party and may exist on-premises, or off-premises. A private cloud is a service, provided by the service provider which is connected to a hardware and networking components within the organization to share the resources. The private cloud also contains a set of servers and provides multiple applications to run on the virtualized server such as VM ARE, AWS.

10.2.3 COMMUNITY CLOUD

Community cloud falls between the private and public cloud. It is costlier than the public cloud. It allows systems and services to be accessible by the group of organization. Google 'gov-cloud' and NASA 'nebula-cloud' are the examples of community cloud.

10.2.4 HYBRID CLOUD

This infrastructure consists of both functionalities of public and private cloud. Federal agencies opt for private clouds when sensitive information is involved, and they also use the public cloud to share data sets with the general public and other government departments. The activities performed through this model. Basically, noncritical activities are performed through the public cloud model. The critical activities are performed through the public model. EXAMPLE: IT ADMIN.

10.3 CLOUD COMPUTING SERVICE MODELS

The cloud service providers use the cloud service models to control. The service providers provide the services based on the user demand using pay as you go method. Figure 10.3 shows service model on-demand services, network access as a medium, shared the resources at a time to multiple clients.

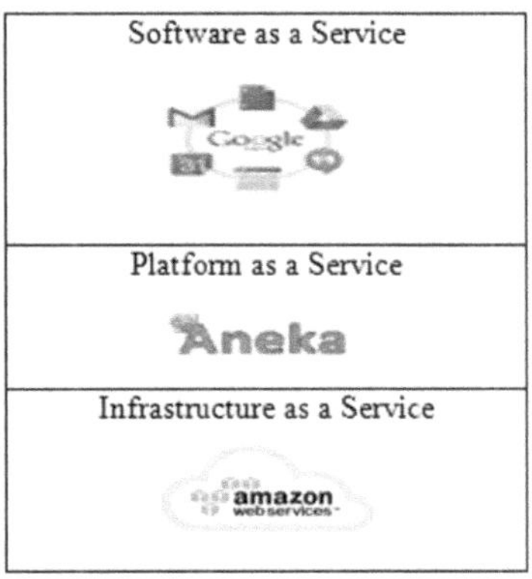

FIGURE 10.3 Service models.

10.3.1 SOFTWARE-AS-A-SERVICE (SAAS)

Software-as-a-service (SaaS) is an independent platform. The service cost is applied based on the applications usage by the user. It is a demand service. It gives the collaboration of working environment. Services can access the services from any computer. The applications are accessed over the internet. Example: Google App Engine.

10.3.2 PLATFORM-AS-A-SERVICE (PAAS)

Platform-as-a-service (PaaS) allows user to create their own cloud applications run on the specific tools and specific language through virtual machine. It provides the environment and the tool to create a new online application in the cloud. It provides cloud platform and runtime environment for developing testing and managing applications, it helps software developers to deploy application without requiring all related infrastructure It provides the rapid application deployment with low cost. It can be deployed in private and public cloud. Example: Aneka.

10.3.3 INFRASTRUCTURE-AS-A-SERVICE (IAAS)

Infrastructure-as-a-service (IaaS) is a fundamental resource sharing the physical machines, virtual machine through the virtual storage. Rather than purchase the huge infrastructure through the cloud IaaS model can share the required resources virtually. It is a fundamental and the basic layer of the cloud computing. It allows the cloud existing applications to be on the run on the specific hardware. Example: Amazon Web Services.

10.4 AWS SERVICES IN CLOUD COMPUTING

AWS is Amazon web services is a global data center. Across the world, AWS is having 20 regions and 61 available zones [4]. Various services are giving accurate responses getting from the AWS servers. AWS regions are the geographical area, and every region consists of two or more zones/data centers for the high availability of the applications supported to the user.

AWS provides more than 300+ services in the cloud environment. In that around 50+ services supported in healthcare.

10.4.1 IOT CORE

AWS IoT integrates with artificial integrate solutions and it will work even without the internet connectivity. It is used mainly for the business purposes. In the healthcare industry, AWS is used to analyze and measure the rate of symptoms of the patients.

10.4.2 AKS (AMAZON KINESIS STREAM)

AKS helps to stream the patient data to store in the data base without internet. Mainly the AKS is used to handle the real-time data in the large file system. It is used to generate the bills daily and weekly. The real-time metrics analyzes and sends the alert messages [5].

10.4.3 EC2

Elastic Cloud Compute increases the efficiency of the system to store huge amount of data and maintain the database. The EC2 provides the elasticity about the patient medicines requirement, database information and the doctor's information in the cloud are maintained by the admin.

10.4.4 EMR (ELASTIC MAP REDUCE)

With the managerial framework of EC2 and S3, AWS provides elastic map-reduce (EMR) to handle the data in large number. It will help to store and maintain the tracking details of the patient through upload, create, and monitor the information of the patient record.

The biggest challenge in the cloud computing is providing digital transmission and storage. The virtualization in the cloud will help to store the data regularly in the cloud. Data maintenance is secure and is assured by the service providers. All healthcare related data will be secure. The data is stored in the third-party server in an encrypted manner to prevent unauthorized access. Cost is affordable; the storage of data is scalable. Since a huge volume of data exists, the healthcare industry can apply prediction algorithms of artificial intelligence (AI) and machine learning (ML) to come up with better healthcare facilities. Even scanned information from scanning machines used in healthcare devices can be stored digitally. In the hospitals the computerized tomography, computerized axial tomography, and MRI scanning information is stored digitally, and the data can be immediately updated in the patient record through the application [6].

Benefits of virtual private cloud:

- It is economically feasible;
- Data privacy and security concerns have largely been mitigated;
- Reduction in operational costs for healthcare providers;
- It supports IT technologies, provides data analytics for improved decision support systems and therapeutic strategies advances in clinical research. The cloud is scalable and connects the care provider to the patient despite location issues and thus cloud is an economical solution.

10.5 PRIVATE CLOUD WORKING IN HEALTHCARE

Private cloud provides limited access to computing resources in terms of scale and the critical need for security and privacy protections have often made it difficult for healthcare systems and life sciences companies to translate these rich data sets into meaningful improvements. Restricted area of operations in private cloud is limited access. It is not globally deployable. If we want to use from others, we must access other operations. Price is more, the price of private cloud increases when the third party develops the private cloud and when new hardware is added to the cloud. Scalability is limited. It depends on the number of resources used in the cloud which is directly proportional to the cost. Along with the other programming language developers, the cloud developers are also required [7].

10.6 HEALTHCARE RELATED TO CLOUD

In 2004, the first whole human genome was sequenced. It cost almost 3 billion dollars. The cost has come down radically to under 1,000 dollars, but that has generated a tsunami of data. The data gives a challenge, when comparing one DNA with another we can see 5 million differences [8]. The challenge is to take a data set of 5 million to figure out what are the differences or the mutations that are important, which of them causes rare diseases, causes cancer and how to treat patients [9, 10]. HIPAA compliance on Google cloud platform-medical billing information and patient histories is shared between the user and the cloud provider.

10.7 LIMITATIONS OF CLOUD WITH HEALTHCARE

- Security and privacy: The data stored in the cloud are prone to data theft and lost;
- Interoperability: The healthcare organizations needs proper communication, collaboration, and coordination between them [11];
- Portability: The data in the cloud can be accessed in different platforms;
- Service quality: The service should be fast and highly secure with good quality;
- Computing performance: The accessing performance should be high.

10.7.1 APPLICATION

Healthcare providers and insurer organizations want to provide clinical and operational solutions for their teams while improving data security [12]. AWS has scalable and secure HIPAA eligible services that enable innovation while reducing complexity risks and costs [13]. Across the healthcare industry, AWS has an ecosystem of partners working with organizations to develop services like advanced ML to help predict potential health risks, develop personalized medicine, and coordinate care improving outcomes for patients around the world. AWS provides secure, cost-effective and scalable solutions [14, 15].

10.8 IMPLEMENTATION AND RESULTS

The healthcare application is developed to track the patient movement to avoid the infections to others. Once the patient is registered through this application, the admin can track the patient movement.

Figure 10.4 shows the mobile application for the patient tracker. This application requires the internet connectivity and sends the information to the cloud.

Figure 10.5 shows the login page of the patient once the patient is registered through the ID generated can login for details. If the user is new, then he or she must register by creating a new account.

Figure 10.6 shows the initial location of the patient is traced through the phone number of the patient; and Figure 10.7 shows the patient movement and the area surrounded to be captured.

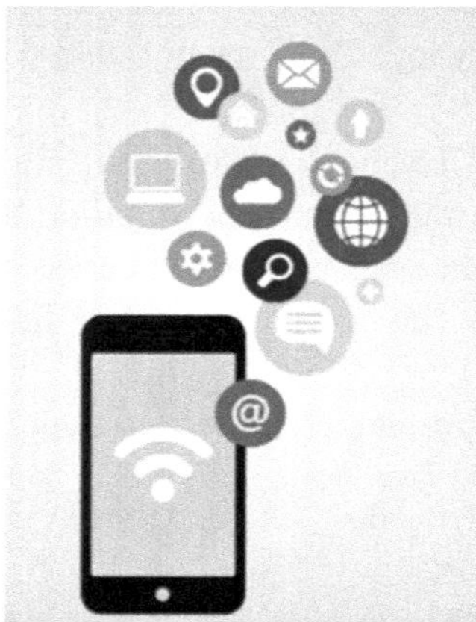

FIGURE 10.4 Mobile application.

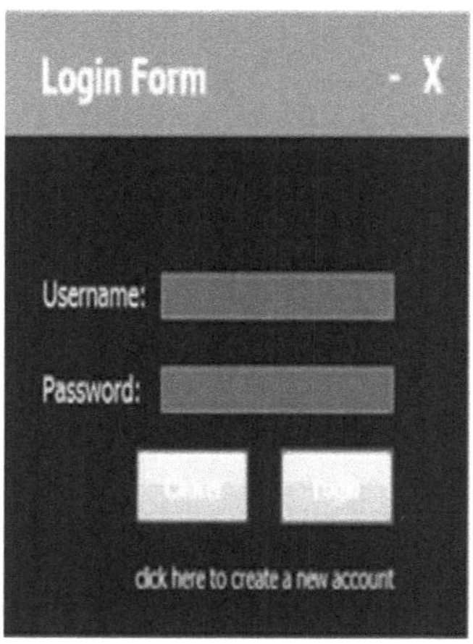

FIGURE 10.5 Login form.

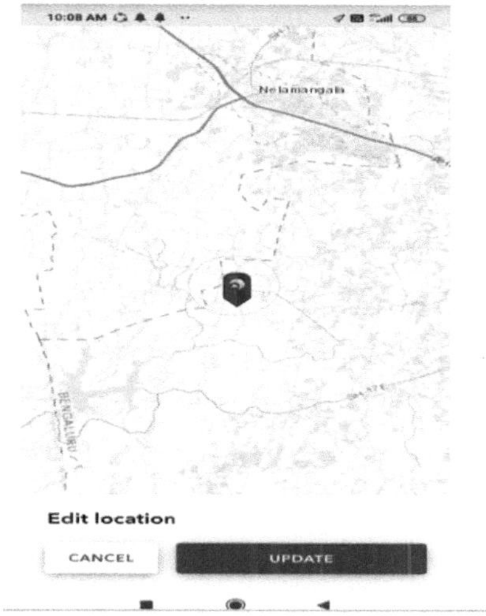

FIGURE 10.6 Initial location of the patient.

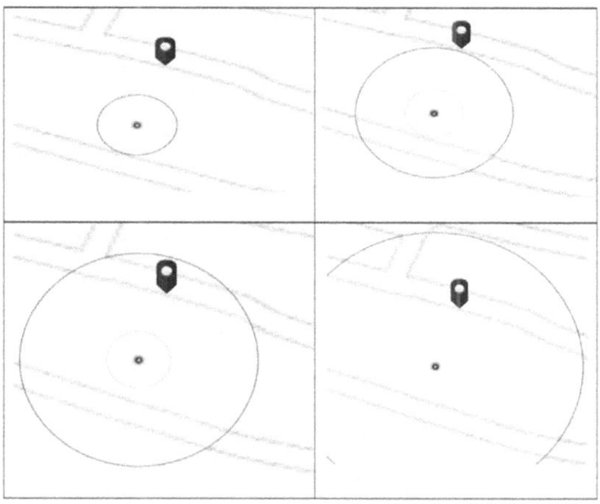

FIGURE 10.7 Movement of patient.

10.9 CONCLUSION

The healthcare application is useful to the administrator to keep track of the patient movement as it results in community issues and spread. Patient movement is tracked through a registered mobile number. This application mitigates the disease spread from one patient to another. The admin can track the patient and suggestions can be recorded. The application can be deployed on a private cloud of an organization and benefit with low cost and minimal infrastructure in the cloud. The capability of a real-time, mobile, and location-tracking application for patients by integrating GPS (global position system) with Cloud Technology is an accuracy of a few centimeters.

KEYWORDS

- **Amazon Kinesis stream**
- **cloud computing**
- **EC2**
- **elastic map-reduce**
- **infrastructure as a service**
- **platform as a service**
- **software as a service**

REFERENCES

1. Usha, J., Jayasimha, S. R., & Srivani, S. G., (2017). Automata approach to reduce power consumption in smart grid cloud data center. In: *3rd International Conference, Cognitive Computing, and Information Processing-CCIP2017* (Vol. 801, pp. 248–257). JSS Academy of Technical Education, Bengaluru.
2. Jayasimha, S. R., Usha, J., & Srivani, S. G., (2018). Efficient power management using fuzzy logic for cloud computing environment. In: *IEEE, 3rd International Conference on Computational Systems and Information Technology for Sustainable Solutions, CSITSS* (pp. 35–40). Bengaluru, India, ISBN: 978-1-5386-6078-2 © 2018 IEEE.
3. Mahmud, S., Iqbal, R., & Doctor, F., (2016). Cloud-enabled data analytics and visualization framework for health-shocks prediction. *Future Generation Computer Systems, 5*, 169–181.
4. Manogaran, G., Varatharajan, R., Lopez, D., Malarvizhi, P., Sundarasekar, R., & Thota, C., (2018). A new architecture of the internet of things and big data ecosystem for secured smart healthcare monitoring and alerting system. *Future Generation Computer Systems, 82*, 375–387.
5. Fabian, B., Ermakova, T., & Junghanns, P., (2015). Collaborative and secure sharing of healthcare data in multi-clouds. *Information Systems, 48*, 132–150.

6. Paper, P., (n.d.). *The Case for Designing Data-Intensive Cloud-Based Healthcare Applications* (pp. 1–6). CEUR-WS. ORG Publication.
7. Calabrese, B., & Cannataro, M., (2015). *Cloud Computing Healthcare in Biomedicines* (Vol. 16, No. 1, pp. 1–18). ISSN 1895-1767.
8. Bahga, A., Madisetti, V. K., & Tech, G., (2015). *Integration and Informatics in the Cloud.* Cover Feature Computing in Healthcare Publication.
9. Jemal, H., Kechaou, Z., Ayed, M. B., Alimi, A. M., & Computing, A. C., (2015). Cloud computing and mobile devices-based system for healthcare applications. *IEEE International Symposium on Technology and Society (ISTAS)* (pp. 1–5).
10. Lq, V., Hdowkfduh, R. I. R. U., Lq, L., Grpdlq, K., Lpsuryhg, L. V., & Sdwlhqw, D. V., (2016). *Security Issues in Cloud Computing for Healthcare* (pp. 1231–1236). 978-9-3805-4421-2/16/2016 IEEE.
11. Singh, I., Kumar, D., & Khatri, S. K., (2019). Improving the efficiency of e-healthcare system based on cloud. *Amity International Conference on Artificial Intelligence (AICAI)* (pp. 930–933).
12. Taher, C., Mallat, I., Agoulmine, N., & El-mawass, N., (n.d). An IoT-cloud based solution for real-time and batch processing of big data : Application in healthcare. In: *3rd International Conference on Bioengineering for Smart Technologies (BioSMART), 2019* (pp. 1–8).
13. Daman, R., Tripathi, M. M., & Mishra, S. K., (2016). *Cloud Computing for Medical Applications & Healthcare Delivery: Technology, Application, Security and SWOT Analysis,* 155–159.
14. Hanen, J., Kechaou, Z., & Ayed, M. B., (2016). An enhanced healthcare system in mobile cloud computing environment. *Vietnam Journal of Computer Science, 3*(4), 267–277.
15. Pouladzadeh, P., Vijay, S., Peddi, B., Kuhad, P., Yassine, A., & Shirmohammadi, S., (2015). A virtualization mechanism for real-time multimedia-assisted mobile food recognition application in cloud computing. *Cluster Computing, 18*(3), 1099–1110.

CHAPTER 11

PROBABILISTIC DETECTION AND PREVENTION OF COVID-19 USING SMARTPHONES

MANISH KUMAR[1] and DIWAKER[2]

[1]*Associate Professor, Department of CSE, CEC-CGC, Landran, Mohali, Punjab, India, E-mail: manish.4379@cgc.edu.in*

[2]*Assistant Professor, School of Computing, DIT University, Dehradun, Uttarakhand, India*

ABSTRACT

This chapter presents the preventive, precautionary, and some control measures to reduce the threat of viable disease transmission of the deadly COVID-19 pandemic. The virus causes illness in human beings, some species of animals and birds like camels, cattle, cats, bats, etc. The origin of this virus COVID-19 is confirmed in Wuhan city of China, because the first patient was recognized in Wuhan by clinical practitioners there itself. However, within a few days it has covered almost all countries in over the globe, so it is declared as pandemic by WHO (World Health Organization). Although scientists across the globe are continuously contributing their best towards the development of foolproof medicine or vaccine, but unfortunately, they are not able to find any solution till date. So, the whole world is left with only one way to overcome this pandemic disease, which is by taking preventive measures to stop transmission. As time passes nowadays, there are various means to identify whether a person is infected

IoT and Cloud Computing-Based Healthcare Information Systems. Anand Sharma, PhD, Hiren Kumar Deva Sarma, PhD & S. R. Biradar, PhD (Eds.)

from COVID-19 or not. We can use clinical analysis of blood test results and chest CT scan images. Common symptoms, including high fever, tiredness, and dry cough can be seen as primary alarm in the infected patients of COVID-19. In particular, many types of equipment and various ways have been emerged nowadays to identify the preliminary symptoms of the virus. However, the high cost of pre-installation before use has emerged as major limitations of these efficient equipment and various devices. We have proposed a way by means of which people will get conscious of the symptoms of COVID-19 over and above they will be able to know how far they are from this virus. To detect novel coronavirus (COVID-19) using smartphone, a new framework is proposed in our work. Our proposed framework is an inexpensive solution, because every second person is using smart phones now a day for their daily routine work. After installation of our proposed framework in smartphone every user will become capable of diagnosing the virus.

11.1 INTRODUCTION

As of late 2019, another pandemic disease, COVID-19 has developed as revile to the entire world. The first patient infected with the said virus was recognized in Wuhan, a city of China by a medical practitioner in October 2019. After quite a while, since the recognizable proof of first patient in start of December 2019, the world-leading organization in health sector, WHO admitted that the infection can harm respiratory system with fever, manifesting pneumonia, and cough. After a few days of declaration, the so called COVID-19 has inculcated all most whole world inside their giant mouth. Due to carelessness and improper organization by the Government of China, it has spread in China, and travelers/tourists become the carries of this virus in many countries internationally [1, 2]. Initially WHO has not shown their interest to stop the virus. Because of which it spread from one individual to another, seeing the outstanding speed of transmission, on January 30, 2020, COVID-19 was confirmed as a pandemic by the Emergency Committee of WHO. This virus has shown an adverse effect on people having poor immunity.

The COVID-19 is a common disease in some of the class of animals like bats, cats, cattle, and camels, but unfortunately, it has transmitted to human beings. The first patient infected with the novel virus was found in a city of China which is now supposed to be the epicenter of this novel virus. Since China has also declared many species of animals and birds as their national property and a bunch of literature also provides evidence of live animals and seafood markets, resulting in animal-to-person spread of said virus. After that exponential growth of infected people, those who are not in direct contact with said carrier animals from COVID-19 indicates that virus is expanding their area using person-to-person spread [3]. This virus has taken the lives of more than 4,000 people and infected a large group of people over the globe before the world-leading organization in healthcare WHO has declared it a pandemic on March 11, 2020 [4].

Human coronaviruses and COVID-19 belong to the same family of viruses known as Coronaviridae. In Ref. [5] authors described the symptoms like sensible cold middle east respiratory syndrome (MERS), or severe acute respiratory syndrome (SARS) can be seen in infected person. Some of the times it may come about that person is infected, but due to strong immune system of infected person it may take more than 3 weeks to show the symptoms, and this is one of the main reasons because of which it becomes very difficult to control the speed of increasing cases. There are other viruses also like SARS and MERS, which has taken the thousands of lives of people across the world. The very first case of SARS-CoV (SARS-associated coronavirus) was found in Southern China in 2003 and swallowed many countries worldwide in a very short span of time. It has also affected the respiratory system of affected persons. Moreover, the first case of MERS affected person was reported in Saudi Arabia and taken the lives of nearly 858 people out of 2,494 affected persons. As per an examination dependent on infection genomes, it was discovered that the infection first began in bats [6]. Although the medical analysis of novel COVID-19 is quite complex, time consuming and can be seen as symptoms like high fever, dry cough initially and sometimes relentless headache.

There are numerous approaches to diagnose and detect COVID-19, here two most generally used techniques like nucleic acid test (NAT) and computed tomography (CT) are discussed. The first technique CT scan is used to detect lung inflammation and severity of COVID-19. Whereas the second technique, NAT is used to detect a sequence of specific nucleic acid that may infect blood tissue [7]. In Hubei Province, China itself confirmed the inclusion of radiographic presentation of pneumonia with the help of National Health Commission in the country [8].

Very quickly COVID-19 virus has pretentious almost all countries worldwide, specifically in the situation is quite panic due to large no affected people. Initially, the administration was not able to read the situation properly, so now a days, when thousands and thousands of affected cases are coming, hospitals are only admitting only critically ill people [9]. The high demand for diagnosis to determine infected people-driven researchers, academicians, and various leading companies in the medical sector to design and device intelligent, responsive, and more efficient methods and equipment. PING a renowned name in health sector has come up with a quick and intelligent method for COVID-19, "smart CT image reading system" which processes the analyzed results in nearly 16 seconds with highest accuracy rate above 90% [10]. Other detection kits are also available for detection of COVID-19. But these devices/kits are quite costly and installation results again results as time consuming process. In our proposed work, modern smart phones containing a variety of specialized sensors with prevailing computation capabilities are used to detect the symptoms of COVID-19. Since it does not involve complex equipment and installation, it is efficient and cost effective. The remaining title is structured as: In Section 11.2 impact of COVID-19 pandemic with respect to India is discussed. Section 11.3 describes the various detection systems developed so far for the detection of COVID-19. Section 11.4 describes the result, and finally, Section 11.5 concludes the work.

11.2 COVID-19 PANDEMIC IN INDIA

In our country the first case was reported on 30 January 2020, who visited India from China. On 26 March 2020 by Indian Council of Medical Research and the Ministry of Health and Family Welfare declared that total of 649 cases, 42 recoveries, 1 migration and 13 deaths in the country. As per analysis at this stage the infection rate of 1.7 was reported in India, significantly lower than in the worst affected countries.

In the current situation has been declared a pandemic in more than a dozen states and union territories. It is decided by the GOI to reduce the speed and community transmission of all educational institutions in the states and many commercial establishments have been completely closed.

India has observed a 14 hour voluntary public curfew on 22 March 2020 as declared by the Hon'ble Prime Minister of India as a preventive measure against COVID-19. Later, on 24 March, the Prime Minister Mr. Narendra

Modi ordered a nationwide lockdown for 21 days in India, affecting the entire population of India. As the cases are increasing day by day and to prevent it from spreading in the community, on 14 April, he further announced nationwide lockdown till 3rd May 2020 (Table 11.1 and Figure 11.1).

TABLE 11.1 India's State/UT wise Record of Cases due to COVID-19 as on 14/04/2020

SL. No	Name of State/UT	Identified Positive Cases	Recovery Cases	Causalities
1.	Arunachal Pradesh	1	0	0
2.	Mizoram	1	0	0
3.	Nagaland	1	0	0
4.	Manipur	2	1	0
5.	Tripura	2	0	0
6.	Goa	7	5	0
7.	Pondicherry	7	1	0
8.	Andaman and Nicobar Islands	11	10	0
9.	Ladakh	15	10	0
10.	Chandigarh	21	7	0
11.	Jharkhand	24	0	2
12.	Assam	31	0	1
13.	Chhattisgarh	31	10	0
14.	Himachal Pradesh	32	13	1
15.	Uttarakhand	35	5	0
16.	Odisha	54	12	1
17.	Bihar	65	26	1
18.	Punjab	167	14	11
19.	Haryana	185	29	3
20.	West Bengal	190	36	7
21.	Karnataka	247	59	6
22.	Jammu and Kashmir	270	16	4
23.	Kerala	379	198	3
24.	Andhra Pradesh	432	11	7
25.	Gujarat	539	54	26
26.	Uttar Pradesh	558	49	5
27.	Telangana	562	100	16
28.	Madhya Pradesh	604	44	43
29.	Rajasthan	873	21	3

TABLE 11.1 *(Continued)*

SL. No	Name of State/UT	Identified Positive Cases	Recovery Cases	Causalities
30.	Tamil Nadu	1,173	58	11
31.	Delhi	1,510	30	28
32.	Maharashtra	2,334	217	160
Total Number of Confirmed Cases in India		**10,363***	**1,036**	**339**

Source: https://www.mohfw.gov.in/.

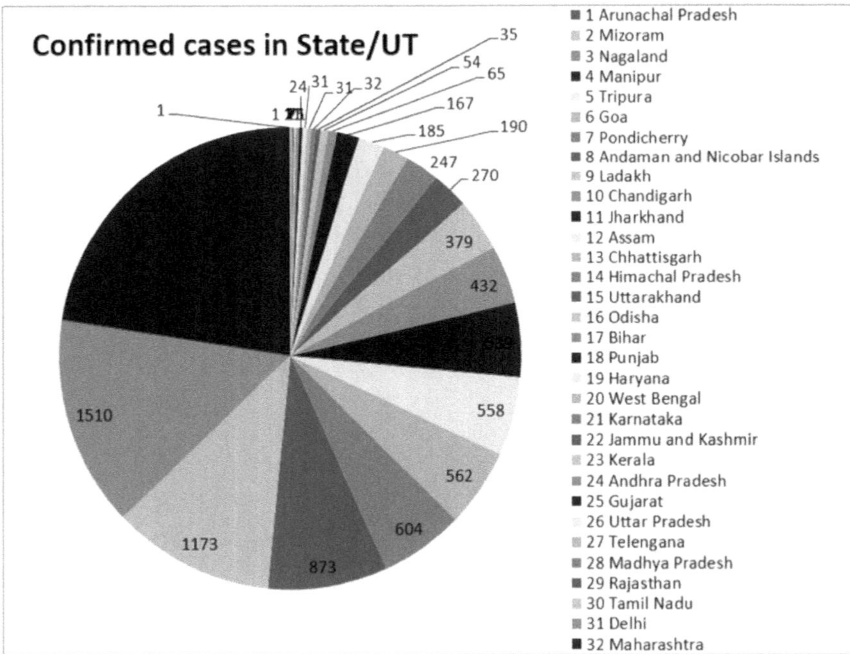

FIGURE 11.1 Confirmed cases state/UT wise.

India is taking every precaution from the very first instance to tackle the COVID-19 pandemic. Government of India is finding a way to guarantee that we are arranged well to confront the test and danger presented by the developing pandemic of COVID-19 the Corona Virus. The individuals of India have been capable of taking each alert with the goal that virus won't spread in our nation at any expense. The main factor in forestalling the spread of the virus locally is to enable the residents with the correct data and avoiding potential risk according to the warnings being given by the Ministry of Health and Family Welfare. Although, every country is trying to develop a vaccine for this virus but still not able to find a solution. The condition of European countries and the USA is worst in case of death and spread of this pandemic. In this situation, India is helping the various nations by proving them hydroxychloroquine tablets to the most affected countries. But still the best way to tackle this problem is the awareness among the citizen and social distancing. Further, the government is getting contributions concerning people and organizations who have created advancements and inventive arrangements, Apps for diagnosis and so on that can be utilized for fortifying the battle against COVID-19.

11.3 PROPOSED FRAMEWORK

In this section, our proposed framework is presented, and a description of each segment is provided. Our proposed framework is sufficient enough to describe the method of designing and implementing a smart phone-based application, which will be able to diagnose the disease. This app will be helpful and able to detect the personal health status.

1. When the user launches the app, he is prompted to provide his/her mobile number and then OTP is being sent to his mobile number for verification. On successful verification of mobile number, the user is being redirected to the dashboard (Figures 11.2 and 11.3).

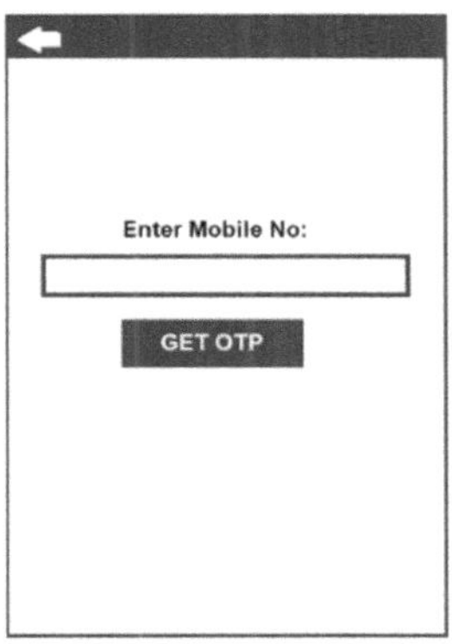

FIGURE 11.2 Mobile number verification model.

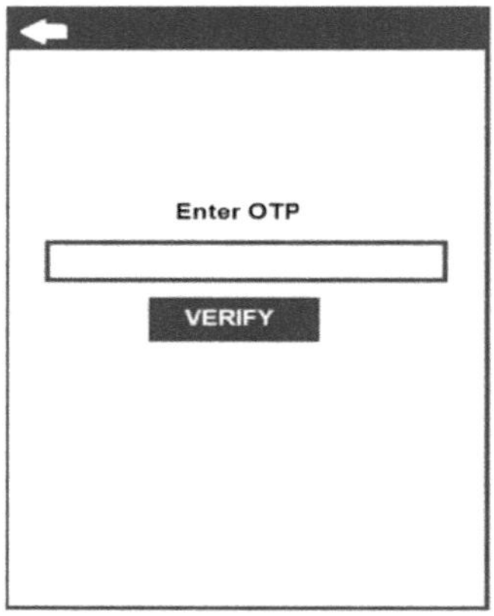

FIGURE 11.3 OTP verification.

2. In the dashboard, the user has an option to answer some questionnaire related to the various symptoms he might be anguish due to CORONA virus (Figure 11.4).

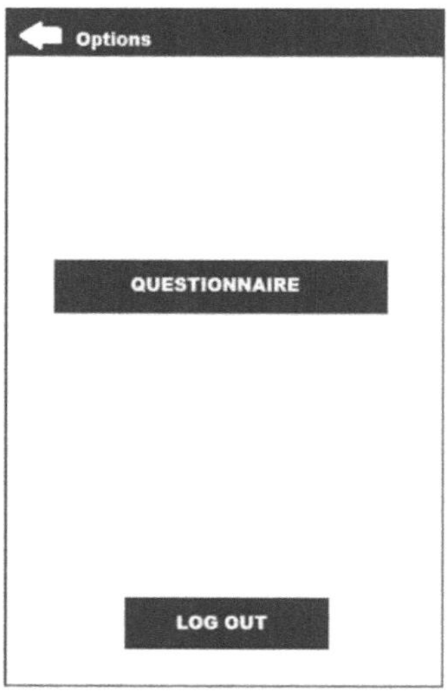

FIGURE 11.4 Questionnaire entry window.

3. Here, the user is being prompted to mark few questions in Yes or No, where every question will be provided some weight

considering their probability of contribution in transmission. The questions are being marked on the basis of some point system given in Table 11.2; Figures 11.5 and 11.6.

TABLE 11.2 Questionnaire and Their Corresponding Weight as per the Probability of Contribution

SL. No.	Question Asked to Person in Doubt	Weighted in Points
1.	Do you have a cough?	1
2.	Do you have colds?	1
3.	Are you having diarrhea?	1
4.	Do you have sore throat?	1
5.	Are you experiencing body aches or myalgia?	1
6.	Do you have a headache?	1
7.	Do you have a mild fever	1
8.	Are you having difficulty breathing?	2
9.	Are you experiencing Fatigue?	2
10.	Have you traveled during the past 14 days?	3
11.	Do you have gone through to a corona infected area?	3
12.	Do you have direct contact or are taking care of a COVID-19 patient?	3

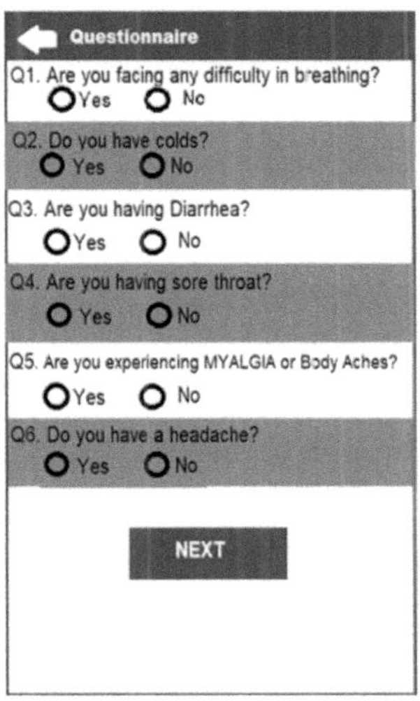

FIGURE 11.5 Questionnaire 1–6.

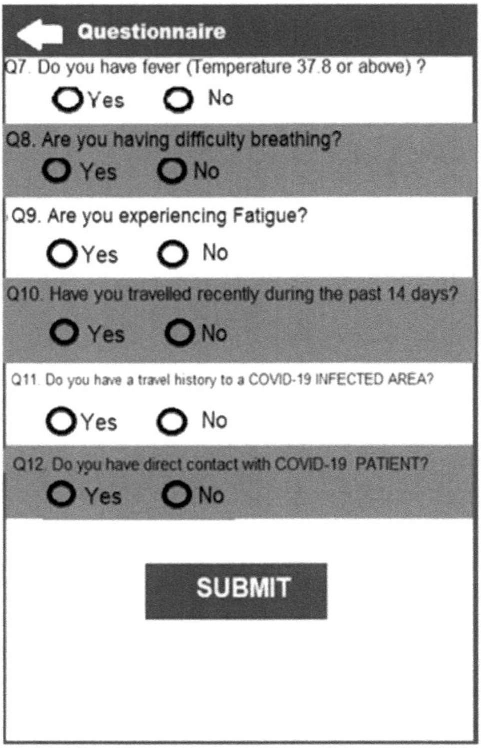

FIGURE 11.6 Questionnaire 7–12.

11.4 RESULT DISCUSSION AND SUGGESTIONS

The score is computed average of total points scored is computed and in the event that the score is in the reach 0–2, at that point, the patient is told that he/she may be experiencing stress. On the off chance that the score is in the reach 3–5, the patient is encouraged to hydrate properly and keep up legitimate individual cleanliness, Observe, and Re-evaluate following 2 Days. In the event that the score is in the reach 6–12, the patient is encouraged to look for a discussion with a doctor. In the event that the score is in the reach 12–24 patient is encouraged to visit the closest medical clinic and get tested for COVID-19. The nearest hospital also receives a notification about that user to get him tested for COVID-19 (Figure 11.7).

As per the result, the user will get the suggestion whether he/she has to consult a doctor and a nearby location and address of the hospital/Diagnosis center will be updated and the same information may be sent to nearby local authority so that necessary action could be taken care.

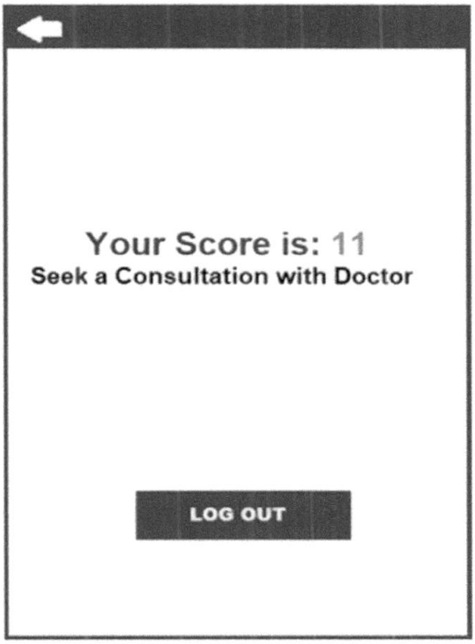

FIGURE 11.7 Result and suggestion.

11.5 CONCLUSION AND FUTURE SCOPE

Although the researcher is searching the effective and suitable vaccines and therapeutics for controlling the deadly COVID-19 as such till now there are no effective vaccines or specific antiviral drugs for COVID-19. Hence, we have to rely exclusively on enforcing strict preventive and control measures that minimize the risk of possible disease transmission. The proposed app will be helpful in providing the information regarding the probable health problem and suggest accordingly. The same information is passed to the nearest government hospital if he/she is suspected to coronavirus. The project can be further improved to gather essential data of regular activities through inbuilt sensors and even visual data using onboard smartphone sensors.

KEYWORDS

- **computed tomography**
- **computed tomography**
- **corona**
- **COVID-19**
- **middle east respiratory syndrome**
- **middle east respiratory syndrome**
- **nucleic acid test**
- **severe acute respiratory syndrome**

REFERENCES

1. Xu, X. W., Wu, X. X., Jiang, X. G., et al., (2020). Clinical findings in a group of patients infected with the 2019 novel coronavirus (SARS-Cov-2) outside of Wuhan, China: Retrospective case series. *BMJ, 368*, m606.
2. Chen, J., Wu, L., Zhang, J., Zhao, Y., Hu, S., Wang, Y., et al., (2020). *Deep Learning-Based Model for Detecting Novel Coronavirus 2019 Pneumonia on High-Resolution Computed Tomography: A Prospective Study*. MedRxiv.
3. Zhang, L., & Liu, Y., (2020). Potential interventions for novel coronavirus in China: A systemic review. *J. Med. Virol*. https://doi.org/10. 1002/jmv.25707.
4. Chang, D., Xu, H., Rebaza, A., Sharma, L., & Dela, C. C. S., (2020). Protecting health-care workers from subclinical coronavirus infection. *Lancet Respir Med.* https://doi.org/10.1016/S2213-2600(20)30066- 7.
5. Zeng, L. K., Tao, X. W., Yuan, W. H., Wang, J., Liu, X., & Liu, Z. S., (2020). First case of neonate infected with novel coronavirus pneumonia in China. *Zhonghua Er Ke Za Zhi, 58*, E009.
6. Li, J., Li, J., Xie, X., et al., (2020). Game consumption and the 2019 novel coronavirus. *Lancet Infect. Dis*. https://doi.org/10.1016/ S1473-3099(20)30063-3.
7. Huang, P., Liu, T., Huang, L., et al., (2020). Use of chest CT in combination with negative RT-PCR assay for the 2019 novel coronavirus but high clinical suspicion. *Radiology*. https://doi.org/10.1148/radiol. 2020200330.
8. Michelle, L. H., Chas, D., Scott, L., Kathy, H. L., John, W., Hollianne, B., Christopher, S., et al., (n.d.). *First Case of 2019 Novel Coronavirus in the United States*. Available at: https://pubmed.ncbi.nlm.nih.gov/32004427/ (accessed on 6 December 2022).
9. Zhao, J. P., Hu, Y., Du, R. H., et al., (2020). *Expert Consensus on the Use of Corticosteroid in Patients with 2019-nCoV Pneumonia, 43,* E007.
10. Holshue, M. L., DeBolt, C., Lindquist, S., et al., (2020). First case of 2019 novel coronavirus in the United States. *N. Engl. J. Med.* https://doi. org/10.1056/ NEJMoa2001191.

11. Government of India. https://www.mohfw.gov.in/ (accessed on 13 June 2022).
12. Purswani, J. M., Dicker, A. P., Champ, C. E., Cantor, M., & Ohri, N., (2019). Big data from small devices: The future of smartphones in oncology. In: *Seminars in Radiation Oncology* (Vol. 29, No. 4, pp. 338–347). Elsevier.
13. Singh, R. K., Dhama, K., Chakraborty, S., Tiwari, R., et al., (2019). Nipah virus: Epidemiology, Pathology, Immunobiology and advances in diagnosis. vaccine designing and control strategies a comprehensive review. *Vet. Q., 39*(1), 26–55. doi: 10.1080/ 01652176.2019.1580827.
14. Yang, Z. Y., Kong, W. P., Huang, Y., Roberts, A., Murphy, B. R., Subbarao, K., & Nabel, G. J., (2004). A DNA vaccine induces SARS coronavirus neutralization and protective immunity in mice. *Nature, 428*(6982), 561–564. doi: 10.1038/nature02463.

CHAPTER 12

TUMOR EXTRACTION SYSTEM USING ELM AND MODIFIED K-MEANS CLUSTERING

SUNEETHA RIKHARI[1] and K. MOHANA LAKSHMI[2]

[1]*Department of Electronics and Communication Engineering, Mody University of Science and Technology, Laxmangarh, Rajasthan, India, E-mail: suneetha.rikhari@gmail.com*

[2]*Department of Electronics and Communication Engineering, CMR Technical Campus, Hyderabad, Telangana, India*

ABSTRACT

The healthcare industry is one of the significant business sectors which are thriving to connect technology with the medical field. This idea has opened the door for technological innovations in the field of biomedical imaging. Internet of things (IoT) and artificial intelligence (AI) using machine learning (ML) are the primary areas of concern in the biomedical field. This chapter focuses on tumor detection and extraction system using extreme learning machine (ELM) and modified K-means clustering. Tumor detection and extraction are very useful for the diagnostic analysis of patient's disease. The use of an automated tumor detection system aids clinicians in detecting the tumor. The strategy utilized in this technique has three modules. The primary module is the pre-processing module in which non-local and local smoothing techniques are utilized to take out the commotion parts. In the next module, classification is finished

IoT and Cloud Computing-Based Healthcare Information Systems. Anand Sharma, PhD, Hiren Kumar Deva Sarma, PhD & S. R. Biradar, PhD (Eds.)

by acquiring highlight vectors from the ELM. The third module portrays the growth recognition stage, where the tumors are portioned utilizing a changed K-implies grouping calculation. Magnetic resonance (MR) tumors pictures are utilized in the proposed work. The results obtained proved that the proposed method is effective for automatic tumor detection.

12.1 INTRODUCTION

Recent developments in the biomedical field have directed to the arrival of the internet of things (IoT) and artificial intelligence (AI). This is one of the fields where IoT and AI together or individually making significant impact in the medical field. IoT is no longer restricted to industrial consumer and public sector applications, IoT is emerging into the healthcare field with AI by providing smart devices for healthcare monitoring, medical data analysis, assisting the doctors with the diagnosis of the patient's disease, etc.

AI is the key factor in producing a smart healthcare device. AI uses ML algorithms to build a mathematical configuration of training data. This training data is used to make predictions or decisions without being explicitly programmed to accomplish the task.

12.1.1 IOT AND AI IN MEDICAL FIELD

IoT has been successfully employed in the commercial areas like smart parking [1], precision agriculture [2], traffic congestion and minimization [3], smart grids [4], water management [5], etc. The application of IoT and AI in these areas has proven that remote monitoring of these devices is practically achievable. Hence, this can be adapted and extended to remote health monitoring of people. This can be very helpful to the people in rural areas, where the clinical details can be reported to the healthcare centers and doctors for necessary action.

In Ref. [6], a system is developed to generate a treatment plan by comparing the patient's present condition with the data base of previous patients. The system generated treatment plan is approved by doctors in 87.9% of cases. In Ref. [7], a mathematical model is proposed for the measurement of joint angles in Physical Hydrotherapy devices. The joint movement is continuously tracked throughout the therapy. In Ref. [8], an

IoT system is developed for monitoring Parkinson's disease using wearable sensors. These sensors observe the gait patterns and tremors. The general activities are monitored using smart cameras. The use of ML algorithms may produce improved results.

A device for monitoring the blood glucose levels of a diabetic patient is proposed in Ref. [9]. Heart attack detecting system was developed in Ref. [10]. This detecting system uses an ECG sensor, microcontroller, and a specially devised antenna. ECG sensor measures the activity of the heart which is then processed by a microcontroller. The processed data is then sent to a smart phone via Bluetooth through an antenna. Another system described in Ref. [11] measures the respiratory rate and provides a system to predict the heart attack. In Ref. [12], the SPHERE system is described which uses wearable sensors and cameras for managing the general day to day activities and health monitoring of old people and ill people.

One of the stimulating areas in the medical field is the extraction of the regions of interest from images. This can be done by image segmentation and is especially employed for tumor tissues segmentation. In general, tumor extraction is performed manually by the medical experts, which is not always obvious due to the high assortment in the appearance of tumor tissues. The tumor tissues appear different for different patients and hence exact position and size of the tumor must be identified for the removal of the tumor tissues. Automatic medical image segmentation using computer-aided tools is still a challenging task in the medical field. The proposed work is concentrated on tumor extraction using ML algorithm and K-means clustering technique.

12.1.2 MEDICAL IMAGING METHODS FOR TUMORS

Magnetic resonance imaging (MRI) is utilized to explore the human body actions and elements of life forms. MRI produces excellent images of the anatomical structures. These structures provide rich data for medical image analysis and diagnosis of the disease. MRI is a non-invasive procedure that can deliver two-dimensional (2D) and three-dimensional (3D) images of the human body organs. Brain Tumor is the presence and development of anomalous cells in the brain. The tumors are classified into two types: benign and malignant. Benign have homogeneous structure type and do not contain any harmful cells, whereas malignant tumors are heterogeneous structure type and contain harmful cells. The benign tumors can be removed by radiological means or by surgery. These tumors once removed do not grow back. Malignant tumors are treated by radiotherapy and chemotherapy.

MR images are widely used for determining the existence of tumors in the scan report. The brain tumor existence would be generally confirmed by the physician by analyzing the MR scan report. The treatment process gets started by the physician based on his knowledge and expertise in the specified field. Hence, there is a requirement to devise a computer aided system which can automatically discover the tumor from the MR image to ease the task of the physician.

For feature extraction, many training algorithms were developed using neural networks. These neural networks are trained in real-time using finite training data set. A single hidden layer feed-forward neural network (FNN) is proposed in Ref. [13] used finite data training set to produce an approximating function. This approach has N neurons and upon considering any non-linear activation function, it can learn N discrete observations with zero error. The weights which are between the input layer and the first hidden layer are to be adjusted as per the existing research works of feed FNNs.

Hence, all the weights and the biases which need to be altered are dependent on the parameters of the individual layers. One of the mostly used learning algorithms is Gradient Descent learning method. But these methods are slow and may get converged to the local minima. So far, many methods have been devised for automatic tumor detection. In this work the segmentation of tumor is done by training an ELM algorithm. It is a single layer feed-forward neural network (SLFN) in which the inverse of the hidden layer output matrices is calculated to determine the output weights. This method is not only producing minimum training error but also consists of the smallest norm of weights. The ELM is fastest learning algorithm when compared to learning algorithms with back propagation (BP) and produces improved generalization presentation.

12.1.3 RELATED WORK

In the recent days enormous number of readings and experiments have been done based on this research topic. Cellular automata-based fuzzy

C-means (FCM) is presented in Ref. [14] for brain tumor segmentation which uses gray level co-occurrence matrix (GLCM) for segmenting the tumor. A novel strategy which uses wavelets and support vector machine (SVM) for classification is explained in Ref. [15]. This approach has yielded good classification rate. Orthogonal discrete wavelet transforms (DWT) named as Slantlet transform (ST) is used in Ref. [16] on MR images for the classification of images. The intensity histogram of the input MR image is connected to ST as its histogram flag and element vector is obtained with respect to the size of the ST. The extracted element vectors are applied to a neural system-based classifier. This method has given good results for Alzheimer's sickness. A combination of DWT and FNN is proposed in Ref. [17]. DWT is used to extract the features and then principal component analysis (PCA) is applied to limit the feature space. The diminished features extracted from the PCA algorithm are applied to FNN and to sustain a strategic distance from overfitting, K-fold cross-validation technique is used.

The decision tree classification algorithm is employed in Ref. [18] to improve the classification efficiency of CT scan images. Automated brain tumor detection was proposed in Ref. [19], where area and circularity features are used for extracting the tumor. A semiautomatic technique for segmenting the MR brain images is discussed in Ref. [20]. In this an active contour model is used to get a segmented area from the fused feature map. Multispectral MRI image segmentation using Markov random field (MRF) model is utilized in Ref. [21]. Initially for extracting the features a wavelet-based method is used and then MRF is employed for segmentation of MR images. An MR image segmentation method using probabilistic neural network (PNN) is described in Ref. [22]. Rough set theory feature extraction with Feed-FNN classifier is explained in Ref. [23]. The FNN classifier efficiently discriminates the abnormal features and the normal features thus resulting in 90% accuracy. PNN with PCA is employed in Ref. [24] for the classification of brain tumor. The PCA generates the features, and the classification is done using PNN. back-propagation neural network (BPNN) with PCA is demonstrated in Ref. [25] for classification of MR brain images. The features are extracted using PCA and then these features are connected to BPNN for classification. This classifier has produced an efficiency of 96.33% with respect to the classification of MR images of the brain. Classification of computed tomography (CT) images using Convolutional Neural Networks is presented in Ref. [26].

The CNN with construction of tri-planar is used in Refs. [27, 28] for voxel classification. This method has greatly reduced the computational time. An automatic segmentation method is presented in Ref. [29] where CNN with 3×3 kernels are used for segmentation. The CNN uses convolution and pooling layers for getting the spatial information related to the pixels of the input image. These two procedures work on consecutive layers of the network in the background. The round up operations and the features obtained increase the classification rate. The disadvantage with the CNN is it needs more training time, and it is confined to a single solution in the course of the training process.

In order to overcome the shortcomings of the BP algorithm [30], in the recent years ELM algorithm is proposed. ELM is less complex and is the fastest learning algorithm. An alternative model to the CNN is proposed in Ref. [31] which use ELM-LRF. In this structure the information from LRF is combined with the ELM.

In this work, the features are extracted using ELM algorithm and a modified K-Means algorithm is employed to extract the tumor. Finally, the volume of the extracted tumor is calculated. The objective of the proposed work is to develop an efficient system for tumor extraction using learning algorithms.

12.2 EXPERIMENTAL METHODS AND MATERIALS

12.2.1 ELM METHOD

In this work, we propose a new methodology for brain tumor segmentation using ELM and hybrid clustering algorithm. ELM is a feed forward single hidden layer learning algorithm used for classification. With ELM training algorithm, the hidden layer node numbers can be set adaptively. The weights of the input and the hidden layers are assigned randomly, and least-squares method is used to obtain the weights of the output layer. The weights and biases need not be adjusted, and hence the ELM is said to have low training speed when related to customary feed FNNs such as BP [32]. BP algorithms employ training using gradient based learning algorithms. Multiple iterations are required for the BP algorithms to obtain better performance. At each iteration are weights are adjusted adaptively. Another disadvantage of BP algorithm is that it converges to local minima.

As depicted in Figure 12.1, ELM is a single hidden layer FNN [30] with N number of training samples and $\tilde{N}$ number of hidden layers where $N \geq \tilde{N}$.

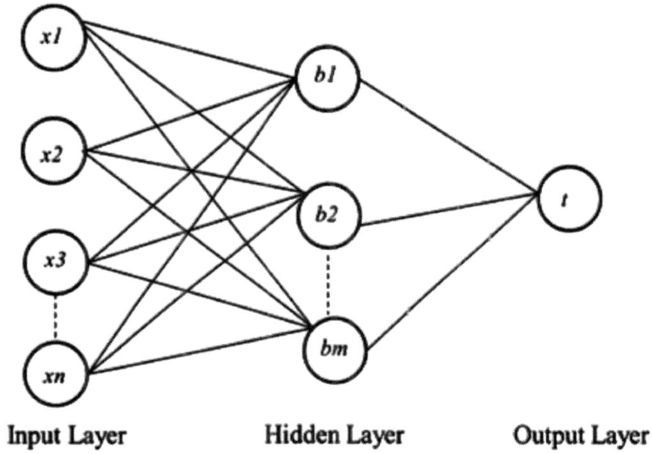

FIGURE 12.1 ELM single hidden layer FNN.
Source: Adapted from Ref. [37].

Let x_i is the input vector given by $x_i = [x_{i1}\, x_{i2}\, x_{i3} \,\ldots\ldots\ldots x_{in}]^T \in R^n$ and the output denoted by 't' as shown in Figure 12.1 is defined as $t_i = [t_{i1}\, t_{i2}\, t_{i3} \,\ldots\ldots\ldots t_{im}]^T \in R^m$. With $g(x)$ as the activation function the standard single Hidden layer FNN is mathematically modeled by the equation:

$$\sum_{i=1}^{\tilde{N}} \beta_i g\left(w_i . x_j + b_i\right) = O_j, j = 1,2,\ldots N \tag{1}$$

where; $w_i = [w_{i1}\, w_{i2}\, w_{i3} \,\ldots\ldots\ldots w_{in}]^T$ is the weight vector which connects the input layer and the hidden layer. $\beta_i = [\beta_{i1}\, \beta_{i2}\, \beta_{i3} \,\ldots\ldots\ldots \beta_{in}]^T$ is the weight vector which connects the hidden layer and the output layer. $w_i . x_j$ is the inner product of w_i and x_j and b_i is the threshold of the ith hidden layer.

The N samples can be approximated with zero error means such that $\sum_{i=1}^{\tilde{N}} \left\| O_j - t_j \right\| = 0$, therefore the values of b_i, w_i, and β_i exists such that:

$$\sum_{i=1}^{\tilde{N}} \beta_i g\left(w_i . x_j + b_i\right) = t_j, j = 1,2,\ldots, N \tag{2}$$

The N equations of Eqn. (2) can be written in the compact form as:

$$H\beta = T \tag{3}$$

where; H is called the output matrix of the hidden layer.

$$(w_1\, w_2 \ldots w_{\tilde{N}}, b_1 b_2 \ldots\ldots b_N, x_1 x_2 \ldots\ldots x_N) = \begin{bmatrix} g(w_1.x_1 + b_1)\cdots & \cdots & g(w_{\tilde{N}}.x_1 + b_{\tilde{N}}) \\ & \vdots\vdots & \\ g(w_1.x_N + b_1)\cdots & \cdots & g(w_{\tilde{N}}.x_N + b_{\tilde{N}}) \end{bmatrix} \tag{4}$$

The size of H matrix is $N \times \tilde{N}$ and,

$$\beta = \begin{bmatrix} \beta_1^T \\ \vdots \\ \vdots \\ \beta_{\tilde{N}}^T \end{bmatrix} \text{ of size } \tilde{N} \times m \tag{5}$$

$$T = \begin{bmatrix} t_1^T \\ \vdots \\ \vdots \\ t_{\tilde{N}}^T \end{bmatrix} \text{ of size } N \times m \tag{6}$$

The advantage of ELM is that the input vectors and the biases of the hidden layer can be randomly selected and further tuning of these parameters is not necessary. To train the network, a least-squares solution for $\tilde{\beta}$ of the linear system $H\beta = T$ has to be solved by Eqn. (7) given by:

$$\left\| H(w_1, w_2 \ldots\ldots w_{\tilde{N}}, b_1, b_2 \ldots b_{\tilde{N}})\beta - T \right\| = \min_{\beta} \left\| H(w_1, w_2 \ldots\ldots w_{\tilde{N}}, b_1, b_2 \ldots b_{\tilde{N}})\beta - T \right\| \tag{7}$$

The worst-case solution for this is:

$$\tilde{\beta} = H^{-1}T \tag{8}$$

The training error can be minimized by the following alternative least-squares solution:

$$H\tilde{\beta} - T = HH^{-1} - T = \min_{\beta} H\beta - T \tag{9}$$

➢ **Algorithm 1:** Assuming an input data set x and activation function g(x) and $\tilde{N}$:

1. Allocate random input weight w_i and bias b_i, where; $i = 1, 2, \ldots, N$.
2. Compute hidden layer output matrix H.
3. Compute the weight of the output, i.e., β from $\beta = H^{-1}T$.

12.2.2 TUMOR SEGMENTATION

The input images may be affected by noise during acquisition or transferring the image data. The noise is removed by adapting a non-local means and smoothing methods [33]. This is called the pre-processing action on the data images. In the proposed work, the clustering operation is enhanced by improved K-Means clustering.

12.2.3 IMPROVED K-MEANS CLUSTERING

K-Means is an unsupervised ML algorithm. It segments the data into k clusters which are mutually exclusive. After partitioning the data, it yields the index of the cluster for each observation. It operates on actual observations rather than on large dissimilarity measures [34]. When compared to hierarchical clustering methods K-Means produces good results for large amounts of data. The algorithm is separated into two distinct modules. In the first one, the value of k is fixed, and k centers are randomly selected. In the second module, the data object which is nearest to the center is taken. In general, Euclidean distance is used as the criterion function to check the distance between the data object and the cluster. This process is repeated iteratively with respect to all the data objects by simultaneously calculating the average of the primarily made clusters. This is repeated until the criterion function is given in Eqn. (10) is minimized.

$$E = \sum_{i=1}^{k} \sum_{x \in C_i} \left| x - \overline{x_l} \right|^2 \tag{10}$$

where; x represents the input object; $\overline{x_i}$ is the average of cluster C_i and E is the sum of squared error of all the objects. The Euclidian distance between two objects x and y is defined as:

$$d = \sqrt{\sum_{i=1}^{n} (x_i - y_i)^2} \tag{11}$$

The traditional K-Means clustering method is time consuming because at each iteration, it calculates the distance of each object from the center of each and every cluster. This algorithm increases the computation time for large data base. In the suggested work, a modified K-Means algorithm is used to improve the computational efficiency. The input to the algorithm is the number of desired clusters k and an input data $x = \{x_1, x_2, \ldots, x_n\}$, where n is the number of input data objects. The output of the algorithm gives k clusters $C_j \ (1 \le j \le k)$.

➢ **Algorithm 2:**

1. Select k objects as initial cluster centers from the input data x.
2. Calculate the Euclidian distance between each x_i and C_j and accordingly allocate the data to the nearest cluster.
3. For each x_i find the nearest center.
4. Store the nearest centers in the form of an array called cluster array *C*[ ] and the distance in *D*[ ] array.
5. Calculate the center of each cluster again and repeat the process.
6. For each x_i, compute the Euclidian distance from the center of the current nearby cluster.
7. If the distance is ≤*D*[i] the data object belongs to the same cluster else for every C_j compute distance between x_i and C_j with respect to all the centers assigned to the data object x_i. Set *C*[i] = j and set *D*[i] = distance between x_i and C_j.
8. Recalculate the cluster centers again until a convergence criterion is met.

This algorithm uses two arrays *C*[ ] and *D*[ ]. The array *C*[ ] stores the labels of the nearest center and *D*[ ] stores the distance of x_i to the closest center.

12.2.4 SIZE OF THE TUMOR

The segmented output image can be represented as a summation of the total number of white and black pixels, i.e.,

$$M = \sum_{x=1}^{L}\sum_{y=1}^{L}\left[f_{x,y}(0) + C\right] \tag{12}$$

where; L = 1 to 256; and $f_{x,y}(0)$ is the black pixel having the value '0;' $f_{x,y}(1)$ is the black pixel having the value '1.'

Hence, the total number of white pixels can be obtained using Eqn. (13):

$$P = \sum_{i=1}^{L}\sum_{j=1}^{L} f_{x,y}(1) \tag{13}$$

where; P represents a number of white pixels.

According to typography and advanced imaging unit's one pixel is equivalent to 0.264583 millimeters, i.e., 1 pixel = 0.264583 mm. Hence, the area or size of the tumor can be calculated as follows:

$$\text{Area or size of the tumor } A = \sqrt{P} \times 0.264583\, mm^2 \tag{14}$$

12.3 RESULTS AND DISCUSSION

All the images used in this work were obtained from publicly available source, and the experiments were performed using MATLAB software. The features are extracted using ELM learning algorithm and a modified K-Means clustering algorithm is used to segment the tumor.

The proposed method is compared with the existing segmentation methods like FCM clustering [35] and traditional K-Means algorithm [36]. The input data set used in this work is depicted in Figure 12.2. The results are depicted in Figure 12.3. The results depicted that the proposed method has given efficient segmentation results in terms of visual quality.

The size of the segmented tumor is calculated by using Eqn. (14) and is shown in Table 12.1. The computational time T_c of the proposed method is compared with the methods FCM and K-means in Table 12.2.

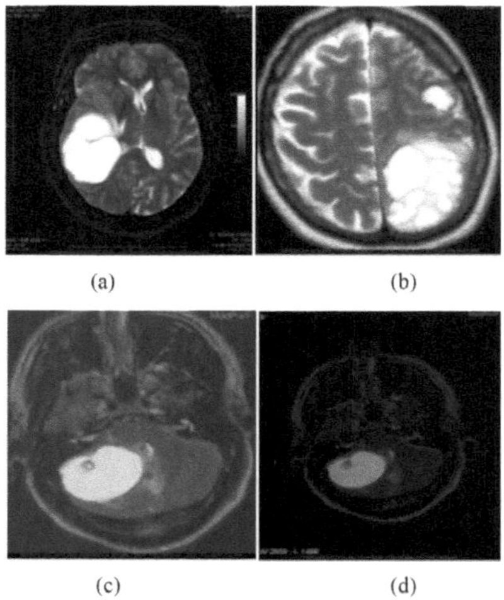

FIGURE 12.2 Input data.

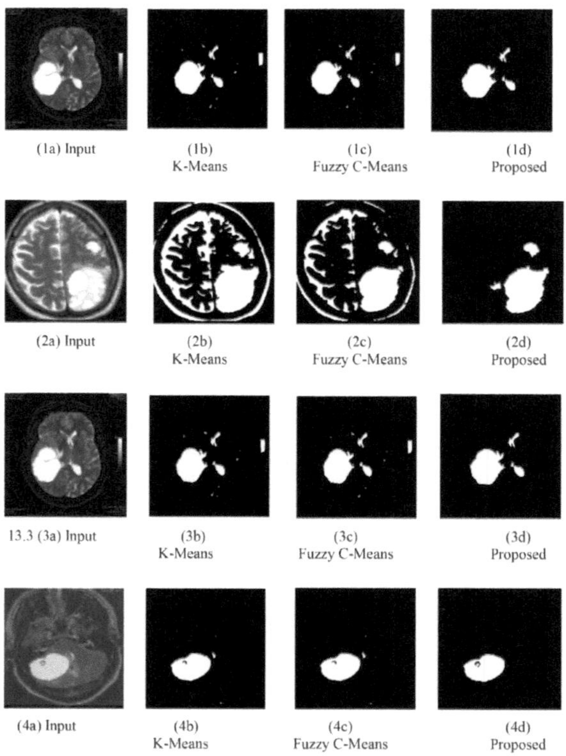

FIGURE 12.3 Segmented tumors.

TABLE 12.1 Calculated Size of the Tumor

Input Image	Size of the Tumor (mm^2)
Figure 12.2(a)	18.5101
Figure 12.2(b)	37.768
Figure 12.2(c)	17.0908
Figure 12.2(d)	16.1790

TABLE 12.2 Computational Time

Input Image	Computational Time (Seconds)		
	K-Means	FCM	Proposed
Figure 12.2(a)	1.6875	2.6250	0.9531
Figure 12.2(b)	1.6406	3.4844	0.3750
Figure 12.2(c)	1.5781	2.8125	0.3125
Figure 12.2(d)	2.3906	2.6719	0.3906

As depicted in Table 12.2, the suggested algorithm is time-efficient with respect to the other methods, and it has efficiently segmented the tumor information compared to K-Means and FCM. The output images depicted in Figure 12.3 clearly shows the segmented tumors are having less distortion. Hence it can be concluded that the proposed algorithm has outperformed the existing methods with respect to the overall execution time and visual quality.

12.4 CONCLUSION

In this work, a new approach for segmentation of tumor is explained. The ELM algorithm is used with a modified K-Means algorithm for classification and detection of tumor. Traditional leaning algorithms like CNN requires multiple hidden layers for training the data set, but ELM is a single hidden layer FNN. ELM is widely preferred for short data training sets. The time required for training is less compared to CNN. The modified K-means algorithm is used for segmenting the tumor from the obtained weight vector. Unlike the popular K-Means algorithm, the computational time of the modified K-means algorithm is less. The blend of both ELM and modified K-Means has yielded better segmentation results in terms of visual quality and less computational time. The proposed method is compared with K-Means and FCM and it is observed that the segmented tumor is more noise-free and qualitatively efficient for calculation of its size. Finally, after segmentation, the size of the tumor is calculated.

KEYWORDS

- **artificial intelligence**
- **extreme learning machine**
- **fuzzy grouping**
- **internet of things**
- **K-means algorithm**
- **magnetic resonance**
- **single layer feed-forward neural network**

REFERENCES

1. Smart Parking, (2017). SmartEye, SmartRep, and RFID Technology-Westminster City Council-London. https://www.westminster.gov.uk/parking (accessed on 13 June 2022).
2. University of New England, SMART Farm, (2017). http://www.une.edu.au/research/research-centres-institutes/smart-farm (accessed on 13 June 2022).
3. El-Sayed, H., & Thandavarayan, G., (2017). Congestion detection and propagation in urban areas using histogram models. *IEEE Internet Things J., 5*(5), 3672–3682.
4. Tan, S., De, D., Song, W. Z., Yang, J., & Das, S. K., (2017). Survey of security advances in smart grid: A data-driven approach. *IEEE Commun. Surveys Tuts., 19*, 397–422.
5. Sensus, (2017). *Smart Water-Smarter at Every Point.* http://www.sensus.com/internet-of-things/smart-water (accessed on 13 June 2022).
6. Fan, Y. J., Yin, Y. H., Xu, L. D., Zeng, Y., & Wu, F., (2014). IoT-based smart rehabilitation system. *IEEE Trans. Ind. Informat., 10*(2), 1568–1577.
7. Alves, R. C. A., Gabriel, L. B., Oliveira, B. T. D., Margi, C. B., & Santos, F. C. L. D., (2015). Assisting physical (hydro)therapy with wireless sensors networks. *IEEE Internet Things J., 2*, 113–120.
8. Pasluosta, C. F., Gassner, H., Winkler, J., Klucken, J., & Eskoer, B. M., (2015). An emerging era in the management of Parkinson's disease: Wearable technologies and the internet of things. *IEEE J. Biomed. Health Inform., 19*, 1873–1881.
9. Chang, S. H., Chiang, R. D., Wu, S. J., & Chang, W. T., (2016). A context aware, interactive m-health system for diabetics. *IT Prof., 18*, 14–22.

10. Wolgast, G., Ehrenborg, C., Israelsson, A., Helander, J., Johansson, E., & Manefjord, H., (2016). Wireless body area network for heart attack detection [education corner]. *IEEE Antennas Propag. Mag., 58*, 84–92.
11. Cretikos, M. A., Bellomo, R., Hillman, K., Chen, J., Finfer, S., & Flabouris, A., (2008). Respiratory rate: The neglected vital sign. *Med. J. Austral., 188*, 657–659.
12. Zhu, N., et al., (2015). Bridging e-health and the internet of things: The sphere project. *IEEE Intell. Syst., 30*, 39–46.
13. Huang, G. B., & Babri, H. A., (1998). Upper bounds on the number of hidden neurons in feed forward networks with arbitrary bounded nonlinear activation functions. *IEEE Transactions on Neural Networks, 9*, 224–229.
14. Sompong, C., & Wongthanavasu, S., (2016). Brain tumor segmentation using cellular automata-based fuzzy c-means, In: *13th International Joint Conference on Computer Science and Software Engineering (JCSSE)* (pp. 1–6).
15. Chaplot, S., Patnaik, L. M., & Jagannathan, N. R., (2006). Classification of magnetic resonance brain images using wavelets as input to support vector machine and neural network. *Biomed. Signal Process Control, 1*, 86–92.
16. Maitra, M., & Chatterjee, A., (2011). A slantlet transform based intelligent system for magnetic resonance brain image classification Biomed. *Signal Process Control, 1*, 299–306.
17. Zhang, Y., Wu, L., & Wang, S., (2011). Magnetic resonance brain image classification by an improved artificial bee colony algorithm. *Progress Electromagnetic Resolution, 116*, 65–79.
18. Naik, J., & Patel, S., (2013). Tumor detection and classification using decision tree in brain MRI. *IJEDR*. ISSN:2321-9939.
19. Sehgal, A., Goel, S., Mangipudi, P., Mehra, A., & Tyagi, D., (2016). Automatic brain tumor segmentation and extraction in MR images. In: *Conference on Advances in Signal Processing (CASP)* (pp. 104–107).
20. Banday, S. A., & Mir, A. H., (2016). Statistical textural feature and deformable model-based MR brain tumor segmentation. In: *6th International Conference on Advances in Computing, Communications, and Informatics (ICACCI)* (pp. 657–663).
21. Ahmadvand, A., & Kabiri, P., (2016). Multispectral MRI image segmentation using Markov random field model. *Signal, Image, and Video Processing, 10*, 251–258.
22. Pankaj, S., Rupinderpal, S., & Shivani, K., (2013). Brain tumor detection using neural network. *International Journal of Science and Modern Engineering, IJISME, 1*(9).
23. Rajesh, T., & Suja, M. M. R., (2013). Rough set theory and feed-forward neural network-based brain tumor detection in magnetic resonance images. *IEEE International on Advanced Nanomaterials & Emerging Engineering Technologies*
24. Mohd, F. O., Mohd, A., & Mohd, B., (2011). Probabilistic neural network for brain tumor classification. *IEEE International Conference on Intelligent Systems, Modeling and Simulation.*
25. Walaa, H. I., Ahmed, A. R. A. O., & Yusra, I. M., (2013). MRI brain image classification using neural networks. *IEEE International Conference on Computing, Electrical and Electronics Engineering, ICCEEE.*
26. Gao, X. W., & Hui, R., (2016). A deep learning-based approach to classification of CT brain images. In: *SAI Computing Conference (SAI)* (pp. 28–31). London, UK.

27. Gao, X. W., Hui, R., & Tian, Z., (2017). Classification of CT brain images based on deep learning networks. *Comput. Meth. Prog. Bio., 138*, 49–56.
28. Zhao, L., & Jia, K., (2015). Deep feature learning with discrimination mechanism for brain tumor segmentation and diagnosis. In: *International Conference on Intelligent Information Hiding and Multimedia Signal Processing (IIH-MSP)* (pp. 306–309). Adelaide, Australia.
29. Pereira, S., Pinto, A., Alves, V., & Silva, C. A., (2016). Brain tumor segmentation using convolutional neural networks in MRI images. *IEEE T. Med. Imaging, 35*, 1240–1251.
30. Huang, G. B., Zhu, Q. Y., & Siew, C. K., (2006). Extreme learning machine: Theory and applications. *Neurocomputing, 70*, 489–501.
31. Huang, G. B., Bai, Z., Kasu, L. L. C., & Vong, C. M., (2015). Local receptive fields based extreme learning machine. *IEEE Comput. Intell. M., 10*, 18–29.
32. Deng, W., Zheng, Q., & Chen, L., (2010). Research on extreme learning of neural networks. *Chin. J. Comput., 33*(2), 279–287.
33. Buades, A., Coll, B., & More, J. M., (2005). A non-local algorithm for image denoising. In: *2005 IEEE Computer Society Conference on Computer Vision and Pattern Recognition (CVPR)*. San Diego, USA.
34. Shi, N., Liu, X., & Guan, Y., (2010). Research on k-means clustering algorithm an improved k-means clustering algorithm. *Third International Symposium on Intelligent Information Technology and Security Informatics* (pp. 63–67). IEEE; IITSI.
35. ZulaikhaBeevi, S. M., & Mohamed, S., (2010). An effective approach for segmentation of MRI images: Combining spatial information with fuzzy C-means clustering. *European Journal of Scientific Research*, 437–451.
36. Mary, P. S., & IlaVennila, (2010). Optimization fusion approach for image segmentation using K-means algorithm. *International Journal of Computer Applications, 2*, 0975–8887.
37. Xiao, D., Li, B., & Mao, Y. (2017). A multiple hidden layers extreme learning machine method and its application. Mathematical Problems in Engineering, 2017.

CHAPTER 13

MACHINE LEARNING MODEL TO DETECT CANCEROUS CELLS THROUGH IMAGE PROCESSING

SHWETA NAIK,[1] ANITA DIXIT,[2] and S. R. BIRADAR[2]

[1]*Department of Computer Science and Engineering, Girijabai Sail Institute of Technology, Karwar, Karnataka, India*

[2]*Department of Information Science and Engineering, SDM College of Engineering and Technology, Dharwad, Karnataka, India, E-mail: anitadixit@sdmcet.ac.in (A. Dixit)*

ABSTRACT

Cancer is an irregular growth of cells and one of the commonly found diseases in India, which has caused the death of 0.3% of the total population yearly. It takes various forms and makes it difficult to detect at early stages. Getting a clean classification from a biopsy image is troublesome as the pathologist must know the comprehensive features of an ordinary and the affected cells. Identifying the cancerous cells from the microscopic biopsy images is very much time consuming and requires good expertise. The proposed system gives an overview of the detection of breast cancer with microscopic biopsy images. It concentrates mainly on image analysis where the input image is processed by using image processing. To predict whether the cancerous cells are present or not, we use a machine learning (ML) approach.

IoT and Cloud Computing-Based Healthcare Information Systems. Anand Sharma, PhD, Hiren Kumar Deva Sarma, PhD & S. R. Biradar, PhD (Eds.)

13.1 INTRODUCTION

Cancer is a harmful disease which has led to millions of deaths every year. It is difficult to discover cancer in the early stages, because when it reaches the last stage, it cannot be cured. Detecting cancer is a challenging task as it consists of several features which are taken into consideration. Cancer is originated by a single living cell during the initial stage. The cells are expanded abnormally and the person experiences certain symptoms. At this stage, an individual should undergo certain tests in order to know whether the person has cancer.

It is studied that in India, about 32% of the population suffers from cancer in their lifetime. This is because of daily habits which include consumption of tobacco, alcohol, and food habits. The chances of curing cancer are increasing day by day due to development in medical and engineering fields. The primary detection of cancer can help in curing and preventing the disease. Malignancy levels help in choosing the type of treatment. Medical expertise uses various familiar techniques for cancer detection. Detection of cancer basically consists of radiological imaging. This imaging technique helps to monitor the spread of the disease and the advancement of the treatment. Oncological Imaging provides very accurate and more varied results. Different imaging methods are used to get sufficient information to decide suitable treatment.

13.2 MATERIALS AND METHODS

13.2.1 DIGITAL IMAGE PROCESSING

Image processing performs operations on an image and provides an enhanced image which intern yields some useful information. It is a sort of signal processing in which input is an image and output contains an image or features associated with that image. It supports broad scale of algorithms and has the ability to remove noise, distortions than signal processing.

Digital image processing supports various types of transformations namely:

- Filtering;
- Image padding;

- Affine transformations;
- Identity;
- Reflection;
- Scale;
- Rotate;
- Shear.

Applications of image processing:

- Image rebuilding;
- Blurring and sharpening of images;
- Encoding;
- Transmission;
- Robot visions;
- Medical field;
- Digital cameras.

In this chapter, image processing is used to calculate the average percentage of cancer type. The given input image is chopped into 12 segments and the cell features are studied and compared with normal cell images.

13.2.2 CONVOLUTIONAL NEURAL NETWORK (CNN)

Basically, a normal neural network is featured as a mathematical structure, and it is prompted by human nervous structure or system. The nervous system receives the information, processes it, and generates suitable responses. Brain in humans is responsible for emitting electric charge when it encounters any stimulus. This network coordinates and handles all the tasks of the body.

CNN is a network of deep learning motivated by biological procedures. It is established by a heap of different layers which changes the input to output. Figure 13.1 shows the typical structure of CNN.

Establishment block of CNN is a convolution layer. The parameters of each layer consist of kernels which act as a receptor. Filters in each layer are convolved to the features like height and width of the input. Activation maps are built for each stack which contains the filters. The magnitude of output volume in spatial arrangement is calculated.

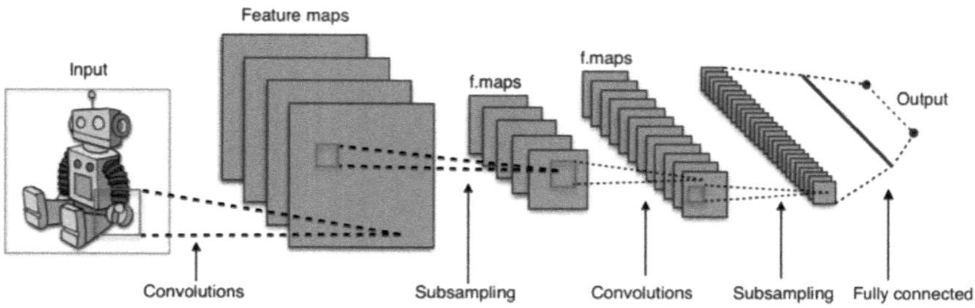

FIGURE 13.1 Architecture of CNN.

Source: Created by Aphex34. https://creativecommons.org/licenses/by-sa/4.0/

13.3 NEED FOR RESEARCH

Cancer has high death rates compared to other diseases. Almost 57% of new cancer patients and 65% of deaths have been encountered in recent days. Immediate action is required to reduce deaths caused by this disease and to overcome the burden of treatment costs.

13.4 A BRIEF SURVEY ON EXISTING SYSTEMS

Belsare et al. [1] give a detailed classification of histopathology images. The biopsy images are placed onto the glass slides and are studied by keeping them at different magnification levels, such as 40X, 100X, and so on. By using computer-assisted diagnosis (CAD), image processing techniques are analyzed, which include segmentation, feature extraction, and classification of the images. Segmentation separates the required objects from the base object. In segmentation, the normalization of colored images, and noise dismissal is carried out to upgrade the image quality. Features are extracted by taking the dependencies and various cell characteristics. Finally, depending on the extracted features, the malignancy levels are classified. They have used statistical study of features to classify the images.

Rajesh et al. [2] depict the clear-cut classification of cancerous and normal cells. They have also used the biopsy images where the tissue parts are tinged with stains and observed for better contrast. The main features used to classify the cells include the shape of the cells and nucleus. They have also used the Automated Cancer Detection model which classifies the normal and cancerous cells. The mechanized detection of cancerous tissues from biopsy helps in upholding the problems faced by early existing technologies. Segmentation approaches used here include K Means, C Means, and also the surface-based segmentation which predicts the performance of the techniques. The parameters included sensitivity, false-positive rate (FPR), precision, probability random index (RI), error rate and variance of information (VOI). It provided better performance results of the tissue classification and detection.

Ahmed et al. [3] depict the classification using feature extraction. The extraction is carried out by taking magnetic resonance (MR) images. In this study, various classification methods were used to classify breast tumors using contrast MRI. The data set included 20 themes categorized into two groups: benign and malignant type. Preprocessing of MRI is done to extract features. For classification, firstly they have used K-nearest neighbor (KNN) and secondly, they have used linear discriminant analysis (LDA). They draw image histograms which makes the classification task easier. By observing the histograms and the contrast scans the parameter called region of interest (ROI) is picked for further study. This setup gives accurate results and calculates the error rate.

Anuranjeeta et al. [4] depict the classification of cancer cells using morphological characteristics. Detecting and classifying cancer disease manually was a very hectic and difficult task. Here the classification is done by considering tissue features, cell distributions, cell shapes and size. They use a computer aided diagnosis system for accurate detection of cancer tissues. Feature extraction is done by image segmentation which includes interactive object extraction, TWS, RATS, and model thresholding methods. The performance is calculated using certain error rates which include global consistency error (GCE), variation, and Index values. For image enhancement they have used CLAHE as it depicts better results.

Gerald et al. [5] depict the use of thermography in order to classify breast cancers. Thermography is a science that helps in the detection of infrared (IR) images which use electromagnetic spectrum within a certain range. They produce images of certain radiations, and these output images are called thermograms. Thermal imaging is a process where it uses a camera. In this study, a sequence of statistical features is combined with a particular classification technique. The technique used is fuzzy rule-based classification where a bilateral imbalance is encountered. This technique gives accurate results when compared to mammography using thermograms.

Bailing et al. [6] depict various diagnosis techniques to give accurate and reliable results. Instead of using mammography, they have used a fine needle biopsy technique. In this chapter they have combined texture features and curvelet transform to give a cascade resemblance model with rejection choices. A combined model provides diverse image features by considering their comprehensive strengths. There are two associations for classification reliability. The first one contains SVM classifiers and the second contains a random subspace class which has the rejection choice. SVM's are used to acquire high accuracy rates for the given input dataset.

Features are defined on the basis of local binary pattern (LBP) which defines the gray level structure of a given image. Binary code is assigned as 0 and 1 to the features of neighbor cells. After LBP, curvelet transform is applied which provides limited representation of an image. Finally, the two classifications are cascaded in order to get the results. This chapter gives the classification accuracy of 97%, and it also depicts the error rate and rejections of the given images.

Ghongade et al. [7] give us a brief description on PC related analysis and framework for the disease with the help of measurable parameters and neural networks. They use a classifier and a selector for feature extraction. The classifier used is multi-layer perception (MLP). MLP is a feed-forward network which is used to plot the given input data to appropriate output. It is usually represented as a directed graph where each node is connected to other nodes. For the selection purpose they have used CFS classifiers. The images are directed towards differentiation and smoothened to encounter the area for feature analysis.

Some important steps carried out in this chapter are (a) differentiation; (b) extraction; (c) pre-handling; (d) positioning; and (e) execution. This chapter uses the CAD framework which categorizes mammograms. After getting computerized mammograms, area of choice (ROI), extraction, and classifying the images, the results are predicted. Picture division technique can be carried out to get better results.

Puman et al. [8], in their study, depict various neural systems or the networks which are created as false networks. Directed mechanism called back spread is used to create a false neural network. As earlier paper, it also has a handling system in each layer. In each layer there will be weights associated with the input and they are given to a handling model in a feed forward manner. RBF method is used to calculate the output data. The summations of all the weights are obtained with the help of yielding units. Gaussian output is used for grouping which returns a non-negative value for x.

13.5 METHODOLOGY

Figure 13.2 shows us the steps followed in the detection of cancer. Functions in each step are explained as follows:

1. **Biopsy Images:** In this step, the images are extracted from the tissues after undergoing microscopic biopsy. Processing: Pre-processing is mainly done to get rid of particular degradation like noise reduction, contrast settings, and image enhancements. The extracted biopsy images may be defective in some aspects such as low contrast and irregular staining. These images require enhancements to increase background and foreground features.
2. **Segmentation:** Various segmentation methods are carried out for the cytoplasm, nuclei, and cells. They are segmented using certain algorithms which include region based, threshold, and clustering algorithms. But the algorithms are selected based on the features preserved and extracted.

   RoI is segmented using K-means clustering algorithms which preserve the required information. Ground truth (GT) images are generated to check out the accuracy of trained data sets. Finally, the ROI pictures are compared with GT images for further analysis.
3. **Feature Extraction:** In this phase, biological features and clinically acceptable morphological features are extracted from segmented images. These images contain wavelet features, texture features, gray level features and LTE features. Finally, it is sent to the classification phase where it has several classifiers like NN (nearest neighbor), Fuzzy NN and SVM's.
4. **Classification:** Due to cluster formation and overlapping objects, the images are blurred, and this becomes a huge problem in extracting required features. The methodology uses various methods like enhancement, background cell segmentation, extraction, and classification. For contrast enhancement, histogram equalization is done and for segmentation k-means algorithms may be used.

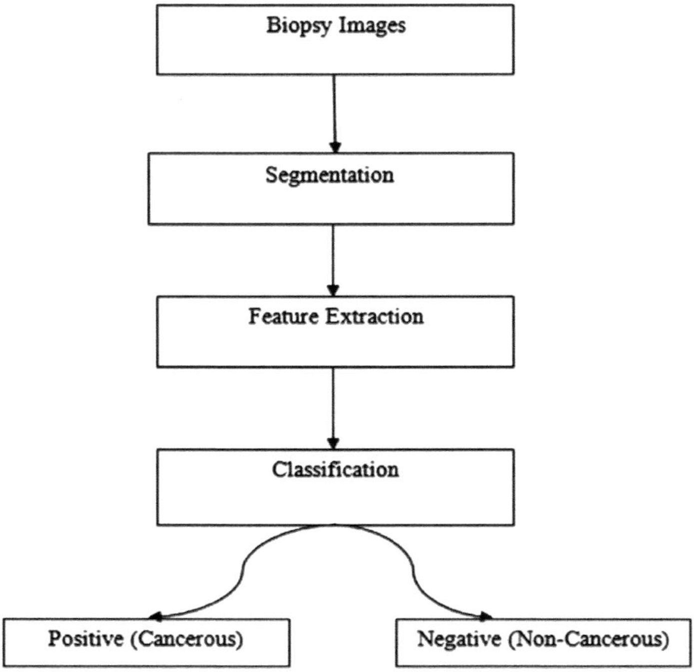

FIGURE 13.2 Architectural diagram of cancer detection.

13.6 IMPLEMENTATION

The implementation phase has two stages:

1. **Image Processing:** In this stage, CNN (convolution neural network) is used. Image is divided into 12 segments, shown in Figure 13.3. From each segment, percentages of different types of breast cancer cells are detected using CNN. Then finally the average is calculated and written to the file. This file is taken for testing with machine learning (ML) phases.
   Snippet to crop an image: The given image sample is cropped by using getCropImage. Percentage of each segment is calculated by,
   $[(\text{Segment } n)/(12 \text{ Segments})] \times 100$
   where; $n = 1, 2, \ldots, 12$
   In Figure 13.4 extracted results are presented.

2. **Machine Learning (ML):** In the ML part, there are two stages, one is training and the other is testing. In the training phase, the intervening result produced is taken from the Image processing stage and Naive Bayes theorem is adapted. This algorithm will be trained with the given data. Huge variants of images are processed and will be given to Naive Bayes algorithm for the purpose of training. In the next testing stage, trained data is taken to classify the image as positive or negative.
   Pseudo code for Naive Bayes:
   Input given:
   Training the data set,
   $F = (f_1, f_2, f_3, \ldots, f_n)$
   Output:
   A category of testing dataset.

Steps:

1. Read training dataset T;
2. Compute the mean. Also calculate the standard deviation of predictor variables in each category;
3. Repeat – compute the chances of blending the gauss destiny equation in each class till the possibility of all predictor variables (f_1, f_2, f_3, …, f_n) has been calculated.
4. Compute the likelihood for each category.
5. Fetch the greatest likelihood.

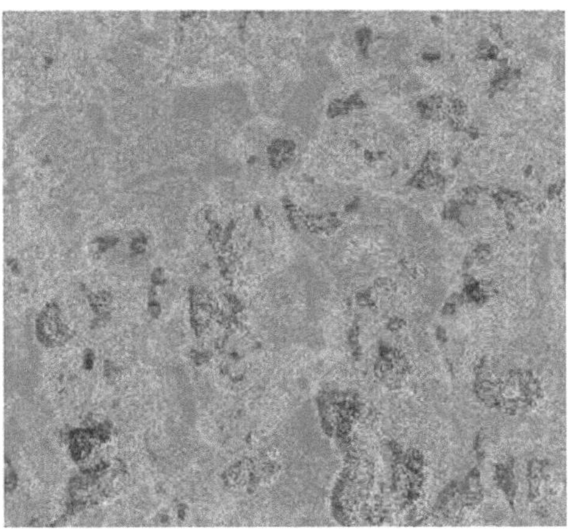

FIGURE 13.3 Segmented image.

Benign : 17.4894%

InSitu : 17.4893%

Invasive : 47.533%

Normal : 17.4883%

FIGURE 13.4 Extracted features.

13.6.1 EXPERIMENTAL RESULTS

The image processing module takes the image as input. This particular image is broken into 12 segments. To each of the segment, CNN is employed. There are totally four types or options considered in detecting breast cancer which is listed down as follows:

i. Benign cancer;
ii. *In situ* cancer;
iii. Invasive cancer; and
iv. Normal cancer.

The CNN helps to get the percent of each variety of Cancer cell present in this each image segment. After extracting the required information, it calculates the average of those 12 segments. The output of this will be stored as an intermediate file. This file is given to ML stage for prediction.

Intermediate Steps:

Analyze the percentile of each variant of cancer cell in each segment.

Image is segmented after feature extraction.

In this step, the average value of all the 12 segments will be written to file (Figure 13.5). Finally, trained data is used to categorize the image as positive or negative.

13.6.2 DISCUSSIONS

Figure 13.6 illustrates the complete process of cancer detection. In our project, we have taken the samples of breast cancer cells, and hence the diagram depicts the process in detection of breast cancer. We can use the same methods to detect other types of cancer by collecting cell samples from various parts of the body.

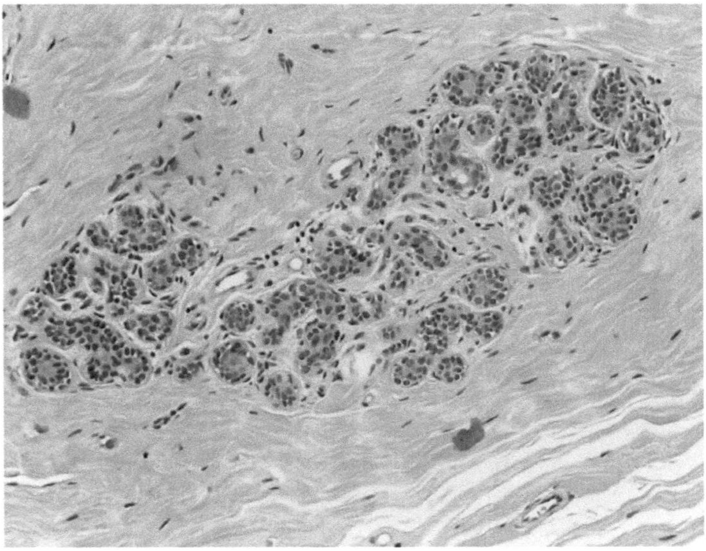

FIGURE 13.5 Cell image.

From Figure 13.6, microscopic biopsy images will be placed from a file in the program. In this process, images will be read and segmented using CNN algorithm. The CNN algorithm segments the given image into 12 parts. For every part it detects the percentage of the type of cancer cell present. Then finally, the average is calculated for 12 parts. Thus, this average is written to the output file. The segmented image thus given as input to feature extraction gives us intermediate output. The completion of the image processing phase shows the average output of all the 12 parts and the segmented image. After getting the average output and segmented image, ML technique is used to train and test the given images.

In predicting results, ML is used. ML part detects the type of cancer for a particular image using the intermediate output based on the Naive Bayes Algorithm. The Naive Bayes algorithm is trained using the same type of data as in intermediate code. The result is displayed as positive or negative after undergoing all the processes. Experimental results are presented in Table 13.1.

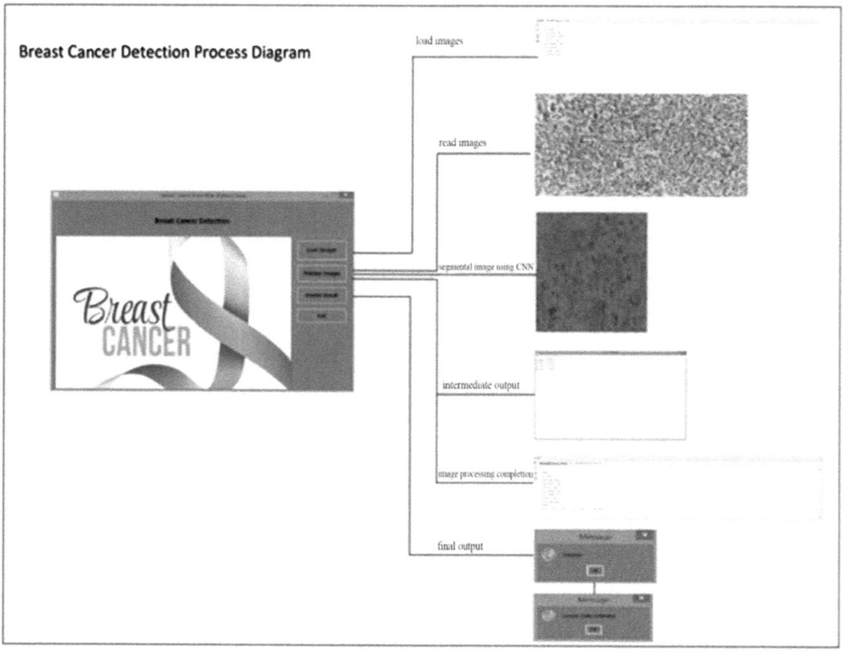

FIGURE 13.6 Cancer detection progress diagram.

TABLE 13.1 Experimental Results

Type	Benign	In Situ	Invasive	Normal	Total
Benign	9	1	0	0	10
In situ	2	8	0	0	10
Invasive	0	0	10	0	10
Normal	0	0	0	10	10
Total	11	9	10	10	40
Accuracy Calculation (%)	9/10 × 100 = 90%	8/10 × 100 = 80%	10/10 × 100 = 99%	10/10 × 100 = 99%	

13.7 CONCLUSION

Every year many people die due to cancer, and the number of death percentages is escalating day by day. This is because there is no healing assurance of the disease. Scientific associations are continuously researching various cancers. In our system, we collect microscopic images, and they are subjected to different enhancement techniques to get a clear image. The biopsy image is subjected to processing techniques where image restoration and image enhancement are done. Then it is sent to the segmentation phase in which the area of interest is featured and separated. In the next step, the required features are extracted by using suitable algorithms. The input file is dropped, and the image is divided into 12 segments. In each segment, the average percentile of cancer cells and the cancer type is calculated. Here we use the Naive Bayes classifier to detect and classify the cancer type. It determines and displays whether it is positive or negative. This project ensures accuracy in providing results and also takes less time in detection, which helps in the fast treatment of patients.

KEYWORDS

- **computer-assisted diagnosis**
- **convolutional neural network**
- **false-positive rate**
- **image processing**
- **linear discriminant analysis**
- **machine learning**

REFERENCES

1. Belsareand, D., & Mushrif, M. M., (2011). *Histopathology Image Analysis Using Image Processing Technique.* Publisher Research Gate.
2. Bailing, Z., (2011). Breast cancer diagnosis from biopsy images by serial fusion of random subspace ensembles. In: 4th *International Conference on Biomedical Engineering and Informatics (BMEI).*
3. Mahin, G., & Hamed, K., (2015). *Role of Biotechnology in Cancer Control.* Publisher Research Gate.
4. Mitko, V., Josien, P. W. P., Paul, J. V. D., & Max, A. V., (2014). *Breast Cancer Histopathology Image Processing.* Publisher IEEE.
5. Rajamanickam, B., Kuo, A. L., Richard, Y., & Kheng, W. Y., (2012). *Cancer and Radiation Therapy: Current Advances and Future Directions.* Publisher Ivy spring International.

6. Yapeng, H., & Liwu, F., (2012). *Targeting Cancer Stem Cells: A New Therapy to Cure Patients, 2*(3), 340–356.
7. Landini, G., Randell, D. A., Breckon, T. P., & Han, J. W., (2010). Morphologic characterization of cell neighborhoods in neoplastic and preneoplastic epithelium. *Analytical and Quantitative Cytology and Histology, 32*(1), 30–38.
8. Sinha, N., & Ramkrishan, A. G., (2003). Automation of differential blood count. In: *Proceedings of the Conference on Convergent Technologies for Asia-Pacific Region (TINCON '03)* (pp. 547–551). Bangalore, India.
9. Kasmin, F., Prabuwono, A. S., & Abdullah, A., (2012). Detection of leukemia in human blood sample based on microscopic images: A study. *Journal of Theoretical & Applied Information Technology, 46*(2).
10. Srivastava, R., Gupta, J. R. P., & Parthasarathy, H., (2011). Enhancement and restoration of microscopic images corrupted with Poisson's noise using a nonlinear partial differential equation-based filter. *Defense Science Journal, 61*(5), 452–461.
11. Pisano, E. D., Zong, S., Hemminger, B. M., et al., (1998). Contrast limited adaptive histogram equalization image processing to improve the detection of simulated speculations in dense mammograms. *Journal of Digital Imaging, 11*(4), 193–200.

CHAPTER 14

5G TO 6G IN ROBOTIC TELESURGERY

AMIT KUMAR VERMA

Faculty, Department of Pharmacy, MJP Rohilkhand University, Bareilly, Uttar Pradesh, India,
E-mail: professoramitmjpuniversity@gmail.com

ABSTRACT

Telesurgery or remote surgery is defined as the branch of medicine where surgeries are conducted by doctors remotely – a doctor performs surgery located miles away for their affected patient. A Telerobotic surgical system consists of one or multiple arms managed remotely by a doctor, a master console and sensing system works in combination with the robotics communication (4G, 5G) technologies and the element of management information. Latency tends to exist when the data is sent across a network either through a cable or wireless to a robot arm or machine. The higher the latency longer the instructions or messages take to send or reach. By decreasing these latency characteristics, time risk of the mistakes can be minimized, and absolute precision can be assured. It is necessary for the surgeon to have excellent image quality for real-time surgical work. The limitations during telesurgery, such as latency problem, slow data speed, poor image quality, etc., can be overcome by the use of high emerging networks technology 5G network and 6G network technology. 5G network technology can move more data (20 Mbps to 250 Gbps), quickly, and reliably than existing 4G networks by operating at higher frequency, 30 GHz to 300 GHz from anywhere. However, any limitation of this network

IoT and Cloud Computing-Based Healthcare Information Systems. Anand Sharma, PhD, Hiren Kumar Deva Sarma, PhD & S. R. Biradar, PhD (Eds.)

related to infrastructure and rolling out exists. The term 6G refers to the sixth generation of wireless technology. Through which it is proposed to integrate advanced features into existing 5G technology with the objective of advanced surgeries or maybe Robot performing surgery by incorporating AI. 6G-enabled network technology will have a great advance in the area of image analysis presents technology and location awareness. 6G connectivity will have a speed of 1 terabyte per second and very low latency. 6G will certainly revolutionize the healthcare sector that fill the barrier of time and space through remote surgery and guaranteed optimization of medical care workflow. 6G systems are the new generation of wireless networks bridging demands of connected, intelligent Digital World. News spectrum, novel PHY techniques, innovative network architecture, and intelligent network are the challenges for the 6G enabled technologies in the telesurgery area. The objective of this chapter is to highlight the limitation of conventional surgery operation and demonstrate the application of the new emerging 5G and 6G enabled technologies in the telesurgery area of medical science.

14.1 INTRODUCTION

It is defined as branch of medicine or telemedicine in which distant surgical procedure or surgery is performed by surgeon or surgical team on a patient located remotely [1]; therefore, it is also called remote surgery. Besides ignoring geographical boundaries, this distant technology ensures the timely availability of surgeons. It utilizes the base of wireless networking and robotics [2]. Through the use of a variety of the communication modalities, doctor for 150 years have tried to transmit medical information to provide consultation to their patients situated remotely via teleconsultation.

In 1970 with the introduction of da Vinci surgical and the Zeus system, the concept of telesurgery was evolved. United State space agency, National Aeronautics and Space Administration (NASA) explored the concept of Telesurgery with a vision to be used for astronauts in orbit or space. Machine having surgical instrument can perform surgical procedures for astronauts located on the space station and controlled by a surgeon on the planet earth. Similarly, the United States Defense Advanced Research Projects Agency (DARPA) advocated the development of telesurgery unit through which surgical procedures can be performed on the fierce battlefields.

In 1985 during a stereotaxic operation the first surgical robot, PUMA 560 perform biopsy by inserting a needle into the brain to avoid error from hand tremor as did frequently by humans. In 1988 PROBOT was used to perform transurethral prostate surgery, a procedure that involved a multiple repetitive cutting motion. In 1992 IBM and an integrated surgical system Ins (ISS) developed ROBODOC which was used to develop a cavity in the femur for hip replacement in patients with greater precision and accuracy. In the late 1990s to carry out minimum invasive surgery. Three system were designed:

- The da Vinci surgical system designed by California intuitive surgical Inc, California;
- AESOP robotic surgical system, Computer motion Inc, California; and
- Zeus robotic surgical, Computer motion Inc, California.

Zeus robotic surgical system performed laparoscopic fallopian tube reanastomosis (Fallopian tubes are reconnected after cutting) and laparoscopic cardiac revascularization procedure in closed chest-beating heart operation where chest was not surgically opened.

In 2003, da Vinci robotic surgical system used work on the advanced technology. It consists of a surgeon, console, instrument that resemble human wrist with a vision system. The surgeon operates from the remote surgeon console where the Master controller were adjusted to control the direct movement of the binocular camera and wrist mimicking instruments. The robotic system was joined to cast positioned adjacent to the patient. The 3D surgical view was recreated at a monitor the computer system visualizes the image and a spatial attachment of the system in a virtual surgical field visualized by the surgeon at the console. The removal of the unwanted motion minimally invasive access mimicking the movement of human hands and 3D visualization with binocular camera system are the advantages over the other robotic surgical system.

Robotic telesurgery opens new ways to provide an urgent extreme health service. A tele surgical system may consist of: (i) master console; (ii) slave robot (teleoperator) one or more arms controlled remotely by the surgeon; (iii) sensory system thus telesurgery works in combination with robotic communication technology and elements of management information system:

1. **Master Console:** This is a human system interface HSI consisting of the device based on haptic feedback for positioning orientation input, for display purpose a video screen output and for video voice feedback at phone is required.
2. **Slave Robot (Teleoperator):** It consists of a 3D video camera, a microphone, and sensors.

For delivering of real-time manipulation commands and multimodal sensory data high speed communication network is required which provides the basis for the interconnection of the master console and the slave robot.

14.2 COMMUNICATION QOS REQUIREMENTS FOR ROBOTIC TELESURGERY

The communication requirement consists of forward link, feedback link, real-time multimedia streams, video display devices, physical vital signs, and haptic data technology.

14.2.1 FORWARD LINK

It delivers real-time manipulation instruction to control the rotation and movement of the robotic arm at teleoperator with the assistant voice stream from the surgeon or doctor to communicate with the surgical team remotely (Figure 14.1).

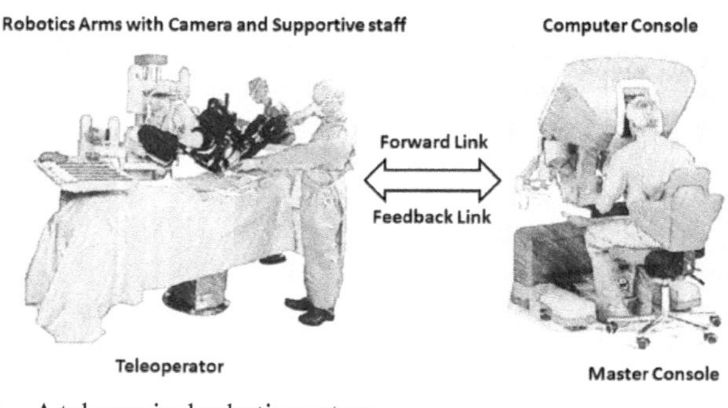

FIGURE 14.1 A telesurgical robotic system.

14.2.2 FEEDBACK LINK

This provides real-time multimodal sensory feedback from the 3D video display force feedback examples – pressure, tissue mechanical properties, patient respiration rate (RR), ECG accompanying voice assistant from healthcare staff.

14.2.3 3D VIDEO DISPLAY DEVICES

The specifications of two high-definition video streams are resolution of 1920 × 1080 pixels having 32 bits per pixel and 30 frames per second fps/60 fps/120 fps is the frame rate for the 3D display device.

Medical video compression rate must be in the range of 1:229 to 1:15, 137 Mbps to 1.6 Gbps is required data rate. Video conferencing system requires jitter within 30 ms and below 1% is packet loss rate.

14.2.4 HAPTIC DATA TRANSMISSION

One kHz is the sampling rate of uncompressed haptic signal. The data rate varies from 128 to 400 kbps, jitter requirement is below 2 ms and latency demands below 50 ms.

14.2.5 REAL-TIME MULTIMEDIA STREAM [3–5]

This involves 2D camera flow data type which requires latency below 150 ms, jitter in between 3 and 30 ms, packet loss rate $<10^{-3}$ with data rate less than 10 Mbps whereas 3D camera flow data type requires latency below 150 ms, jitter in between 3 and 30 ms, packet loss rate $< 10^{-3}$ with data rate in between 137 Mbps and 1.6 Gbps. Audio flow demand latency below 150 ms, jitter below 30 ms, packet loss $< 10^{-2}$ with data rate of 22–200 Kbps.

14.2.6 PHYSICAL VITAL SIGNS [6]

These data types such as temperature, blood pressure, heart rate (HR), RR, EEG, ECG EMG all require latency below 250 ms with packet loss $<10^{-3}$. Temperature, blood pressure, HR, and RR requires data rates of <10 Kbps.

The data rate requirement for ECG data type is 72 Kbps, for EEG data type is 86.4 Kbps and for EMG data type is 1.536 Mbps.

Doctor tends to be positioned at a console (usually in the same room) and distantly manage four robotic arms in the Da Vinci Robotic Surgical System. The only drawback is the surgeon is unable to get his sense of touch (TecTile, haptic feedback). With introduction of 5G technology having real-time haptic feedback which makes it possible to control surgical robots more precisely for diagnosis and treatment. The introduction of haptics provides more feel and control to the surgeon who is managing the robotics distantly. By wearing a special glove with sensors, the surgeon can feel the depth of a tumor, or any unusual cyst touched by robots arm during the operation.

14.2.7 NETWORK ARCHITECTURE

Boot enhanced mobile broadband (eMBB) for 3D video streaming and ultra-low-latency communications (uRLLC) for hepatic feedback are essential for communication networking. The master console and teleoperator access the network through the radio access network of D-RAN or C-RAN.

14.3 LIMITATION OF CURRENT ROBOTIC SYSTEM

The current robotic arrangement faces various limitations which are discussed in subsections.

14.3.1 LACK OF EFFECTIVE HAPTIC FEEDBACK

Both tactile and force feedback are present. Tactile feedback sensing explains the viscosity and surface texture of the tissues, which in turn helps the surgeon to accurately determine the margin of the abnormally to perform better subsequent dissections. Force-feedback aids in improving the operation precision (coronary artery bypass grafting) and decreasing unavoidable injuries during dissection methods [7].

14.3.2 LATENCY

Another important obstacle of limitation is latency. It is defined as the technology which mediates the transmission of the tactile information to the teleoperator it causes the teleoperator to feel the tissue consistency and the tension within the sutures during operation. Latency is the time from the surgeon's initiation of the operation to the corresponding operation displayed on the surgeon's screen. Latency is a function of the distance between the master and slave units [8, 9].

Global network of telesurgery is difficult to attain without the solving the problem of latency. According to the researchers, latencies less than 200 ms are ideal for the telesurgeries and latencies up to 300 ms are suitable [10]. However, task completion time increases at >500 ms, but the error rate remains low. Robot telesurgery works on a predictive algorithm that incorporates useful data about the environment with the doctor's movement. Telesurgeries can be performed to the moon, at such large distances, light-speed data transmission results in latencies of 500–2,000 ms.

14.3.3 BANDWIDTH

It is defined as the amount of data transmitted per given amount of time insufficient bandwidth causes buffering and incomplete transmission leading safety concern.

14.3.4 HIGH COST

ATM (asynchronous transfer mode) lines cost $100,000 to $200,000 and telerobotic surgical range from $1–2 million [11].

14.4 NECESSITY OF 6G NETWORK TECHNOLOGY

From the first to the 5th generation of the mobile technology, the advancement results in the successful completion of telesurgery. Nowadays, data-centric, data dependent, attainment of global networking in telesurgery and telemedicine is a challenge. The success and performance of remote surgery mainly depends on the network performance, as stability of the system depends on the latency, jitter, and packet loss and their ignorance result in the low performance of the system. Sutures haptic data requires less than 10 ms latency and packet loss of $<10^{-4}$. The communication networks can be assumed as the nervous system of telesurgery network must be such that it can transfer a much greater amount of data at much higher speeds and the trend already started in four generation and five generation, sixth-generation connection will work with realization of the internet of thing paradigm connecting patients, computing resources, surgeon, and robotic agent. To attain high surgical precision and accuracy of automated robotic surgical system requires a data rate in the order of terabits per second, a latency of hundreds of microseconds and 10^7 connections per km^2 may limits even the capabilities of new 5G system however low latency is tried by providing novel additional wireless tracts through new millimeter wave spectrum and redesigning of core network. It is known that 5G Network operate at higher frequencies of order mm-wave band in NR. 6G will operate through terahertz and optical communication. It operates between 100 gigahertz and 10 terahertz enabling data rates in the order of hundreds of Gbps which may revolutionize the field of telesurgery. Future 6G different architectures may provide three-dimensional (3D) coverage thereby connecting terrestrial infrastructure with non-terrestrial platforms hence telesurgery can be performed at space station also. 6G may cause disaggregation to the extreme by virtualizing Medium Access control (MAC) and physical layer component (PLC). This will reduce the cost of networking equipment making the development of networking infrastructure economically valid, a limiting factor in telesurgery operations whereas 5G is silent on challenges related to the development of disaggregated architectures, in addition to this 6G is planned to install energy circuits harvesting circuits to make devices self-powered.

14.5 QOS PROVIDED BY 6G COMMUNICATION TECHNOLOGY IN FUTURE

14.5.1 VIRTUAL COMMUNICATION

The virtual communication such as augmented and virtual reality (VR) and holographic communication which require very high speed, low latency for maintaining virtual presence, force feedback, tactile feedback needed in robotic telesurgery, such QoS will be provided by 6G communication technology.

14.5.1.1 HOLOGRAPHIC COMMUNICATION

High data rates and high-definition streaming videos are the requirement of Holographic communication, in addition to this, it requires very low latency for real-time voices and spontaneous control responses to provide excellent QoS. Overall satisfaction level will be high [12, 13]. 6G will be capable of satisfying all the requirements. Holographic communication will use the core service of combined and enhanced eMBB and URLLC will be used by holographic communication providing breakthrough during 6G Holographic communication which will make communication similar to face-to-face interaction and this is possible because of high speed data, low latency resulting in uninterrupted communication making the physical presence of surgeon or doctor during ongoing surgical operation not compulsory.

14.5.1.2 AUGMENTED REALITY (AR) AND VIRTUAL REALITY (VR)

Similar requirements needed for augmented reality (AR) and virtual reality (VR) as in the case of holographic communication. The core service of combined and enhanced eMBB and URLLC is used by augmented and VR maintenance of high data rates, very low latency, jitters, packet loss, etc., are essential for real-time voices and immediate control responses needed for real-time surgical procedures remotely [14].

14.5.1.3 PEAK DATA RATE

The peak data rates requirement of AR and VR is 1 Tbps and user experience of >10 Gbps with >0.1 ms latency which can be provided by MBBLL [15]. AR can provide visibility inside the human body anatomy without separating the different components of the different organs. For example, various components of the brain are visible without removing its parts, beside this the depth of the visibility can be changed, i.e., the user can view deeper and deeper inside the brain (physical depth). Zooming can be done to view different parts of the brain such as the cerebellum, medulla oblongata, amygdala, hippocampus region, etc., for better visibility. Artificial environment of neuronal networks of the brain can be created to know the physiology and anatomy of the brain. Better collaborative works can be achieved with the combined use of the holographic communication, AR, and VR through 6G communication network technology.

14.5.1.4 TACTILE/HAPTIC INTERNET

Tactile Internet requires ERLLC and high-speed communication to grab the tactile in real-time. Usually, the doctor or surgeon performing surgery in remote area sends the signal to another human or robot or robot surgical system. This technology is incorporated where a physical presence is compulsory to perform a surgical procedure. Usually, this task requires precise work and robots cannot always be trained to perform such tasks. During such remote telesurgery, the surgeon can use tactile technology to perform a surgery using a human or a robot. As per the movement or directions of the remote surgeon or doctor, the robot will move or perform surgical procedures. 6G communication technology with its high-speed data rates resulting in uninterrupted and high-speed Internet will provide great support in achieving these tasks of telesurgery.

14.5.2 INTELLIGENT HEALTHCARE

QoL will be the greatest contributor in the application of intelligent healthcare. It is assumed that 6G communication technology will revolutionize healthcare sector. In the near future, 6G will be able to overcome the limitation of time and space barriers of healthcare. In addition to the application in robotic telesurgery 6G driven. Intelligent healthcare will help in the implementation of hospital-to-home (H2H) service through intelligent hospital vehicle. Thus, the concept of mobile hospital will soon replace ambulance services in the coming time.

Hospital to home services will also implement real-time accident detection and automatic emergency detection. Diverse intelligent wearable devices and sensors will help in the tracing of accidents remotely automatically Also, needle-free blood sample reader (BSR) sensor [15] will greatly help in the detection of communicable and non-communicable diseases automatically and are very useful in pandemic like COVID-19. Further to the surprise, BSR sensor will read the blood sample and report it to the pathologies. Therefore, intelligent wearable devices (IWD) reduce the contamination risk of medical staff from bacteria, viruses. Such type of devices has an important role to play in pandemic like COVID-19. The travel risk of the patient to the hospitals for regular checkup, pathological testing can be minimized.

14.5.3 INTELLIGENT INTERNET OF MEDICAL THINGS (IIOMT)

Newly arrived concept of intelligent internet of medical things (IIoMT) will help in nullifying the time and space barriers [16]. For example, surgeon located remotely can perform surgical operations using telesurgery which requires QoS from 6G communication technology. The surgeon can manage the telesurgery through verbal, telestration or tele-assist. For verbal, the surgeon will take help of holographic communication. This helps the surgeon in the movement to have a better visual of the surgery area during robotic telesurgery. For telestration, doctor(s) will use AR and VR technology, further the doctor(s) can tele-assist the surgery using tactile/haptic technology. All the requirements needed to fulfill these tasks will be managed by 6G communication.

14.5.4 ARTIFICIAL INTELLIGENCE (AI)

If we talk about artificial intelligence (AI) then convolutional neural network and deep learning has an important role to play role in telesurgery. In order to enhance precision, accuracy, security, safety, various tools based on AI can be applied which contribute to the stability of haptic control and decrease the traffic in the core network, thus enhancing the overall latency and reliability.

To improve the safety and accuracy, the force and position signals created by software can be obtained and applied to human operators. For example, around anatomical structure a virtual wall can be placed to keep the surgical instrument from contacting it [16]. In order to reduce the latency and packet loss impact on haptic control instability the various predictive and interpolative/extrapolative modules may be applied on edge cloud [17]. If the AI software predicts the risks of a manipulation error, then warning provisions are suitably placed, e.g., due to the delayed display of video stream, the robotic arm will cut an artery by mistake then a warning can be issued to the surgeon with the help of software. This will allow the surgeon to hold on the movement, thereby avoiding the operation errors caused by the delayed arrival of the sensory data feedback. With the help of AI, real-time verification of the manipulation can be achieved.

14.6 CONCLUSION

Telesurgery enables medical practitioners to perform surgeries via robotic surgical system, thus providing improved patient access to surgical support. Application of remote surgery extends from aquanauts in underwater to astronauts in space station. Latency is the biggest challenge for telesurgical operations; beside this, networking infrastructure requirements and high investment cost are other limitations in its global implementation. High generation communication technologies such as 5G and 6G are the lifeline and fate decider of telesurgery and will surely see a lot of surprises in this area.

KEYWORDS

- **6G network**
- **artificial intelligence**
- **latency**
- **physical layer component**
- **robotics**
- **telesurgery**
- **virtual reality**

REFERENCES

1. Schreuder, H. W. R., & Verheijen, R. H. M., (2009). Robotic surgery. *BJOG, 116*, 198–213.

2. Raison, N., Khan, M. S., & Challcombe, B., (2015). Telemedicine in surgery :what are the opportunities & hurdles to realizing the potential ? *Curr. Urol. Rep., 16*, 43.
3. Perez, M., Xu, S., Chauhan, S., Tanaka, A., Simpson, K., Abdul-Muhsin, H., & Smith, R., (2015). Impact of delay on telesurgical performance: Study on the robotic simulator dv-trainer. *International Journal of Computer Assisted Radiology and Surgery, 11*, 581–587.
4. Eid, M., Cha, J., & Saddik, A. E., (2011). Admux: An adaptive multiplexer for haptic-audio-visual data communication. *IEEE Transactions on Instrumentation and Measurement, 60*(1), 2131.
5. Cizmeci, B., Xu, X., Chaudhari, R., Bachhuber, C., Alt, N., & Steinbach, E., (2017). A multiplexing scheme for multimodal teleoperation. *ACM Trans. Multimedia Comput. Commun. Appl., 13*(2), 128. [Online]. Available: http://doi.acm.org/10.1145/3063594.
6. Patel, M., & Wang, J., (2010). Applications, challenges, and perspective in emerging body area networking technologies. *IEEE Wireless Communications, 17*(1), 8088.
7. Konstantinova, J., Jiang, A., Althoefer, K., Dasgupta, P., & Nanayakkara, T., (2014). Implementation of tactile sensing for palpation in robot-assisted minimally invasive surgery: A review. *IEEE Sensors Journal, 14*(8), 24902501.
8. Haidegger, T., Sándor, J., & Benyó, Z., (2011). Surgery in space: The future of robotic telesurgery. *Surgical Endoscopy, 25*(3), 681–690. doi: 10.1007/s00464-010-1243-3.
9. Stern, J. A., Walrath, L. C., & Goldstein, R., (1984). The endogenous eyeblink. *Psychophysiology, 21*(1), 22–33. doi: 10.1111/j 1469-8986.1984.tb02312.x.
10. Xu, S., Perez, M., Yang, K., Perrenot, C., Felblinger, J., & Huburt, J., (2014). Determination of the latency effects on surgical performance and the acceptable latency levels in telesurgery using the DV-Trainer® simulator. *Surgical Endoscopy, 28*(9), 2569–2576. doi: 10.1007/s00464-014-3504-z.
11. Marescaux, J., Leroy, J., Rubino, F., Smith, M., Vix, M., Simone, M., & Mutter, D., ((2002).). Transcontinental robot-assisted remote telesurgery: Feasibility and potential applications. *Annals of Surgery, 235*(4), 487–492. doi: 10.1097/00000658-200204000-00005.
12. Giordani, M., Polese, M., Mezzavilla, M., Rangan, S., & Zorzi, M., (2020). Toward6g networks: Use cases and technologies. *IEEE Communications Magazine, 58*(3), 55–61.
13. Calvanese, S. E., Barbarossa, S., Gonzalez-Jimenez, J. L., Ktenas, D., Cassiau, N., Maret, L., & Dehos, C., (2019). 6G: The next frontier: From holographic messaging to artificial intelligence using subterahertz and visible light communication. *IEEE Vehicular Technology Magazine, 14*(3), 42–50.
14. Gui, G., Liu, M., Tang, F., Kato, N., & Adachi, F., (2020). 6G: Opening new horizons for integration of comfort, security, and intelligence. *IEEE Wireless Communications*, 1–7.
15. Nayak, S., & Patgiri, R., (2020). 6G communications: A vision on intelligent healthcare. *IEEE Internet of Things Journal, Under Communication.*
16. Okamura, A. M., (2009). Haptic feedback in robot-assisted minimally invasive surgery. *Current Opinion in Urology, 19*(1), 460473.
17. Aijaz, A., Dohler, M., Aghvami, A. H., Friderikos, V., & Frodigh, M., (2017) Realizing the tactile internet: Haptic communications over next-generation 5G cellular networks. *IEEE Wireless Communications, 24*(2), 8289.

CHAPTER 15

MUSIC RECOMMENDATION SYSTEM BASED ON USERS' RATING AS A CLOUD-BASED HEALTHCARE INFORMATION SYSTEM

SUDIPTA CHAKRABARTY,[1] MD. RUHUL ISLAM,[2] and HIREN KUMAR DEVA SARMA[3]

[1]*Department of Computer Application, Techno India Salt Lake, Kolkata, West Bengal, India*

[2]*Department of Computer Science and Engineering, Sikkim Manipal Institute of Technology, Sikkim, India*

[3]*Department of Information Technology, Sikkim Manipal Institute of Technology, Sikkim, India, E-mail: hirenkdsarma@gmail.com*

ABSTRACT

There has been a significant rise in the available music in general, and songs in particular in digital format. Such music and songs are available mostly in cloud platform. The relevance and importance of music recommendation system (MRS) have increased in recent times. A MRS is helpful for the listeners in order to choose desirable music, from within a huge collection of music available in the cloud (cloud as storage). In this chapter, a MRS has been presented. The proposed system creates a list of music that has been recommended automatically, based on users' rating

IoT and Cloud Computing-Based Healthcare Information Systems. Anand Sharma, PhD, Hiren Kumar Deva Sarma, PhD & S. R. Biradar, PhD (Eds.)

of music piece. The system can create a personalized favorite music list, based on users' feedback ratings considering different songs available in the storage. Furthermore, a learning model has been implemented that is based on star rating feedback of different users considering the question "whether a particular song is the most appropriate for a particular mood, like Happy, Sad, Angry, Scared, Tender, Excited, etc.?" A MRS can also be applied in music therapy and in than case it will have greater impact to the overall development of the human society. The possibilities of applying such a MRS in music therapy have been explored. A web-based software application has been developed to validate the concept.

15.1 INTRODUCTION

In recent time, music information retrieval (MIR) has attracted many researchers, and it is an emerging research area of Computer Science and Engineering. MIR produces required information from different music pieces. A music recommendation system (MRS) is an effective software tool that is used to help users to find certain music pieces from large databases of music pieces, based on the user's preference. Normally, music recommendation depends on collaborative filtering mechanism or content-based mechanism to satisfy users' requirements. A MRS may be implemented based on feedback of different users with respect to the question, "whether a particular song is appropriate for a particular mood, like Happy, Sad, Angry, Scared, Tender, Excited, etc." Further, a MRS may be applied in music therapy; and in that case it will have a greater impact on development of the human society as a whole.

In this chapter, an architecture of a MRS has been proposed. The basic features of the proposed MRS are:

- The system sorts the music playlist based on the user's rating of music piece, and user's browsing behavior; star rating by the user on a particular mood of a music has also been considered as input in preparing the play list.
- User can register in the system, and after login, they can play the music, which are currently stored on the cloud, and then they can give their ratings and reviews.
- According to their ratings, music will be sorted and ordered so that new users can get appropriate music as per their requirements. New

users can also give feedback and can also make their favorite music list.

- The system is web-based; it consists of music, where users can give their ratings and also can set favorites music list.
- Users can compare different music after listening to the music online, through cloud technology.
- Users' can view available music, can set their favorites, and also categorizing the music as per their judgment.
- The MRS sorts the music, prepares a playlist based on the users' rating against the music items.

Users' star rating feedback is used to determine the mood of the music. The system can create a personalized mood-based music/song list depending on that feedback. Therefore, a specific music/song that is applicable for the treatment of various health and mind disorders as per music therapy can be made available through this music recommendation system. Such a system can be helpful in the field of healthcare.

15.2 RELATED WORK

There are research works available in the areas of application of computing technologies in the field of music. Computational musicology is an emerging area that heavily relies on different concepts of computer science. Indian Classical Music (ICM) is complicated in its structure, also difficult and a very large area to explore. However, application of computing science in ICM, in particular, is relatively unexplored.

ICM consists of Raga. There is a specific relation between Raga and Rasa. Raga means music origin and rasa means music emotions. Therefore, music, and emotions are directly related to each other. In Ref. [3] this relationship has been exploited and a content-based culture-specific MRS model has been developed. In Ref. [4], effort has been made to develop a music analysis system applicable for clinical music therapy. In Ref. [5], it is stated that music is a very effective mode of mental treatment, and human mental state can be controlled by Indian Music Therapy.

Different raga names and their corresponding healing powers are enlisted in Ref. [6]. A music recommendation using content and context information mining is reported in Ref. [7]. A context-aware mobile music recommendation for daily activities is reported in Ref. [8].

A music modeling technique and a useful tool that formalize the music composition rules have been reported in Ref. [9]. The techniques proposed in this chapter increase music analysis speed; the technique exploits music Petri nets and Schoenberg's rules. Pearson's Correlation of Coefficient has been utilized to determine the similarities between songs in Ref. [10]; fundamental frequencies of the songs are considered for computing the similarity levels. A context aware music recommendation system has been developed in Ref. [11]. Depending on the age group of the listeners, suitable songs from within the music library are recommended by the system.

A model of musical creativity is proposed in Ref. [12]. The complexity of songs are measured through statistical techniques in Ref. [13]. An approach for improving the quality of music composition is presented in Ref. [14]. An approach to improve Music Rhythm is presented in Ref. [15]. How similar the two songs are in terms of embedded raga in the songs may be an important problem to address. A method to determine the similarity between songs has been proposed in Ref. [16]. The proposed method is based on analysis of fundamental frequencies. Statistical concepts like Coefficient of Concurrent Deviation are used in the method.

15.3 PROPOSED METHODOLOGY

The objective is to create a web-based application for as a MRS. The ratings and feedback given by users against different songs are considered as input. Star rating feedback given by the users is considered as a parameter to set the mood of a song. A song of a particular mood is helpful for different mind issues. Music has great healing power and may be used to eliminate mind hazards, like depression, loneliness, and various differently able symptoms. The prescription of appropriate music to listen for different issues related to health and mind is extremely important, and this is the basis of music therapy.

The various steps involved in this MRS, as workflow of a user, are as follows:

- **Step 1:** Open the website of the music recommendation system.
- **Step 2:** Register on the home page and click the "submit" button; registration details are stored.
- **Step 3:** Options mentioned below are available on the website: Login as users

- **Step 4:** Provide the registered email-id, password to Sign-In; validation takes place.
- **Step 5:** In User page click on "Select Singer" and also "Select Particular Song."
- **Step 6:** Play the song and then "Give Rating."
- **Step 7:** User can compare among different input music.
- **Step 8:** User can also provide feedback.
- **Step 9:** Then add songs to favorite and create different personalized mood-based music list.
- **Step 10:** Log out from the system.

This system has been implemented by using could technology and the required steps to follow in order to connect with the cloud server are as follows:

- **Step 1:** Open cloud server (web page).
- **Step 2:** Login with username and password.
- **Step 3:** Create the database.
- **Step 4:** Connect with the local host with IP address.

The use case diagram of 'Admin' and 'User' of the work is depicted in Figure 15.1.

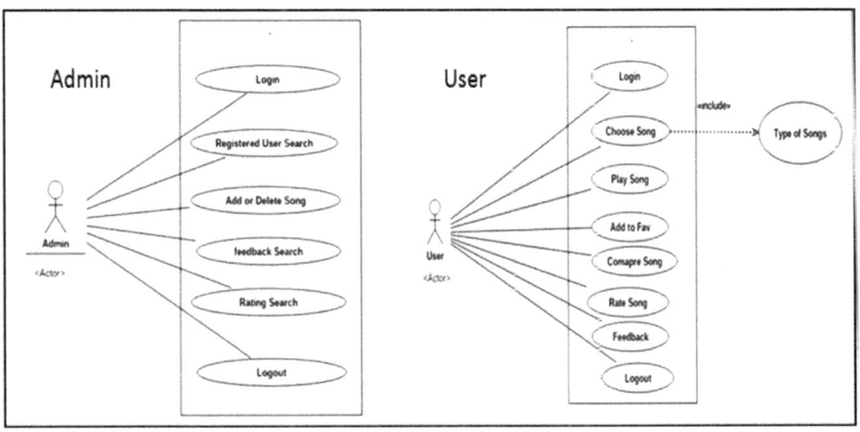

FIGURE 15.1 Use case diagram of 'admin' and 'user.'

The activity diagram of the system has been depicted in Figure 15.2.

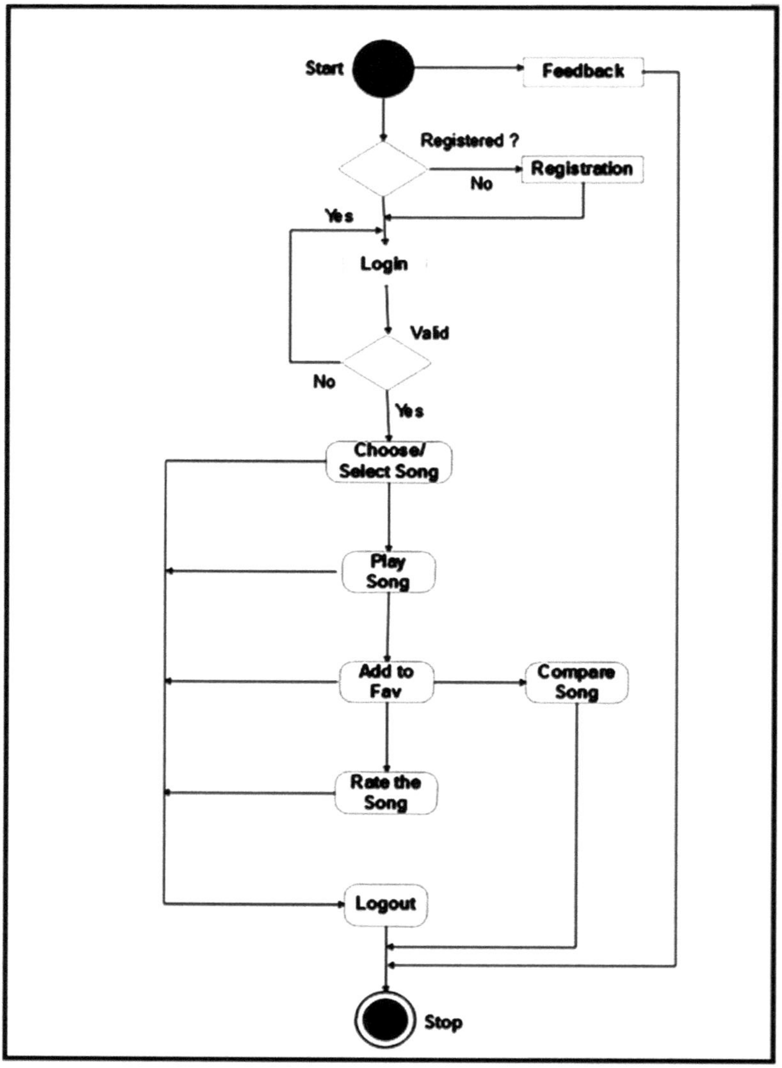

FIGURE 15.2 Activity diagram of the system.

15.4 RESULTS AND DISCUSSION

Various snapshots of the system are reported in this section. Different steps of the workflow presented in the previous section are realized through these snapshots (Figures 15.3–15.5).

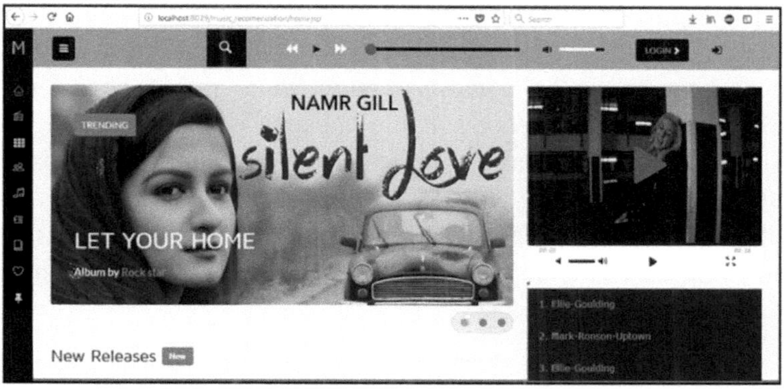

FIGURE 15.3 Website of the music recommendation system.

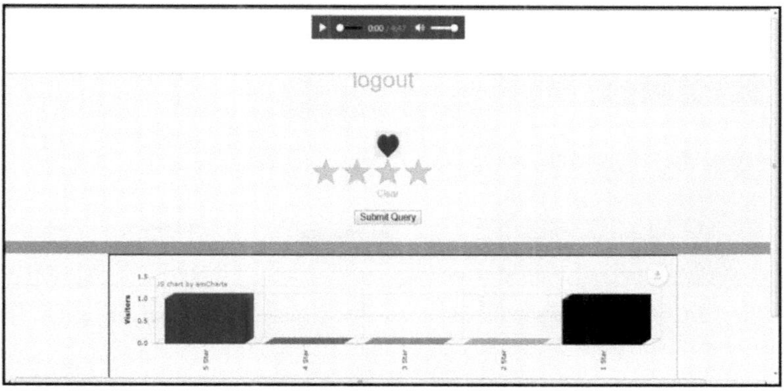

FIGURE 15.4 User can give rating against different song (Step 6).

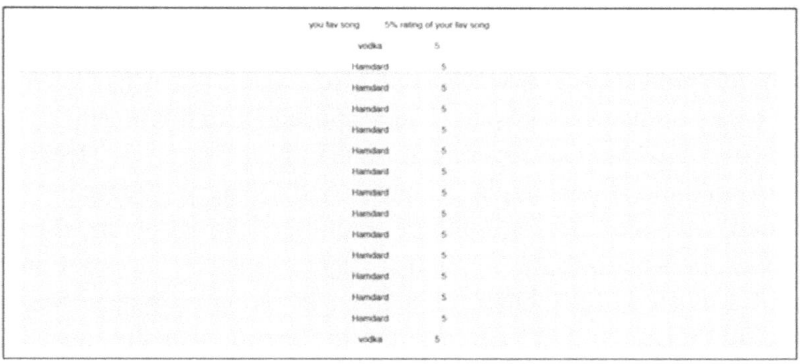

FIGURE 15.5 Analysis of user-given 5* rating (Step 7).

From Figure 15.5, 'Hamdard' song is most popular song depending on users' choice; this is because 'Hamdard' song consists of 13, 5* rating, whereas the song 'vodka' consists of only two, 5* rating. Therefore, as per feedback provided by users a suitable sad song is 'Hamdard.'

Then add this 'Hamdard' song is added into the "Sad Playlist;" there are six mood-based playlists (e.g., Happy Playlist, Sad Playlist, Angry Playlist, Scared Playlist, Tender Playlist, Excited Playlist). Users' personalized mood-based music list based on users' feedback against a music has been reported in Figure 15.6.

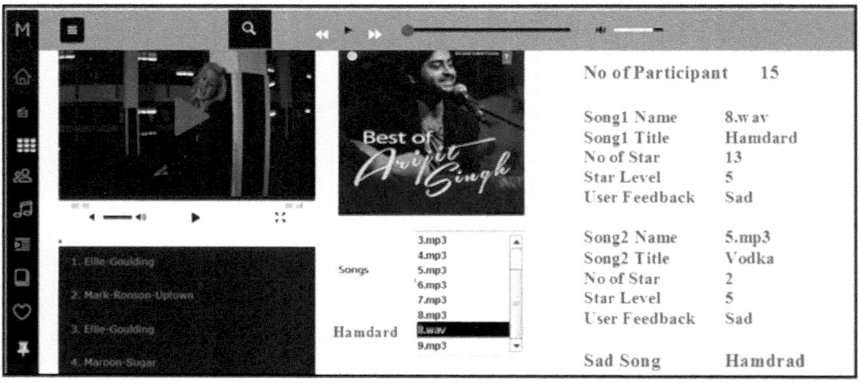
M
Best of Arijit Singh
1. Ellie-Goulding
2. Mark-Ronson-Uptown
3. Ellie-Goulding
4. Maroon-Sugar
Songs
Hamdard
3.mp3
4.mp3
5.mp3
6.mp3
7.mp3
8.mp3
8.wav
9.mp3
No of Participant 15
Song1 Name 8.wav
Song1 Title Hamdard
No of Star 13
Star Level 5
User Feedback Sad
Song2 Name 5.mp3
Song2 Title Vodka
No of Star 2
Star Level 5
User Feedback Sad
Sad Song Hamdrad

FIGURE 15.6 Users' personalized mood-based music list based on users' feedback against a music (Step 9).

15.5 CONCLUSION

In this work, an innovative web-based application is presented. The proposed application is a web-based MRS. The system has been developed based on users' feedback. The proposed system is a generic framework for MRS that can recommend music based on users' feedback on certain emotions, for example, 'Happy,' 'Sad,' 'Angry,' 'Scared,' 'Tender,' 'Excited,' etc.; after determining the emotion of the music based on users' feedback, personalized music playlist may be created. The emotion detection of a music is fully based on a five-star rating on a particular music given by the users. After determining the emotion of the music by the users given star rating feedback, a personalized mood-based music list can be created. Such a system is applicable for treatment of various health and mind disorders. The knowledge of music therapy is essential for an appropriate recommendation of songs against different health and mind issues. This system is applicable as a cloud-based healthcare system for the aid of the people.

KEYWORDS

- **cloud**
- **healthcare information system**
- **music information retrieval (MIR)**
- **music recommendation system**
- **music therapy**
- **web application**

REFERENCES

1. Sriram, P., (1990). *A Karnatik Music Primer*. Published by The Karnatin Music Association of North America, Inc.
2. Vasudha, J., Iyshwarya, G., Tamarai, S. A., Iniyaa, S., & Jeyakumar, G., (2011). Application of computer-aided music composition in music therapy. *International Journal of Innovation, Management and Technology, 2*(1), 55–57.
3. Gopala, K. K., & Bipin, I., (2010). *A Behavioral Study of Emotions in South Indian Classical Music and its Implications in Music Recommendation Systems*. SAPMIA'10.
4. Erkkila, J., Lartillot, O., Luck, G., Rikkila, K., & Toiviainen, P., (2004). Intelligent music systems in music therapy. *Music Therapy Today, 5*, 1–21.
5. Srilatha, B., Neetha, K., Krishnaveni, V. D., Radha, K. N., & Aparna, V. B., (2014). Indian music therapy: Could it be helpful in the management of mental. *International Journal of Medical Research & Health Sciences*, 354–357.
6. http://www.pilu.in/raga-therapy.html (accessed on 13 June 2022).
7. Su, J. H., Yeh, H. H., Yu, P. S., & Tseng, V. S., (2010). Music recommendation using content and context information mining. *Intelligent Systems, IEEE, 25*(1), 16–26.
8. Wang, X., Rosenblum, D., & Wang, Y., (2012). Context-aware mobile music recommendation for daily activities. In: *Proceedings of the 20th ACM international conference on Multimedia* (pp. 99–108). ACM.
9. Baratè, A., Mauro, A. D., Haus, G., & Ludovico, L. A., (2018). Formalizing Schoenberg's fundamentals of musical composition through Petri nets. In: *15th Sound and Music Computing Conference (SMC 2018)* (pp. 254–258). Limassol, Cyprus.

10. Chakrabarty, S., Islam Md, R., & Sarma, H. K. D., (2018). An approach towards the modeling of pattern similarity in music using statistical measures. In: *The Proceedings of 5th International Conference on Parallel, Distributed and Grid Computing (PDGC).* In JUIT, Waknaghat, Himachal Pradesh.
11. Chakrabarty, S., Banik, S., Islam Md, R., & Deva, S. H. K., (2018). Context aware song recommendation system. In: *The Proceedings of 3rd National Conference on Communication, Cloud, and Big Data (CCB).* in SMIT, Majhitar, East Sikkim.
12. Arutyunova, V., & Averkinb, A., (2017). Genetic algorithms for music variation on genome platform. 9th international conference on theory and application of soft computing, computing with words and perception, ICSCCW 2017. Budapest, Hungary. *Procedia Computer Science, 120*, 317–324.
13. Sudipta, C., Sangeeta, B., Md Ruhul, I., & Deva, S. H. K., (2020). Measuring song complexity by statistical techniques. In: *Proceedings of Second International Conference on Communication, Devices and Computing* (pp. 687–695). Springer Nature.
14. Sudipta, C., Md Ruhul, I., & Hiren, K. D. S., (2020). Intelligent music abstraction tool for improvising the quality of music composition. *International Journal of Advanced Trends in Computer Science and Engineering, 9*(3), 3641–3648.
15. Chakrabarty, S., Bhattacharjee, A., Islam Md, R., & Deva, S. H. K., (2019). Algorithmic improvisation of music rhythm. In: *Proceedings of International Conference on Communication, Devices and Networking* (pp. 323–335). Springer.
16. Chakrabarty, S., Banik, S., Islam Md, R., & Deva, S. H. K., (2019). Music similarity mapping through fundamental frequencies by coefficient of concurrent deviation. In: *Proceedings of International Conference on Computing, Power, and Communication Technologies* (pp. 910–915). IEEE.

CHAPTER 16

IoMusT^2: INTERNET OF MUSIC THERAPY THINGS TO IMPROVE MENTAL HEALTH MANAGEMENT

SUDIPTA CHAKRABARTY,[1] MD. RUHUL ISLAM,[2] and HIREN KUMAR DEVA SARMA[3]

[1]*Department of Master of Computer Application, Techno India Salt Lake, Kolkata, West Bengal, India*

[2]*Department of Computer Science and Engineering, Sikkim Manipal Institute of Technology, Sikkim, India*

[3]*Department of Information Technology, Sikkim Manipal Institute of Technology, Sikkim, India, E-mail: hirenkdsarma@gmail.com*

ABSTRACT

Mental health hazards are great challenges in front of humanity today. A large portion of the entire population of the world is facing different mental hazards, for example, Alzheimer's disease, Parkinson's disease, autism, insomnia problem, dementia, depression, etc. All of the hazards have some specific symptoms. Music therapy may be used to reduce these problems to a certain specific level, without any harmful effects, although harmful effects are very much prominent in the case of several chemical medicines. Computational music therapy heavily borrows principles, and concepts from Computer Science in general, and from the knowledge domains like pattern recognition, machine learning (ML), genetic algorithms (GA),

IoT and Cloud Computing-Based Healthcare Information Systems. Anand Sharma, PhD, Hiren Kumar Deva Sarma, PhD & S. R. Biradar, PhD (Eds.)

Petri nets, different statistical approaches, and especially from internet of things (IoT), etc., in particular. This is an emerging area of knowledge, at the moment. The internet of musical therapy things ($IoMusT^2$) is an emerging research field which includes IoT, new musical expression-based interfaces, networked-based music performance systems, context aware pervasive music, artificial intelligence (AI), human-computer interaction, and participatory art. $IoMusT^2$ is a therapy or treatment that uses a computing device which is capable of sensing data, acquiring data, processing data, actuating data, and exchanging data; the healing power of music is exploited for the therapy. In this chapter, the topic "internet of musical therapy things" is explored.

16.1 INTRODUCTION

Music is a language which is universal (Universal Language). It is a communication medium, which can be pleasant, and at the same time, the listener can also have a healing experience. The world of music and the field of computational science are having several overlapping areas and, therefore, are nearer to each other. Recommendation systems (computer-based) provide suggestions or recommendations to the users regarding various music items that can be useful to them. This software system or tool is gaining popularity in present time. A music recommendation system (MRS) estimates the user's music preferences from within a pool of music which may be a localized collection of music. MRS then generates different songs or music based on such estimates considering a relatively wider music repository. MRS can be classified in two types, primarily. These are content-based recommendations and collaborative filtering-based recommendations. Content-based MRS analyzes music from the music database, and then classifies songs based on different attributes like tempo, instrumentation, or genre. Collaborative filtering MRS is based on collaboration with multi-user utility approach, and their explicit preferences.

Music is the greatest element of the entertainment world that have healing power and that is why music information retrieval (MIR) is an emerging research area of Computational Musicology. MRS is used to create the personalized music lists from the large music databases according to user's preferences; it can be applied in music therapy also that will have greater impact in the society for well-being of the people in the society. MIR is a contemporary computational research area that aims at retrieving musical data from music sources. The background of MIR is signal processing, machine intelligence, human-machine interaction, pattern recognition, audio mining, computational musicology, and combinations of these. MRS depends on various factors, like star rating, seasons, cultures, human mood, places, human behavior, human choices, different time slots, etc. This chapter primarily focuses on the mental healthcare field through IoT-based music therapy applications.

Some of the features of the MRS are:

- MRS can create music playlists depending on the user's star rating of music.
- User can register into the MRS, and after login, user can play music which are stored on the cloud and then can provide the ratings and reviews on different music.
- Depending on the user's ratings, music may be stored in sorted order. In this case, feedback from the new users can also be considered to create favorite music list.
- MRS is normally a web-based application that fully consists of music and its healing power, where users provide ratings that can be used to set favorites list (of music).
- User can also compare different music, and map similarity and dissimilarity among the music available online through the cloud (as storage).
- Users can view a list of music; they also can determine the list of favorite music. Users can also classify various music based on music knowledge.
- MRS may be used for different music therapy applications.
- The overarching challenge for MRS research is comprehensive access to large data sets, including not only user's rating but also contextual information and audio content.

As a summary, MRS, and the therapy based on music known as music therapy, together are applicable for treatment of various health and mind disorders, and thus music therapy is an important dimension of the healthcare field.

Internet of music therapy things ($IoMusT^2$) is the field in which music therapy is combined with IoT and both are exploited in a combined manner for the purpose of mental health management. In this chapter, the basic principles of IoMusT^2 are explored. A (IoMusT^2) based framework is proposed for mental health management. Implementation strategy of the proposed framework is outlined.

This chapter is structured as follows: Section 16.2 presents a relevant literature review. The proposed framework is presented in Section 16.3, followed by Section 16.4, in which the implementation strategy is outlined. Finally, the Section 16.5 concludes the chapter.

16.2 RELATED LITERATURE REVIEW

There are quite a lot of research works available in the area of computational musicology. Computational musicology is one of the most emerging research areas that depends on the different concepts of Computer Science. On the other hand, Indian Classical Music (ICM) is highly complicated, difficult, and vast area and at the same time relatively unexplored from computational musicology perspective. This section of this chapter highlights some relevant literature in the field of computational musicology.

Authors propose a virtual reality (VR) system (virtual harmony) in Ref. [1]. The goal of this system is to reduce anxiety and stress. Music therapy has been adopted to achieve the goal. The proposed system facilitates users to listen to music and also to play different musical instruments in a 3D environment. In this 3D environment, real-world panoramic video is presented in the background scenes. The user shall have a feeling of staying in a musical environment. Music has the capability and can help human beings in activating and shaping the brain. Moreover, mind can be sharpened. Again, music can improve the cognitive ability, ability to hear and interpret speech, and also emotion awakening is possible through music. The memory capability can be enhanced through music. Music has proven to be effective for patients suffering from different health issues, for example, schizophrenia, traumatic brain injury, and even cancer. Music can be used to help patients suffering from sleeplessness, stress, chronic pain, etc. [2]. The online MRS, considers the past listeners and analyzes the historical records. Then analysis of the historical data happens through various statistical means, and finally, the recommendation system recommends appropriate music to the intended users [3]. Authors propose a new recommender system in Ref. [4]. This is an IoT enabled mobile health (m-health) application. The utility of such a system is shown in different specific cases. Different advantages of the proposed recommendation systems are outlined. Moreover, the IoT enabled m-health applications are detailed.

Music therapy can be a promising alternative to various health treatment. The amount of risks and side effects is insignificant. There are studies that suggest that music therapy is effective in improving memory capabilities, familiarity pattern machine capabilities, and also in improving recollection of past events, in individuals [5]. In Ref. [6], authors explored how voice assistants (VA) are used in homes, investigated the role of VAs as scaffolding for IoT device control, and characterized emergent issues of privacy for Voice Assistant users. Thus, music has the capability to serve many different goals. Some of these goals may be individual-oriented and some others may be associated with the social lives of the people. If an individual is considered, music can always provide means for the expression of emotion. Music can help in changing mood, can relax an individual and also can provide stimulation leading to comfort. Thus, people have started believing that music can be used for treatment and in therapy. Music is entertaining, and it provides esthetic enjoyment. Music can even influence in enhancing the impacts of another form of art. Different effects of music on humans are examined in Ref. [7]. Study has been carried out regarding the positive and negative effect of music on an individual, while the performance of the individual against a particular task is being monitored. A review regarding the results of recent clinical studies considering the influence of music therapy on individual patients is presented in Ref. [8]. This review is based on the reports produced by reputed medical journals.

In Ref. [9], the authors claim about the positive impact that music therapy can provide. As per the chapter, music therapy can assist in improving the speech capability of a person, to improve memory, and even it can improve physical balance. Music can also provide emotional healing. It can help people in developing a positive self-image. Music can also help individuals in managing stress and pain. In Ref. [10], the author presents the effectiveness of Internet of Music Therapy Things. In this work, different components of Internet of Music Therapy Things, for example, remote participation, innovative concert experiences, e-learning of music are elaborated. The work also elaborates on co-located participation, and smart applications.

In Ref. [11], the authors proposed an approach to find the complexity of any particular song (as input) based on some statistical measures. In Ref. [12], authors introduced the music editing software that generates different versatile music, which is the combination of both vocal and instrumental. Authors propose technique to create different music rhythms depending on the Memetic Algorithm in Ref. [13]. In Ref. [14], the authors proposed a method to compute the music similarity based on Fundamental Frequencies. The approach was based on the statistical concept, "Coefficient of Concurrent Deviation." In Ref. [15], the author proposed an approach to generate song similarity percentage by the pitch values through Correlation Coefficient. In Ref. [16], authors propose a method to generate personalized song list using user's listening habits, and age factor.

Formal languages can be adopted for representing musical processes. This is an emerging sub-field of computational musicology. Application of machine learning (ML) principles is explored in Ref. [17]. Interactive genetic algorithm (IGA) is a powerful tool for controlling parametric music generation system [18]. In Ref. [19] the issues of Tabla improvisation and evaluation is considered. A linguistic model has been proposed which is derived from pattern languages and the formal grammars. The model is implemented in the bol-processor [19]. In Ref. [20], a study of vocal performance and pitch analysis in Hindustani music is reported. A system for musical pattern recognition is proposed in Ref. [21]. Key sequences of music are processed with Recursive Median Filter in order to recognize the musical patterns. In Ref. [22], three measurement techniques are used for determining rhythm complexity in a system, for musical pattern recognition by machine, and to find pitch and rhythmic error.

In Ref. [23], the authors address the issue of musical pattern recognition by machine. They consider several perceptual issues to recognize the patterns. They also proposed several measures for measuring rhythm complexity. A new method to determine a tonal context which is localized is also proposed. This approach is based on empirically derived key distances.

In Indian Classical Music (ICM), a raga-based composition is a collection of musical notes. These notes are arranged in a manner and order because of which listener achieve a pleasant feeling. Raga is identified by short pieces of taan [24]. In Ref. [25], the author proposes a valuable approach for the classification of automatic musical genre; a MIR system was developed and evaluated various features for any type of content based analysis of musical signals [25]. In Ref. [26], a method has been reported to automatically extract pure and altered notes from 'aalap' portion of 'kheyal' rendering [26]. Genetic algorithm (GA) is one important tool that can be applied in computational musicology and for music composition [27]. In Ref. [28], a new concept of automated generation of realistic drum set rhythm has been proposed. GA was used in order to achieve the goal. GA was applied for the automatic music generation using the calculation of fitness value, with the help of normalized compression distance [29].

In general, a recommendation system can be considered as an information filtering tool. Moreover, it is a customization tool. The recommendation system in this context sorts the music playlist based on the user's rating of music items, similarity of item contents, or user's browsing behaviors. Some recommendation systems are based on the concept of context-awareness [30]. On the other hand, some recommendation systems are based on recommender and constraints [31]. Particle swarm optimization (PSO) is used for generating remixing of music tracks to create new sounds and music, from preloaded sampled sound data [32]. Automatic generation of computer music modular system is a two-level collaborative multi agent approach based on experts systems technology and rule-based system's principles [33]. There are a few music recommender systems developed which are based on the emotion management [34].

In Ref. [35], the author proposes a method to automatically transform Hindustani music into the appropriate acoustic signals. Again in Ref. [36], a new concept is proposed regarding multiple views of Tabla sequence. A variable-length n-gram model was used for this purpose. Tonal modulation by providing musical motivations and interpretations for a selection of mathematical ideas was developed using graph theory [37]. In Ref. [38], the author state that Reflection Rhythm and Toggle Rhythm are the two classes for good rhythm timelines within the context of designing tools for the composition of music by using GA. In Ref. [39], the authors propose a technique that can estimate the fundamental frequency of Carnatic music and also of film songs. This has been achieved using biological mutation theory. GA is one of the most important mechanisms for composing music. In Ref. [40], the authors propose a technique to generate a new rhythm. In this work, a pre-defined rhythm is applied to an initial population to generate a new rhythm. Modified GA operator has been used for this purpose.

Mobile music applications make use of the new interfaces for musical expression (NIME); NIME can support many acoustic musical instruments with respect to their immediate, self-contained, and mobile nature. NIME is much more sophisticated in comparison to the older computer based musical systems. Ubiquitous Drum is a tangible, wearable musical instrument [41]. Drummer thus can have a Drum kit with them all the time and irrespective of wherever they move to. Dastgah classification technique is used in Iranian traditional music [42]. A MRS based on the human behavior is presented in Ref. [43]. A latent Dirichlet allocation (LDA) model is exploited to identify the Raga of South Indian Carnatic music [44]. The LDA is an unsupervised statistical approach used for document classification. Using this technique, one can identify the underlying topics present in a given document.

Hidden Markov models (HMM) is used to identify the Melakartha Ragas [45]. Nearest neighbor (NN) classification focuses on a mechanism to determine the distance between neighbors. It uses CD, earth mover's distance (EMD), etc. Thus, applying these techniques one can identify NNs [46].

Music therapy is an upcoming field. It is part of para medicine, in which music or sound pulses are used to treat patients. Different kinds of music are used for treating patients suffering from different ailments like mesothelioma, depression, asthma, and even asbestos cancer, peritoneal mesothelioma, etc. Thus, identifying different music patterns applicable for different treatments is an important task.

In Ref. [47], computer aided music composition of Carnatic music is explored. The applications of Carnatic music in music therapy are also studied. In Ref. [48], evolutionary music is represented through the executable graph. Here, the nodes execute arithmetic functions. The input nodes supply time variables and abstract control variables. On the other hand, multiple output nodes are mapped to MIDI data. In Ref. [49], a MRS is presented that is based on the daily activities of human beings. In Ref. [50], a music recommendation that is based on the theories of signal property has been reported.

A software than can accompany the singer with normal notes is presented in Ref. [51]. This software can also predict the next note of the singer. This software has been developed using temporal mining algorithms. In the process of identifying the 'nyas' or long note, segmentation method of phrases was introduced [52]. Similarity was computed with respect to the reference characteristic phrase. The same concept of NN classification is used for finding the distance between neighbors. CD, EMD, etc., are used to identify the NNs. Algorithms are developed for identifying Ragas in Ref. [53]. Music semantic annotation generation tool M-SAGT is flexible, and user friendly. In Ref. [54], ontology based semantic annotations are explored and generated. These can be stored in RDF/XML format as discussed in Ref. [54]. Data mining algorithms are used for automatic identification of Carnatic raga in Ref. [55]. The 'Swaram' notes were used for this purpose. A unique Artificial Neural Network (ANN) based approach was introduced in Carnatic classical music in Ref. [56]. The purpose is to study the phenomenon of tonic shifting. The approach uses multi-layer perceptron and linear regression. There is another approach based on the selection of the best distance metrics for nominal, ordinal, numeric, and binary attributes, and that has been reported in Ref. [57].

There are some researchers focused on music discovery with the idea of developing technologies to explore culture specific music audio collections [58].

A new multi objective constraint handling technique is proposed in Ref. [59]. It systematically takes closeness, diversity, and feasibility into consideration and find solutions in each iteration. In Ref. [60], the author proposes a dynamic recommender system (DRS) based on evolutionary clustering algorithm that makes clusters of similar users; this depends on relevant user preferences considered over time. This method performs an optimization of conflicting parameters instead of using GA.

16.3 PROPOSED FRAMEWORK

Today, mental illness is highly common for the people of all age groups. Mental illness signifies either behavioral changes, or emotional changes, or a combination of both, that causes significant changes in human thought processes considering social and behavioral aspects. Some common mental health hazards are Autism, Dementia, Alzheimer's disease, Parkinson's disease, Insomnia problem, etc. As a summary, some common symptoms of all the mental health hazards are enlisted below.

- Stereotypic behavior;
- Socially impaired;
- Repetitive pattern following;

- Sleep difficulty;
- Minimal concentration;
- Decrease ability to think;
- Emotional turmoil;
- Decreased motivation;
- Language problem;
- Problem remembering recent events;
- Language problem;
- Disoriented;
- Unpleasant emotional response to isolation;
- Sensitive to a lack of connection or communication;
- Unenthusiastic feeling;
- Disinterested in activities;
- Sleep disturbance;
- Feeling worthlessness;
- Depressed mood.

The internet of musical therapy things (IoMusT^2) is an emerging research field which includes IoT, new musical expression based interfaces, networked based music performance systems, context aware pervasive music, artificial intelligence (AI), human-computer interaction, and participatory art. IoMusT^2 is defined as therapy treatment using a computing device that is capable of sensing data, acquiring data, processing data, actuating data, and exchanging data serving through the healing power of music. In this chapter, the objective is to highlight the fact that IoMusT^2 is one of the tools in the field of Music Therapy, that can be exploited for Mental Health Management considering several behavioral issues of patients or users.

In the computational science perspective, IoMusT^2 refers to the embedded networks of computing devices in musical physical things applications, dedicated for management of mental health issues using music therapy.

IoMusT^2 presents effectiveness of the internet of music therapy things in the following perspectives:

- Innovative concert experiences;
- Co-located participation;
- Remote participation;
- e-learning of music;

- Music therapy for both therapist and patients;
- Smart application.

Figure 16.1 depicts the overall architecture, and several elementary inter co-related activities of IoMusT^2.

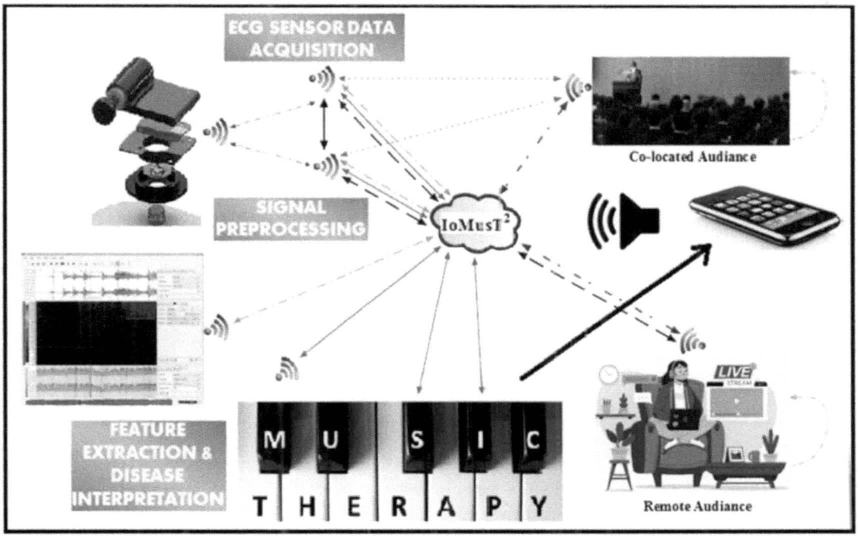

FIGURE 16.1 Overall architecture and different elementary inter co-related activities of IoMusT^2.

User extracted information is the most useful data for IoMusT^2 which can be acquired from different sources, like: (i) ECG data sensors; and (ii) data from signal pre-processing. After that IoMusT^2 analyzes these data through different approaches (applications) and then extracts features for interpreted diseases. Again, IoMusT^2 analyzes the collected, extracted features of disease. The IoMusT^2 also analyzes music things from co-related audiences, and remote audience performers in order to generate the appropriate music therapy, for a particular mental health hazard.

IoMusT^2 based framework can be described through Users' Contextual Input Application based activities. IoMusT^2, in general, have the following components:

1. **Environments:** Environmental factors for the listeners are the temperature, amount of background noise, time of day, etc.

2. **Sensors:** These are used to capture different data to assess the ability to gain contextual information from different environmental sources and deriving the emotional state of mental patients.
3. **IoT:** These are embedded with software, sensors, and other technical devices for the purpose of sensing data, acquiring data, processing data, actuating data, and exchanging data.
4. **Musical Things:** These are, for example, musical smart instruments, connected by an infrastructure with locally and remotely multidirectional communication system.
5. **Music Therapy:** It is an approach toward health treatment by using music; music therapy can address the physical, emotional, cognitive, and social needs of a group of people, or an individual.
6. **Specific IoMusT² for Users:** It means one particular IoMusT² can be applied for a specific mental health hazard issue of a user.

Figure 16.2 depicts the user's contextual input application-based activities of IoMusT².

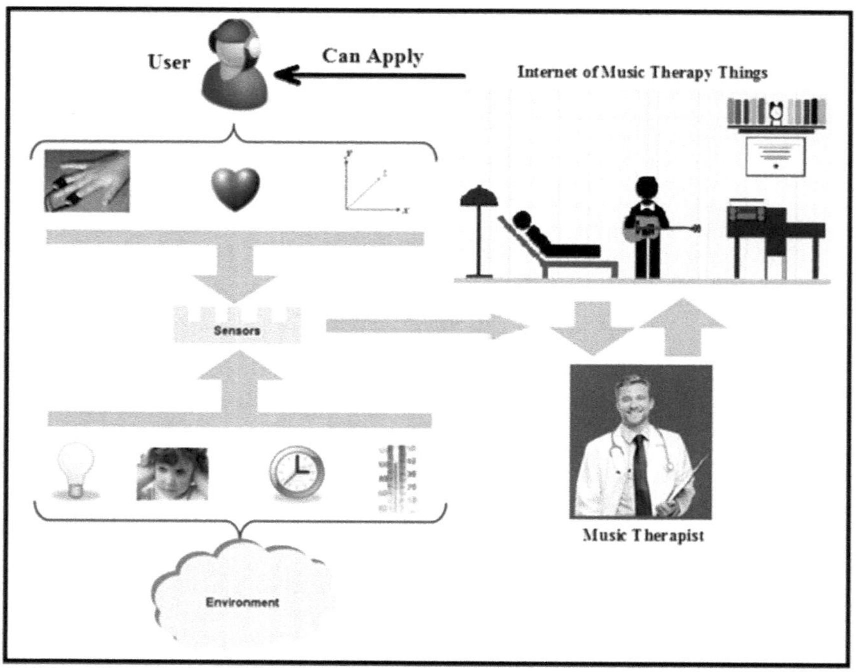

FIGURE 16.2 User's contextual input application-based activities of IoMusT².

16.4 IMPLEMENTATION PLAN

The proposed framework which is basically a system based on IoMusT². In order to implement it needs different IoT devices, along with the availability of the Internet. Raspberry Pi may be used for implementing the IoT part; similarly, an application software to handle the music objects with different music therapy capabilities needs to be incorporated. Moreover, different sensor-based kits available to measure the mood levels of a person, may also be incorporated in the system while testing the effectiveness of the proposed system against different patients facing mental health hazards.

16.5 CONCLUSION AND FUTURE WORKS

In this chapter, IoMusT² is explored; IoMusT² may be applied as one of the efficient tools in the field of music therapy aiming at mental health management. Such a system is applicable for handling several mental and behavioral issues. IoMusT² can improve the behavioral performance level of any mental patient. A framework based on IoMusT² has been proposed for possible application in mental health management. However, the complete implementation and testing of the proposed model/framework may be carried out in future.

KEYWORDS

- **internet of music therapy things**
- **mental health hazards**
- **music information retrieval (MIR)**
- **music recommendation systems**
- **music therapy**
- **web application**

REFERENCES

1. Xiangxu, L., Saifuddin, M., Ethan, J., Alfred, S., Alena, M., Shadi, K., & Jong-Hoon, K., (2020). Virtual reality-based musical therapy for mental health management. In: *10th Annual Computing and Communication Workshop and Conference (CCWC).*

2. Lea, W., Thomas, W., & Wolf, B., (2011). *Music and Health Care.* Available at: https://culturehive.co.uk/wp-content/uploads/2014/01/Music_and_Health_Care.pdf (accessed on 13 June 2022).
3. Ning-Han, L., Szu-Wei, L., Chien-Yi, C., & Shu-Ju, H., (2009). Adaptive music recommendation based on user behavior in time slot. *International Journal of Computer Science and Network Security, 9*(2), 219–227.
4. Erdeniz, S. P., Maglogiannis, I., Menychtas, A., Felfernig, A., & Tran, T. N. T., (2018). Recommender systems for IoT enabled m-health applications. In: Iliadis, L., Maglogiannis, I., & Plagianakos, V., (eds.), *Artificial Intelligence Applications and Innovations: AIAI 2018* (Vol. 520). IFIP Advances in information and communication technology. Springer, Cham. https://doi.org/10.1007/978-3-319-92016-0_21.
5. Patricia, K., (2015). *Alzheimer's Disease and the Importance of Music Therapy.* Available at: https://digitalcommons.augustana.edu/cgi/viewcontent.cgi?article=1001&context=celebrationoflearning (accessed on 13 June 2022).
6. Ammari, T., Kaye, J., Tsai, J. Y., & Bentely, F., (2019). Music, search and IoT: How people (really) use voice assistants. *ACM Transactions on Computer-Human Interaction, 26*(3), 1–28. Article No.: 17 https://doi.org/10.1145/3311956.
7. Gregory, Y., (2003). *Effects of Music on Task Performance.* Available at: http://jclauson.com/msqa/term_papers/effects_of_music_on_task_performance.pdf (accessed on 13 June 2022).
8. Siddiqui, S., Nesbitt, R., Shakir, M. Z., Khan, A. A., Khan, A. A., Khan, K. K., & Ramzan, N., (2020). Artificial neural network (ANN) enabled internet of things (IoT) architecture for music therapy. *Electronics, 9*(12), 2019. https://doi.org/10.3390/electronics9122019.
9. Shivam, D. V., Vaibhav, D. K., Akash, D. S., Omkar, M. V., & Vaishali, M. B., (2017). IoT-BEAT: An intelligent nurse for the cardiac patient with music therapy. *International Research Journal of Engineering and Technology, 04*(12), 1679–1685.
10. Turchet, L., Fischione, C., Essl, G., Keller, D., & Barthet, M., (2018). Internet of musical things: Vision and challenges. In: *IEEE Access (Vol.* 6, pp. 61994–62017). doi: 10.1109/ACCESS.2018.2872625.
11. Sudipta, C., Sangeeta, B., Md Ruhul, I., & Deva, S. H. K., (2020). Measuring song complexity by statistical techniques. In: *Proceedings of Second International Conference on Communication, Devices and Computing* (pp. 687–695). Springer Nature.
12. Sudipta, C., Md Ruhul, I., & Hiren, K. D. S., (2020). Intelligent music abstraction tool for improvising the quality of music composition. *International Journal of Advanced Trends in Computer Science and Engineering, 9*(3), 3641–3648.
13. Chakrabarty, S., Bhattacharjee, A., Islam Md, R., & Deva, S. H. K., (2019). Algorithmic improvisation of music rhythm. In: *Proceedings of International Conference on Communication, Devices and Networking* (pp. 323–335). Springer.
14. Chakrabarty, S., Banik, S., Islam Md, R., & Deva, S. H. K., (2019). Music similarity mapping through fundamental frequencies by coefficient of concurrent deviation. In: *Proceedings of International Conference on Computing, Power, and Communication Technologies* (pp. 910–915). IEEE.
15. Chakrabarty, S., Islam Md, R., & Deva, S. H. K., (2018). An approach towards the modeling of pattern similarity in music using statistical measures. In: *Proceedings*

of the 5th International Conference on Parallel, Distributed and Grid Computing (PDGC) (pp. 436–441). IEEE.

16. Chakrabarty, S., Banik, S., Islam Md, R., & Deva, S. H. K., (2018). Context aware song recommendation system. In: *Proceedings of the 3rd National Conference on Communication, Cloud, and Big Data (CCB)* (pp. 157–165). Springer.
17. Jim, K., & Bernard, B., (1992). Modeling music with grammars: Formal language representation in the Bol processor. *International Journal of Computer Representation and Models in Music*, 207–238.
18. Damon, H., (1994). Generating rhythms with genetic algorithms. In: *Proceedings of ICMA* (pp. 142, 143).
19. Darrell, C., & Ian, H. W., (1995). Multiple viewpoint systems for music prediction. *International Journal of New Music Research*, 51–73.
20. Datta, K., Sengupta, R., Dey, N., & Dipali, N., (1997). Pitch analysis of recorded vocal performances in Hindustani music: Evidence of a personal scale. *J. Acoust. Soc. Ind.*
21. Edward, J. C., & Ilya, S., (1998). A System for machine recognition of music patterns. In: *Proceedings of the Acoustics, Speech, and Signal Processing* (Vol. 3, pp. 3597–3600). IEEE.
22. Shmulevich, D. P., (1998). Rhythm complexity measures for music pattern recognition. In: *Proceedings of IEEE Workshop on Multimedia Signal Processing* (pp. 7–9).
23. Shmulevich, Yli-Harja, O., Coyle, E. J., Povel, D., & Lemstrm, K., (2001). Perceptual issues in music pattern recognition complexity of rhythm and key finding. *Computers and the Humanities* (pp. 23–35). Kluwer Academic Publishers.
24. Dutta, K., Sengupta, R., Dey, N., & Dipali, N., (2001). Studies on identification of raga using short pieces of Taan: A signal processing approach. In: *Proceedings of 6th International workshop on Recent Trends in Speech, Music, and Allied Signal Processing*.
25. George, T., & Perry, C., (2002). Musical genre classification of audio signals. *IEEE Transactions on Speech and Audio Processing, 10*(5), 293–302.
26. Sengupta, R., Dey, N., Dipali, N., & Dutta, A. K., (2002). Automatic extraction of swaras and srutis from kheyal renditions. *Journal of Accustic Society* (p. 30). India.
27. Gartland-Jones, A., & Peter, C., (2003). The suitability of genetic algorithms for musical composition. *Contemporary Music Review, 22*(3), 43–55.
28. Martin, D., (2005). Genetic algorithms as a model of musical creativity–on generating of a human-like rhythmic accompaniment. *Computing and Informatics, 22*, 321–340.
29. Alfonceca, M., Cebrian, M., & Ortega, A., (2006). A fitness function for computer-generated music using genetic algorithms. *WSEAS Trans. On Information Science & Applications, 3*(3), 518–525.
30. Sasank, R., & Jeff, M., (2006). Lifetrak: Music in tune with your life. In: *Proceedings of International workshop on HCM*. ACM.
31. Golden, R., Dan, B., Ted, B., & Eugene, C., (2007). Towards a personal automatic music playlist generation algorithm: The need for conceptual information. In *Proceedings of 2nd International Conference on Audio Mostly Conference: Interaction with Sound* (pp. 84–89).

32. Unemi, T., & Bisig, D., (2008). A generative remixing of music tracks based on an interactive swarm. In: *Proceedings of 11th International Conference on Generative Art* (pp. 388–392).
33. Miguel, T., Worldo, F., & Molina-Solana, M., (2008). Inmamusys: Intelligent multiagent music system. *International Journal on Expert Systems with Applications* (Vol. 36, pp. 1–7). Elsevier.
34. Man-Kwan, S., Fang-Fei, K., Meng-Fen, C., & Suh-Yin, L., (2009). Emotion-based music recommendation by affinity discovery from film music. *International Journal on Expert Systems with Applications, 36,* 7666–7674. Elsevier.
35. Datta, K., Sengupta, R., Dey, N., Dipali, N., & Mukherjee, A., (2010). A methodology of note extraction from the song signals. *Yugoslav Journal of Operations Research, 20*(1), 157–177.
36. Parag, C., Avinash, S., & Aaron, A., (2010). Evaluating multiple viewpoint models of tabla sequences. In: *Proceedings of 3rd International Workshop on Machine Learning and Music* (pp. 21–24). ACM.
37. Adrian, W., (2010). A graph-theoretic approach to tonal modulation. *Journal of Mathematics and Music* (pp. 45–56). Taylor & Francis.
38. Godfried, T. T., (2010). "Generating good" musical rhythms algorithmically. In: *Proceedings of the 8th International Conference on Arts and Heuristics* (pp. 774–791).
39. Rajeswari, S., Karthiga, S., & Geetha, T. V., (2010). *Fundamental Frequency Estimation of Carnatic Music Songs Based on the Principle of Mutation, IJCSI, 7*(4).
40. Dragan, M., (2010). A genetic algorithm for composing music. *Yugoslav Journal of Operations Research, 20*(1), 157–177.
41. Boris, S., & Mark, D. G., (2010). Ubiquitous drums: A tangible, wearable musical interface. In: *Proceedings of CHI.*
42. Sajjad, A., (2011). Iranian traditional music dastgah classification. In: *Proceedings of 12th International Conference on ISMIR* (pp. 275–280).
43. Yajie, H., & Mitsunori, O., (2011). Nextone player: A music recommendation system based on user behavior. In: *Proceedings of 12th International Conference on ISMIR* (pp. 103–108).
44. Rajeswari, S., & Manasa, S., (2011). Latent Dirichlet allocation model for raga identification of Carnatic music. *Journal of Computer Science*, 1711–1716.
45. Tarakeswara, R. B., & Prasad, R. P. V. G. D., (2011). A novel process for melakarta raaga recognition using hidden Markov models (HMM). *International Journal of Research and Reviews in Computer Science, 2*(2), 508–513.
46. Prasad, R. P. V. G. D., Tarakeswara, R. B., Sudha, K. R., Hari, C. H. V. M. K., (2011). K-nearest neighbor and earth mover distance for raaga recognition. *International Journal of Computer Application, 33*(5), 30–38.
47. Vasudha, J., Iyshwarya, G., Tamarai, S. A., Iniyaa, S., & Jeyakumar, G., (2011). Application of computer-aided music composition in music therapy. *International Journal of Innovation, Management & Technology, 2*(1), 55–57.
48. McDermott, J., & Uma-May O'Reilly, (2011). An executable graph representation for evolutionary generative music. *International Journal of GECCO*, 403–410. ACM.
49. Xinxi, W., David, R., & Wang, Y., (2012). Context-aware mobile music recommendation for daily activities. In: *Proceedings of International Workshop on MM.*

50. Olufisayo, O., & Michael, G., (2012). Impact of user context on song selection. In: *Proceedings of International Workshop on MM*. ACM.
51. Yogesh, P. P., (2012). Predicting shrutic in harmonium using temporal mining. *Journal of Engineering Research and Application*, 213–217.
52. Joe, C. R., & Preeti, R., (2012). Detection of raga-characteristics phrases from Hindustani classical music audio. In: *Proceedings of the 2nd Comp Music Workshop* (pp. 133–138).
53. Tarakeswara, R. B., Sivakoteswararao, C., Lakshmi, K. P., & Gargi, M., (2012). Automatic melakarta raaga identification system: Carnatic music. *International Journal of Advanced Research in Artificial Intelligence, 1*(4), 43, 44.
54. Sunitha, A., (2012). Knowledge based semantic annotation generation of music. *International Journal of Computer Applications, 47*(8), 8–12.
55. Priya, K., Geetha, R. R., & Shomona, G. J., (2012). Data mining techniques for automatic recognition of Carnatic raga swaram notes. *International Journal of Computer Applications, 52*(10), 4–10.
56. Srimani, P. K., & Parimala, Y. G., (2012). Artificial neural network (ANN) approach for an intelligent system: A case study in Carnatic classical music (CCM). In: *Proceedings of International Conference on Intelligent Computational Systems* (pp. 101–105).
57. Momfil-Contreras, E. U., Alor-Hernandez, G., Cortes-Robles, G., Rodriguez-Gonzalez, A., & Gonzalez-Carrasco, I., (2013). RESYGEN: A recommendation system generator using domain-based heuristics. *International Journal on Expert Systems with Applications, 40*, 242–256. Elsevier.
58. Xavier, S., (2012). Opportunities for a culturally specific approach in the computational description of music. In: *Proceedings of the 2nd International Workshop of Comp. Music Workshop* (pp. 1–4).
59. Qiang, L., (2014). A constraint handling technique for constrained multi-objective genetic algorithm. *Journal of Swarm and Evolutionary Computation*, 66–79. Elsevier.
60. Chhavi, R., & Sanjay, K. J., (2014). An evolutionary clustering algorithm based on temporal features for dynamic recommender systems. *Journal of Swarm and Evolutionary Computation*, 21–30. Elsevier.

CHAPTER 17

DATA SCIENCE DEPLOYMENT IN HEALTHCARE SYSTEMS TO FIGHT AGAINST THE COVID-19 PANDEMIC

VIBHA OJHA,[1] ANAND SHARMA,[2] POOJA SHARMA,[3] and MEENAKSHI YADAV[4]

[1]*Government Engineering College, Ajmer, Rajasthan, India, E-mail: vibha.ojha@gmail.com*

[2]*CSE Department SET, Mody University of Science and Technology, Laxmangarh, Rajasthan, India*

[3]*IPEM, Ghaziabad, Uttar Pradesh, India*

[4]*Sirifort Institute of Management Studies, Rohini, New Delhi, India*

ABSTRACT

COVID-19 (2019-nCoV, more widely known as 2019 coronavirus disease), brought by SARS-CoV-2 (severe acute respiratory syndrome coronavirus 2), is a rising public health issue compromising the life of over 2.4 million individuals comprehensively. It is a worldwide health crisis of exceptional extents. The WHO (World Health Organization) pronounced the coronavirus 2019 a pandemic on date March 11th, highlighting the more than 118,000 cases in more than 110 nations and regions around the globe. The continuous death toll comprehensively, underscoring the supported danger of further worldwide spread just as explained diversely inside individual

IoT and Cloud Computing-Based Healthcare Information Systems. Anand Sharma, PhD, Hiren Kumar Deva Sarma, PhD & S. R. Biradar, PhD (Eds.)

countries through communities because of asymptomatic transporters, has produced a requirement for interdisciplinary logical research, reaction, and activity through clear, point-by-point informing to worldwide constituencies. Governments around the globe are forcing different control measures while the social insurance framework is preparing itself for tidal waves of contaminated people that will look for treatment.

Since January 2020, a powerful group of research has been rising up out of medical disciplines, for example, virology, the study of disease transmission, immunology, microbiology, radiology, bioinformatics, and phylogeny. Tragically, there is next to zero insightful work rising up out of non-medical disciplines. This work focused on the gaps in the literature by concentrating on the data science deployment to battle against the novel SARS-CoV-2 pandemic. The introduced work looked to decide the utilization of information Science in social insurance frameworks to battle against COVID-19.

17.1 INTRODUCTION

The talk encompassing the pandemic, in any case, has been hazardous and unevenly spread. Reports and conversations about the present circumstance and condition of information, data about dangers and defensive practices, and forecasts of future situations identified with COVID-19 are practically ubiquitous in media nowadays. Political, social insurance, healthcare, and financial concerns have affected the informing objectives of worldwide authorities.

By and large, these vital stories are at chances with the messaging suggested by the WHO and other driving general health authorities, making an irreconcilable circumstance that directly affects open message utilization and public health needs.

Discussions of the effect of COVID-19 have included references to government activity that bear the qualities of wartime talk.

As of recently, these conversations have principally centered around potential over-burdens of the healthcare system just as monetary misfortunes which are strengthened by political measures (for example, lockdowns, curfews, and shutting of not important organizations).

In spite of the fact that not all insights concerning it's the epidemiology are clear yet, deaths identified with COVID-19 essentially influence the old, and fundamentally individuals with attending sicknesses, for example, cardiovascular maladies, respiratory ailments, and diabetes [1].

To address the inquiry that the vast majority might want to ask, "On the off chance that somebody is COVID-19 constructive, how likely is this individual to kick the bucket?" three terms are considered [2–5].

17.1.1 CASE FATALITY RATE (CFR)

One takes the quantity of individuals who have died by COVID-19 and divide it by the absolute number of individuals diagnosed. For instance, if 20 individuals have died and 200 individuals have been diagnosed to have the malady, the CFR is [20/200], or 10%.

In any case, mind that it is the proportion between the quantity of affirmed deaths the quantity of affirmed cases, not absolute cases. That implies that it isn't equivalent to – and in quick-moving circumstances like COVID-19, most likely not in any case exceptionally near the genuine hazard for a contaminated individual.

17.1.2 CRUDE MORTALITY RATE (CMR)

It quantifies the ratio, any person in the populace will pass away from it; not simply the individuals who are tainted or are affirmed as being contaminated. It's determined by dividing the quantity of passings by the absolute population. Such as, if there were 20 passings of 1,000 population, the CMR would be [20/1,000], i.e., 2%, regardless of whether just 100 individuals had been determined to have the disease.

17.1.3 INFECTION FATALITY RATE (IFR)

It's the quantity of passings from an ailment isolated by the absolute number of cases. On the off chance that 10 individuals passed by the disease, and 500 really have it, at that point the IFR is [10/500], or 2%. Two numbers are required to calculate the IFR, the all-out number of cases and the all-out number of passings.

The information on coronavirus is as often as possible changing on regular routine, and it is hard to give real insights to the affected, recovered, and died. In any case, in light of some underlying examinations, a couple of attributes are rising for this infection. It is accounted for that the CFR for it was 2.3%, at first; in any case, the age gathering of 70 to 79 years has 8% CFR, and the CFR is 14.6% for those over 80 years of age [1]. This implies the infection stronger affects the matured populace.

17.2 BATTLE WITH COVID-19

As indicated by real-time data [6], affirmed COVID-19 cases are increasing exponentially in many nations around the globe. In Spain and Italy, the pandemic is as of now overburdening the system of healthcare [7], and will present patterns continue, it won't take some time before these turns into the horrid reality additionally in numerous other Asian, European nations and the United States.

The fight can be won by tending to the two key components:

- In the primary spot medical domain is thought of, to train governments and healthcare proficient what's in store, which measures to force and what kind of treatment a corona positive patient required?
  - With the quick advancement that has been made with indicative reagents, immunotherapeutic methodologies, drug repurposing, and vaccine production as an outcome to the episode of SARS-CoV-2 or COVID-19, it might speak to a quickly developing field of study for remedial mediation with regards to COVID-19 disease.
  - Medical/clinical identification of novel COVID-19 tainted individual through testing the samples go under this. At that point after identification of the patient, the specific clinical treatment will be given.
  - Various drugs that are being utilized, including antimalarials (e.g., chloroquine) and antivirals (e.g., favipiravir, remdesivir, arbidol) [8], or tocilizumab with significant levels of interleukin 6 and bilateral pulmonary lesions.
  - Finally, however, perhaps even more important, measures for ensuring the protection of caregivers in medication and nursing are required. As of now in the beginning times of the pandemic, we are confronting an enormous absence of

individual protective equipment. This isn't just significant for clinical consideration (for example, intensive care units), yet in addition for care of nursing staff and casual caregivers.

- Secondly the social domain, to inspire the more extensive public to stick to the procedures that were forced to break the spreading in case an unfortunate situation will unfurl [9].
    - o The rule of solitary, which is utilized in health insurance. Everyone – formal and casual caregivers, family members and friends – requirements to act in solidarity and obligation regarding securing older, which are a populace at specific risk [10].
    - o Social distancing and isolation (quarantine) are basic to stemming the spread without pharmacological methodologies for anticipation and treatment.
    - o In expansion, there are mental and social long-haul impacts which may happen because of dejection brought about by isolation or lockdowns. In this way, it is exceptionally applicable to rehearse social distancing, however, to maintain a strategic distance from social segregation.

17.3 REMEDIAL MEASURES

This section gives the healing estimates that can be embraced to battle COVID-19.

17.3.1 PREVENTION

The Government has passed another law that expands the limitations forced on residents wherein outside activities and visits to gardens are disallowed. A few locales have passed laws that disallow, with prompt impact, and development of people entering and leaving these areas. Considering the potential introduction to contamination, a quick proportion of a quarantine of 14 days will apply for the individuals who abuse these limitations [11].

17.3.2 INCREASE HOSPITALS AND MEDICAL PERSONNEL

For this, the Government has announced the imminent construction of hospitals, and further, these increased doctors and medical personnel, will be included in duty groups.

17.3.3 INCREASED SUPPLY OF MECHANICAL VENTILATORS AND MASKS

The supply of medical equipment like mechanical ventilators should be increased, and the masks and other wearable kits should be increased.

17.3.4 INCREASED TESTING OF THE FRONTLINE WORKERS

The mortality rate is higher on the grounds. Toward the start of the pandemic, there was falsehood that asymptomatic cases didn't transmit the infection. This announcement is positively erroneous, and the acknowledgment of asymptomatic/somewhat symptomatic cases could diminish the quantity of contamination. [12].

17.3.5 MONITORING OF PATIENTS

These patients can spread the infection SARS-CoV-2, so the patients should be monitored.

17.4 DATA SCIENCE FOR COVID-19

Data science is a developmental extension of statistics fit for managing the massive amounts of data produced today. It adds techniques from computer science to the collection of statistics. The primary things that set a data scientist apart from a statistician are the capacity to work with big data and expertise in ML, computing, and algorithm building.

The key points in data science are:

- Retrieving data;

- Data preparation;
- Data exploration;
- Data modeling or model building;
- Presentation and automation.

The quick spread and worldwide effects of COVID-19 can cause individuals to feel defenseless and terrified as the novel coronavirus raises and forces them to change numerous aspects of their regular daily existences. Nonetheless, individuals can feel hints of something better over the horizon in these uncertain times by seeing increasingly about how data scientists are striving to find out as much about COVID-19 as possible.

The necessary conditions for deployment of data science for the COVID-19 are:

- COVID-19 data, without data we can't in any way, shape, or form how it is progressing;
- Without having data, we cannot react suitably to the risk, and it would not be realized where the countermeasures are working;
- The number of affirmed cases advises us about the improvement regarding the pandemic;
- But the affirmation of case depends on a test. The WHO characterizes an affirmed case as "an individual with laboratory confirmation of COVID-19 contamination;"
- Reliable data on testing is along these lines shows the dependability of the data that educates us about the spread of the pandemic.

The pandemic is making the enormous volume of data, which is used by data scientists to follow the disease, manage the response, and discover treatments. For a common man, the data from pandemics can be difficult to deal with outbreak obvious outcomes – especially at amount.

Data science can be significant and can advise individuals of the number of affirmed cases, fatalities, and recoveries. Medical professionals and others, regardless of whether an individual is on the front lines of the coronavirus battle, or a concerned resident must get right and exceptional information they need in one spot about how the coronavirus circumstance changes step by step.

Effectively, numerous projects are in progress utilizing data analysis to fight the pandemic. It can assume a job over the entire lifespan of the outbreak: starting from expectation, recognition, and reaction, right to recuperation.

17.4.1 DETECTION

Data Science utilizes a sequential procedure to analyze data from large numbers of sources. Those incorporate airline ticketing information, news reports, health data, government notification and ailment systems to identify the rise of new irresistible ailments. It utilizes innovation to take a gander at data without communicating with nearby specialists who might be more slow or hesitant to share data.

17.4.2 SPREAD

In addition to detecting an outbreak, data science can also be useful to predict its spread. Location statistics are used to break down the spread of the infection and help in assigning assets as per populace conveyance. Mobile phone location is used to track the movement of individuals to predict where the disease is about to spread.

Data science driven expectations of disease spread can be utilized by healthcare authorities in their decisions.

17.4.3 MANAGING THE PANDEMIC

Social distancing is key weapon to limit ahead transmission of COVID-19. One of the troubles experienced how and when the imprisonment time frame can be intruded. Lifting the imprisonment too soon could be the result of setting off a subsequent wave significantly wilder than the first. Researchers as of now missing the enormous data on this required to give exact outcomes.

17.4.4 RECOVERY

When the outbreak contained, health specialists can utilize data science to settle on choices about how to manage flare-ups later on. The pandemic data will be important in seeing how best to manage future outbreaks. That will permit authorities to check various situations and results to settle on data-driven decisions on the best moves to make later on.

17.5 DATA SCIENCE DEPLOYMENT IN HEALTHCARE SYSTEMS

Given the worldwide size of the pandemic, innovation will assume a basic role in about each aspect of tending to COVID-19, from utilizing data science to crunch monstrous datasets to examining disease vectors and recognizing treatment impacts (Figure 17.1).

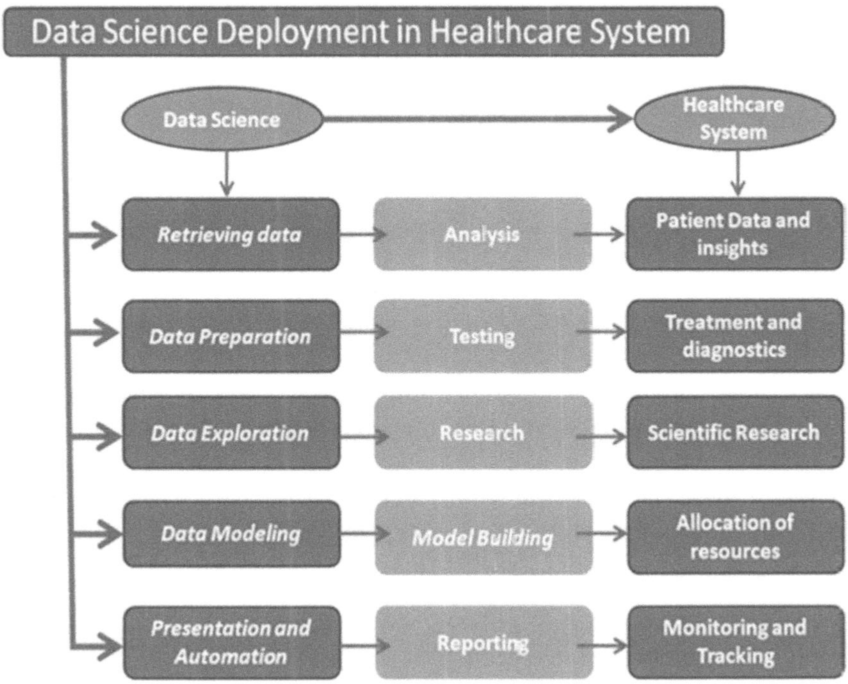

FIGURE 17.1 Data science deployment in healthcare systems.

Knowing however much about the coronavirus as could reasonably be expected will spare lives. Our endeavors to help COVID-19 related research endeavors will concentrate on five regions:

17.5.1 ANALYSIS

This step is to collect and analyze patient data. In this progression information researcher guarantee that he can utilize the data in his program, which means checking the presence of, quality, and access to the data. Data can likewise be conveyed by outsider organizations and takes numerous structures running from Excel spreadsheets to various sorts of databases.

Data scientists examine how data can be gathered from where it very well may be gathered, how much, and why; with the most elevated estimation principles to settle on the most ideal decisions:

- End-to-end patient data collection and analysis;
- Planning, allocation, inventory, and merchandising analysis;
- Performance, and optimization;
- Patient data segmentation, targeting, and automation;
- Patient experience analysis;
- Predictive/prescriptive analytics.

17.5.2 TESTING

In this stage, data scientist upgrades the quality of the data and set it to use in the healthcare system to give the diagnostics and treatment. This phase consists of diagnostics, extracting values from a patient data source and treatment, ensures that the clinical/therapeutic treatment is suitable for the given set of patient data.

This phase offers a wide variety of options for testing the patient data that explore new opportunity and knowledge for diagnostics and treatment:

- Real-time dynamic testing;
- Patient propensity diagnosis;
- Acquisition and engagement strategy for treatment;
- Controlled experimentation for diagnosis;
- Decision sciences for treatment;
- Engagement performance of patient treatment.

17.5.3 RESEARCH

Data exploration is worried about structure a more profound comprehension of patient data. That empowers research to promote the improvement of diagnostics, vaccines, and therapeutics. It further investigates the scientific research to contemplate and comprehend COVID-19.

To accomplish this, data scientists, for the most part, utilize descriptive statistics, visual systems, and straightforward modeling.

Data scientists conduct primary and secondary research to find the solutions for most squeezing COVID-19 inquiries:

- Primary research, patient data;
- Behavioral and psychographic segmentation;
- Market and industry research for medical equipment;
- Social-economic data of patient;
- Products for diagnostics and therapeutics;
- Product equity analysis.

17.5.4 MODEL BUILDING

In this stage data scientist use domain knowledge, models, and experiences about the data found in the past strides to distribute the resource, remembering suggestions for the designation of restricted resources, for example, hospital space and clinical supplies. Data scientists select a method from the fields of machine learning (ML), statistics, operations research, etc. Model building is an iterative procedure that includes choosing the variables for the model, executing the model, and diagnosis of model.

Data scientist can associate the data for effective capacity, access, analysis, and displaying for assignment of healthcare assets, from data investigation to integration, arrangement, and the executives to high-confidence decision-making:

- Data exploration and analysis for resources;
- Big data definition and building data dictionaries;
- Machine learning and automation;
- Forecasting and regression modeling;
- Model building and fitting with maintenance;
- Simulation and risk management;
- Anomaly detection of rare items.

17.5.5 REPORTING

Finally, data scientist presents the results in the form of reports and further monitoring and tracking of COVID-19 patient. These results can take many forms, ranging from presentations to research reports. Sometimes data scientist needs to automate the execution of the process because of the dissemination of accurate information to minimize misinformation sharing. It will also explore the understanding and tracking our progress against COVID-19.

We need the world to all the more likely comprehend COVID-19. Accordingly, we have built up a lot of intuitive visualizations, accessible beneath, so everybody has full straightforwardness into the extent of the issue and the advancement we are making together to recuperate the world. We will proceed to refresh and refine this visualization with new data and bits of knowledge.

The main objective is performance reporting that is exact, convenient, and of high-quality. Data scientist builds altered customized reporting to fit your needs.

- Real-time reporting of patient;
- Data visualization and illustration for patient monitoring;
- Metrics creation and key performance for tracking our progress;
- Configuring web-analytics platforms: Google, Adobe, etc.;
- Tag management, implementation, standardization, and QA.

17.6 ADVANTAGES OF DATA SCIENCE DEPLOYMENT

Research on pandemic procedures has long and productive history in physics [13, 14]. Straightforward numerical models that depict the embodiment of plague spreading can be utilized to fit the data, and the acquired qualities would then be able to be utilized to make educated expectations. As of late, the research community has likewise collected overpowering proof for unpredictable and heterogeneous availability designs in informal communities [15, 16].

It assumes a key role in deciding the conduct of harmony and non-balance frameworks by and large, and the spreading of pandemics and finding ideal optimal methodologies specifically.

From traditional models that expect very much blended populations to the later models that represent conduct criticism and the structure of our informal organizations, we have made some amazing progress in understanding disease dynamics, infection, and transmission. We are presently ready to utilize this information to create effective prevention measures, and all the more extensively, we can utilize the cooperative energies between these various fields of respective research for societies to improve human lives [17].

It can assume a focal role to analyze the enormous scale testing of individuals by connecting those outcomes with health attributes of patients in hospital. This will permit us to comprehend the key risk factor and protect individuals with the most serious risk. Since COVID-19 is new, it is not yet completely comprehended. The more data there we have; the more exact predictions can be made. This will likewise permit us to improve decisions of how and when social separating ought to be lifted.

Data Science is likewise being utilized to quicken drug advancement to treat coronavirus. For instance, Google's DeepMind AI framework is being utilized to distinguish attributes of the infection that may assist with seeing how its capacities. It would be valuable in working out what medications to seek after. Others incorporate Benevolent AI, UK-based, which is utilizing AI to recognize promising existing medicines for different ailments that would be powerful to treat COVID-19.

Data Science can likewise help recognize where the following outbreak will originate from, and which structures will it take. Early knowledge about any outbreak can assume a fundamental role to improve the reaction to the sickness. That makes worldwide illness observation a significant part in the fight against potential pandemics. Data Science is assuming an undeniably significant role in the movement. It can assist analysts with dissecting worldwide data about known infections, human movement, sickness demonstrating, disease modeling, mapping, and visualization to anticipate where the following pandemic will show up and the effect it will have.

17.7 CHALLENGES FOR DATA SCIENCE DEPLOYMENT

Some tools do a great job streamlining the data science deployment process in the healthcare system. However, deploying data science on servers or hardware continues to be a challenge. This section describes the challenges, mainly with respect to COVID-19 data which is faced to deploy data science in healthcare systems:

1. **Data Unavailability – or it is Just Hard to Find?:** A few nations are not giving or not refreshing the official figures. That too it is

similarly significant is to make the accessible data findable at a specific location.

2. **Data References Description – 'Performed Tests' or 'Individuals Tested'?:** Numerous nations report the tests performed, while other nations report only the quantity of people tested. The explanation behind this is that basic for coronavirus testing that a similar individual is tested more than once.
3. **Inclusion of Negative Results and Pending Results Included:** Numerous sources reported the quantity of people who have been precluded or are suspected. To be dependably remembered for test tallies, it should be expressed whether such classes reflect the quantity of individuals who have tested negatively or are anticipating test results.
4. **Data is Complete or Partial:** Figures announced by nations may possibly be halfway if not all the laboratories are answering to authorities. The extent of testing data ought to be made unequivocal by the various sources.
5. **Data Storage:** Front-line workers seldom consider about where data is being put away, yet it's a security, cost, and performance issue for the data science. As the size of COVID-19 data increase exponentially, a few suppliers are not, at this point, ready to deal with the expenses and effects of on premise.

   Numerous associations end up with a half and half methodology of server farms and distributed storage to their information stockpiling programs, which might be the most adaptable and useful methodology for providers with varying data access and capacity needs.
6. **Reliability of Aggregate Data:** So as to evaluate the aggregate data reliability, it should be referenced if heterogeneous data is being added together.

   For example, the COVID Tracking Project of the US clarifies that their sums combined data for tests performed and people tested, contingent upon which is accounted for by singular states.
7. **Data Security:** So as to assess the data, it should be approved and verified by healthcare organizations. From phishing attacks to malware to virus attack, COVID-19 data is subject to a nearly infinite array of vulnerabilities.

8. **Data Publishing Date:** Data about the number of total tests should clarify the date on which the count starts. The key inquiry that should be addressed is that data published incorporate the date of tests conducted.
9. **Comparability of the Data Over Time?:** In the event that we need to see how figures are changed after some time, we have to know the various factors examined above may have been changing as well.
10. **Testing Practices in the Region?:** Knowing how regularly people are tested, will help the clients of these insights to see how estimation performed and people tested may relate with one another.
11. **Data Lost or Misinterpreted by Mistranslating:** People getting data published in alternate languages may misinterpret the data by mistranslation.

17.8 CONCLUSION

Interdisciplinary explorations of factual material science, statistical physics, epidemiology, and network science, the study of disease transmission, driven by gigantic measures of data gathering our health and lifestyle, have offered ascend to computerized epidemiology to the hypothesis of scourge forms on complex systems.

Regardless, in the midst of criticality even the most straightforward model can be excessively entangled, and the little gap between various domains of research can appear gaping openings. "Data and computation will help light the way to moderating the pandemic. It is energetic to point the computing resources and expertise at engaging those with the most encouraging headings, remembering endeavors for biomedicine, epidemiology, logistics, and public health."

A few associations, including Johns Hopkins University, IBM, and Tableau, have released intelligent databases that offer continuous perspectives real-time view on what's going on with the infection.

A significant number of these sources pull from data provided by trusted bodies, for example, the WHO and U.S. Centers for Disease Control and Prevention (CDC). They likewise incorporate direct connections to those spots with the goal that individuals have brisk, simple access to dependable data.

In this work, basic iterative data science is conveyed to fight with COVID-19 with the presumption that administrative data is authentic and truthful. The objective isn't to make progress toward fastidious precision nor to introduce this strategy as the best in class, yet just to give guidelines on elementary principles.

Infectious diseases have consistently existed together with mankind and keeping in mind that advanced life is influential in quickening this pandemic, we never furnished to manage it. Understanding this coronavirus is fundamental in fighting, and obviously, we despite everything have a lot to get some answers concerning COVID-19. The more data we gather, the better it will have the option to support us. The data science arrangements reshape the healthcare systems, reveal new experiences, and transform courageous thoughts into the real world. The opportunities for coordinating data science and healthcare services are extending as the measure of data is developing quicker every day, and the technologies are continually improving.

We will be glad if this work propels further scientific research to yield progressively intricate and precise prediction methods.

KEYWORDS

- **coronavirus**
- **COVID-19**
- **data science**
- **healthcare systems**
- **public health communication**
- **SARS-CoV-2**

REFERENCES

1. World Health Organization, (2020). *Report of the WHO-China Joint Mission on Coronavirus Disease 2019 (COVID-19).* Available online at: https://www.who.int/docs/default-source/coronaviruse/who-china-joint-mission-on-covid-19-final-report.pdf (accessed on 13 June 2022).

2. Taubenberger, J. K., & Morens, D. M., (2006). 1918 influenza: The mother of all pandemics. *Revista Biomedica, 17*(1), 69–79.
3. Jessica, Y. W., Heath, K., Dennis, K. M., Joseph, T. W., Gabriel, M. L., & Benjamin, J. C., (2013). Case fatality risk of influenza A (H1N1pdm09): A systematic review. *Epidemiology, 24*(6).
4. Lipsitch, M., Donnelly, C. A., Fraser, C., Blake, I. M., Cori, A., Dorigatti, I., & Van, K. M. D., (2015). Potential biases in estimating absolute and relative case-fatality risks during outbreaks. *PLoS Neglected Tropical Diseases, 9*(7).
5. Kobayashi, T., Jung, S. M., Linton, N. M., Kinoshita, R., Hayashi, K., Miyama, T., & Suzuki, A., (2020). Communicating the risk of death from novel coronavirus disease (COVID-19). *Journal of Clinical Medicine.*
6. Dong, E., Du, H., & Gardner, L., (2020). An interactive web-based dashboard to track COVID-19 in real-time. *Lancet Infect Dis*. doi: 10.1016/S1473-3099(20)30120-1.
7. Remuzzi, A., & Remuzzi, G., (2020). COVID-19 and Italy: What next? *Lancet*. doi: 10.1016/S0140-6736(20)30627-9.
8. Dong, L., Hu, S., & Gao, J., (2020). Discovering drugs to treat coronavirus disease 2019 (COVID-19). *Drug Discov Ther., 14*, 58–60. doi: 10.5582/ddt.2020.01012.
9. Ippolito, G., Hui, D. S., Ntoumi, F., Maeurer, M., & Zumla, A., (2020). Toning down the 2019-nCoV media hype–and restoring hope. *Lancet Respir. Med., 8*, 230, 231. doi: 10.1016/S2213-2600(20)30070-9.
10. McCloskey, B., Zumla, A., Ippolito, G., Blumberg, L., Arbon, P., Cicero, A., et al., (2020). Mass gathering events and reducing further global spread of COVID-19: A political and public health dilemma. *Lancet, 395*, 1096–1099. doi: 10.1016/S0140-6736(20)30681-4.
11. https://www.regione.calabria.it/website/portaltemplates/view/view.cfm?17173 (accessed on 13 June 2022).
12. Li, R., Pei, S., Chen, B., Song, Y., Zhang, T., Yang, W., et al., (2020). Substantial undocumented infection facilitates the rapid dissemination of novel coronavirus (SARS-CoV2). *Science*. eabb3221. doi: 10.1126/science.abb3221.
13. Pastor-Satorras, R., Castellano, C., Van, M. P., & Vespignani, A., (2015). Epidemic processes in complex networks. *Rev Mod. Phys., 87*, 925. doi: 10.1103/RevModPhys.87.925.
14. Wang, Z., Bauch, C. T., Bhattacharyya, S., D'Onofrio, A., Manfredi, P., Perc, M., et al., (2016). Statistical physics of vaccination. *Phys. Rep., 664*, 1–113. doi: 10.1016/j.physrep.2016.10.006.
15. Boccaletti, S., Latora, V., Moreno, Y., Chavez, M., & Hwang, D., (2006). Complex networks: Structure and dynamics. *Phys. Rep., 424*, 175–308. doi: 10.1016/j.physrep.2005.10.009.
16. Boccaletti, S., Bianconi, G., Criado, R., Del Genio, C., Gómez-Gardeñes, J., Romance, M., et al., (2014). The structure and dynamics of multilayer networks. *Phys. Rep., 544*, 1–122. doi: 10.1016/j.physrep.2014.07.001.
17. Helbing, D., Brockmann, D., Chadefaux, T., Donnay, K., Blanke, U., Woolley-Meza, O., et al., (2015). Saving human lives: What complexity science and information systems can contribute. *J. Stat. Phys., 158*, 735–781. doi: 10.1007/s10955-014-1024-9.
18. *Information is Beautiful.* https://informationisbeautiful.net/visualizations/covid-19-coronavirus-infographic-datapack/ (accessed on 13 June 2022).

19. World Health Organization, https://www.who.int/emergencies/diseases/novel-coronavirus-2019/situation-reports (accessed on 13 June 2022).
20. Hardin, J., Hoerl, R., Horton, N. J., & Nolan, D., (2014). *Data Science in the Statistics Curricula: Preparing Students to Think with Data.* arXiv preprint arXiv:1410.3127.
21. Dhar, V., (2013). Data science and prediction. *Communications of the ACM, 56*(12), 64–73.

CHAPTER 18

INTERNET OF THINGS IN HEALTHCARE: CHANGING THE LANDSCAPE

ANGANA SAIKIA and SANDEEP JAISWAL

Department of Biomedical Engineering, SET, Mody University, Laxmangarh, Rajasthan, India, E-mail: bmejaiswal@gmail.com (S. Jaiswal)

ABSTRACT

Since two decades, we have seen an astonishing pace of technological revolution, including engineering in the field of biology and science, molecular biology tools, tomography tools such as additive and subtractive manufacturing, new manufacturing technologies, robotics, sensor technology, semiconductor chip miniaturization, and energy storage, achieving increased computing power, and parallel advances. Data processing is related to the growth of semiconductor chips, storage, and communication networks. Many of these techniques are quickly transformed into what is called the melodic fourth image [1].

Due to rapid changes in technology, a number of factors have led to the internet of things (IoT). These led to significant improvement in processing power for mobile computing and handheld devices, including the development of "near field communication" (NFC) such as Bluetooth low power technology, high frequency detection (RFID) technology, and finally, storage capacity. It provides integrated circuits (chips) and big data clouds

IoT and Cloud Computing-Based Healthcare Information Systems. Anand Sharma, PhD, Hiren Kumar Deva Sarma, PhD & S. R. Biradar, PhD (Eds.)

like Amazon and Google [2]. The economics of scale, theory of diversity, has created an integration in the networks of "connected computer devices or things" around the world that can be identified with a specific identity. This is called the "internet of things" (IoT). This chapter emphasizes on various aspects of IoT used in healthcare.

18.1 INTRODUCTION

Growth in healthcare across the globe is personal and participatory and at the heart of this trend is the digitization of healthcare growth. In healthcare, IoT is not only able to collect and store information, but it can also connect to networks to analyze data and analyze a variety of physiological data that can send therapeutic images like those of life-form signature and genomics data. Medical Things (IOMT) on the Internet that could describe growing medical products.

The internet of things (IoT) has been a global concern for decades. However, the healthcare industry has realized the benefits in many of the industry's workplaces through the provision of new, better healthcare devices, services, and interactions. IoT award in healthcare began with the adoption of remote patient monitoring (RPM) for data retrieval from bedside devices. It helps physicians and nurses make better treatment decisions and reduce human interaction. The error rate may be over. The quality of IoT services can be improved through healthcare which may reduce the healthcare costs. IoT can change hospitals and healthcare in general [3, 4].

Healthcare IoT has been adopted as a practice among the patients' family members, with various ways patient care has been defined over the past few decades. The healthcare industry is almost giving up hope due to rising healthcare costs, the growing age of the world's population and many chronic illnesses. To protect this, the IoT in healthcare is provided in the form of patient monitoring units and X-ray equipment for hospital meters that help improve surgery and patient care. Internet does not prevent the population from recovering from old age or chronic illness, but it does make a significant contribution to making treatment services accessible, better, and easier. Healthcare IoT is embedded in existing processes and systems, helping to streamline and intersect patient flows at the tissue level, primarily RPM, ope-operability in the context of real-time health data collection and transfer, ultimately eliminating connections that enable data movement, analysis, and Exchange important information, and communicate with machines. For treatment diagnoses, IoT has helped make regular health check-ups more patient and home-focused as opposed to a health-centric approach [5]. Thus, the healthcare IoT has assisted in monitoring, diagnosing, treating, and redefining treatment for general healthcare practices, reducing costs and errors.

IoT has enabled medical sector more useful. Various medical equipment has been added with sensors to monitor the external environment. A faster and more efficient Internet connection for communication, companies can collect information and return reports in real-time. In various global level, IoT demonstrates the growing the use of IoT devices within the healthcare sectors to help track important and expensive devices more effectively.

Some of the examples of IoT in healthcare are as follows [6, 7]:

- Cancer treatment;
- Smart continuous glucose monitoring;
- Closed-loop insulin delivery;
- Connected inhalers;
- Ingestible sensors;
- Connected contact lenses;
- The apple watch application which monitors depression;
- Apple's research kit and Parkinson's disease;
- ADAMM asthma monitor.

The application domains in Smart healthcare system are described in Figure 18.1.

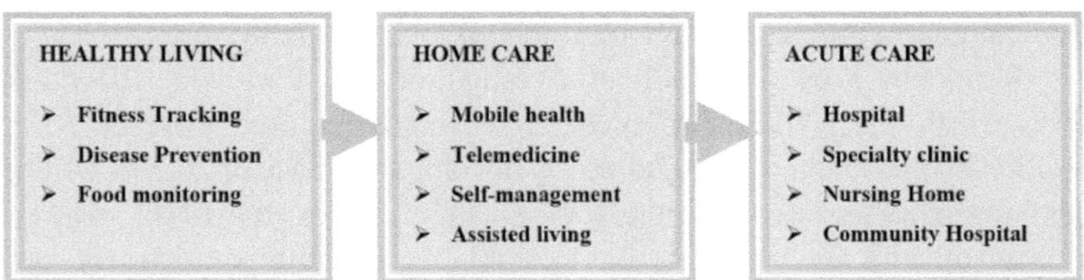
HEALTHY LIVING
➤ Fitness Tracking
➤ Disease Prevention
➤ Food monitoring
HOME CARE
➤ Mobile health
➤ Telemedicine
➤ Self-management
➤ Assisted living
ACUTE CARE
➤ Hospital
➤ Specialty clinic
➤ Nursing Home
➤ Community Hospital

FIGURE 18.1 Domains in smart healthcare system (self-drawn).

18.2 FUTURE SCOPES

Figure 18.2 shows the global market of IoT in the healthcare domain in the near future.

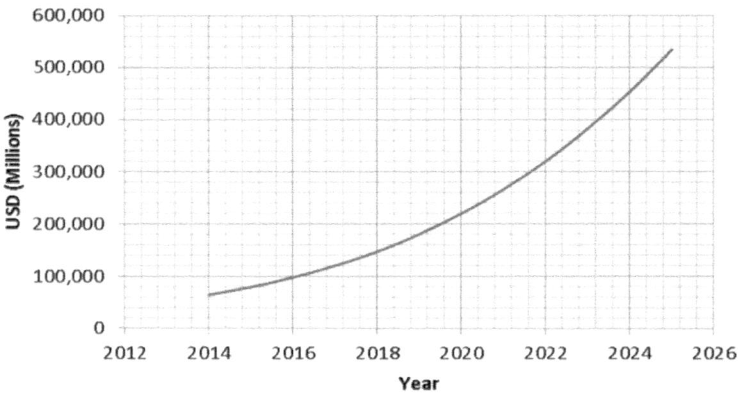

FIGURE 18.2 Global IoT healthcare market (self-drawn).

Despite the fact that the social insurance industry was slower in the underlying stage to embrace the IoT advances when contrasted with different businesses however the internet of medical things (IoMT) is a distinct advantage. It is ready to change how to keep individuals protected and solid that too in a cost-proficient way. Every one of these things demonstrates the general future extent of IoT in the Healthcare space.

IoMT is a combination of clinical gadgets and versatile applications associating human services data innovation frameworks by means of organize advancements. The innovation can decrease superfluous clinic visits alongside reducing the weight on social insurance frameworks by associating patients to their doctors and specialists while permitting the exchange of clinical information that took over a safe system [8].

Report by Frost and Sullivan investigation, the worldwide IoT market was worth $22.5 billion of every 2016 and is required to reach $72.02 billion by 2021, at a compound yearly development pace of 26.2%. Offering extraordinary assistance to the social insurance area, the IoMT market is loaded up with savvy gadgets like wearable's, clinical/imperative screens for health awareness use in the home, network, facility, or medical clinic settings while partner ongoing area, tele-wellbeing, and different administrations.

Moreover, on-body Segment is partitioned into two portions Consumer wellbeing wearable's and clinical/clinical-grade wearable's:

1. **Consumer Health Wearables:** Consumer-grade devices for personal wellness, such as activity trackers, bands, wristbands, sports watches, and smart garments.
2. **Clinical-Grade Wearables:** Regulated devices and supporting platforms that are generally approved for use by o health authorities, like the U.S. Food and Drug Administration (FDA).

Scarcely any instances of such wearable's are savvy belts from Active Protective that distinguishes falls and conveys hip assurance for older individuals. Radiance Neuroscience's Halo Sport headset worn during exercises and physical instructional meetings for animating cerebrum territories answerable for muscle memory, quality, and continuance. Neurometrix Quell, which is a wearable neuromodulation gadget that takes advantage of tactile nerves for giving help from constant torment. Moreover, the on-body Segment is partitioned into two fragments Consumer wellbeing wearable's and clinical/clinical-grade wearable's [9].

18.2.1 FUTURE SCOPE OF HEALTH MONITORING DEVICES BASED ON IOT [10]

1. **Healing at Home:** A couple of years back, checking patients was restricted to the consideration of family or home medical attendants on the off chance that the patient is mending at home. Then again, in the event that a patient chooses to be in the medical clinic, at that point normal observing is a conspicuous undertaking. In any case, with the progression of time and the presentation of instruments based on IoT, the decision of recuperating at household leads out to be simple. Combination of ongoing checking and other distinct modules, patients don't really need to be under the medical clinic rooftop. According to the data given by Grand View Research, the worldwide IoT distant wellbeing checking market is relied upon to make more than $300 billion by 2022. The innovation consequently holds a fortifying future giving free and versatile wellbeing observing while at the same time lessening the worry to visit specialists and wellbeing staff.
2. **Peace of Mind:** It becomes a risky affair if no one is present at home for patient care. The circumstance turns out to be most

exceedingly awful when a patient is experiencing dementia. Fortunately, the circumstance was a strain before that has been wiped out. The expansion of wearable innovation into it makes it significantly more grounded. These wearable gadgets identify the patient's condition alongside sending data to the guardian as well. The data can either be given through content or e-mail while alarming the specialists as well.

3. **Independent Health Monitoring:** In health-related crises, individuals of all ages need quick support from any wellspring of help. The requirement for sending the alert signal to the concerned individual alongside the specialist, IoT home wellbeing observing gadgets are expanding levels of autonomous wellbeing observing. Aside from that, the gadget is a help for the individuals who are distant from everyone else. Perceiving how helpful these IoT observing gadgets are-in future, the quantity of houses will be equipped with sensor arrange. These systems will screen every single action of a disease person using the sensor by sending in alarms in a crisis. These sensors, then again, can be set in fridges, cupboards, restroom entryways or some other aspect of the home.
4. **Medicines on Right Time:** IoT observing gadget that monitors a patient's endorsed medication schedule. The innovation can be demonstrated best for person suffering from dementia or Alzheimer's.

Figure 18.3 shows some of the areas of the healthcare domain which applies IoT.

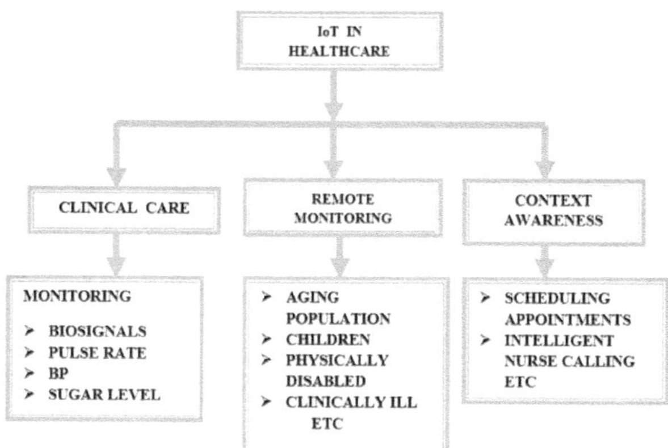

FIGURE 18.3 Subcategories of IoT-based healthcare systems (self-drawn).

The graph in Figure 18.4 shows the estimated IoT devices globally installed for healthcare.

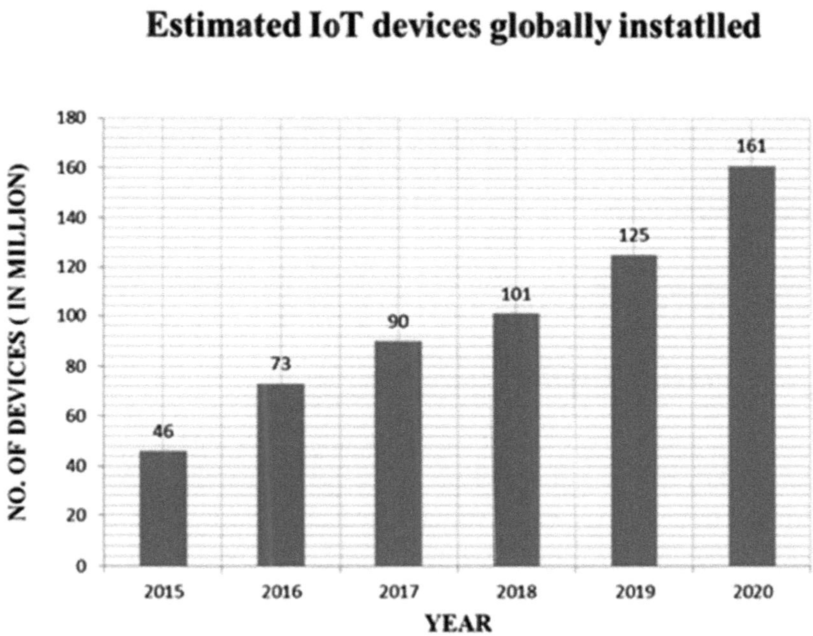

FIGURE 18.4 IoT devices globally installed for healthcare.

m-Health as a standard, basic thing on a worldwide scale, and diminished physical visits to medical clinics. This is just a surmised image of the IoMT achievement. All things considered, as youthful as the idea seems to be, it isn't generally respected to be that novel by dynamic emergency clinics of the now. A huge part of them is either demonstrating major IoT strategies and capacities or as of now have upgraded parts that are in their alignment stage. Needle-less and practical medical services arrangements have consistently been on incredible interest. With huge financing and expanding consideration towards the brilliant medical care space, there are various items also, applications accessible for clients. As smart healthcare has various areas of applications, it offers an extension for analysts to continually develop new items and improve the previously existing designs. The change towards smart medical care administrations, is a gradual cycle. This is principally on the grounds that medical care experts need to be continually instructed and persuaded to adjust to the computerized time. Despite the fact that the keen medical care arrangements supported by the IoT can improve income, and increment personal satisfaction, the advantages can be handily dominated, if security is undermined. Extra estimates should be taken to deal with dangers and make sure about the expected data at both the client and engineer closes. In this way, the vision and long-haul achievement of this progressively developing industry lays in the cooperative energy of analysts, medical services experts, and the general population [11].

18.3 HEALTHCARE APPLICATIONS OF IOT

18.3.1 TELEMEDICINE

Telemedicine for the use of telecommunications and information technology (IT) provides clinical care remotely. It can overcome and improve distance barriers. Access to various medical facilities that are not available in remote rural areas community [12]. Exchange information such as voice, images, videos, graphic, treatment material, etc., commands to surgical robots.

Some features of telemedicine are:

- Remote diagnosis, recording, and transfer of remote patient health parameters;
- Prescription based diagnostics, history records;
- Personal website for patients;
- Management reservations management-patients can check and book treatment schedules;
- Built-in billing function;
- Biosensor for detecting blood pressure, ECG, temperature, etc.;
- Multiple camera options in both non-stop video conferencing-real-time and offline modes.

Patients record questions in the local language and doctors follow up via voice or SMS including treatment information. Education for healthcare providers includes:

- Training materials are created and used for multilingual speech recognition;
- A practitioner of human-like conversation to test knowledge and skills.

18.3.1.1 BENEFITS OF TELEMEDICINE

- Improved access to healthcare in remote areas and new markets;
- Makes the right skills available everywhere and reduces the movement of unnecessary patients;
- Improved access and quality of care at relatively low cost;
- Care Continuity of care, emergency response, public awareness.

18.3.2 OUTPATIENT MONITORING

- Hospital services are available to host model patients;
- Monitoring-patient from a remote patient was discharged from the hospital;
- Surveillance heartbeat monitoring, heartbeat monitoring, heartbeat with hospital alerts;
- 24/7 patient monitoring, real-time tracking of outsiders;
- Geo fence, deviation warning, signs record;
- Alert friends and family, constantly monitoring external ECG;
- Cardiac telemetry, handling important messages.

18.3.3 EXAMPLES OF OUTWARD OBSERVATION

- Chest pain, mild heart failure;
- High blood pressure, weakness, dizziness;
- nausea, mood swings, anemia, mild asthma;
- Back pain, dehydration.

18.3.3.1 ADVANTAGES OF OUTDOOR OBSERVATION

- Reduce the risk of re-entering the watch at high risk;

- The adoption allows the patient to identify the practitioner and take corrective action beforehand;
- Serious medical condition;
- Improve patient information efficiency and safe use of income 24 hours a day;
- A centralized position not only makes treatment staff more efficient, but also enables hospitals;
- Effectively manage the beds and promote the top lines;
- Patient helps to improve patient outcomes and overall satisfaction;
- Improving care planning and seamless delivery.

18.3.4 TELEHEALTH

It is the delivery of medical services and diagnostic information to remote locations. This is an FDA-approved platform that connects patients interactively across the country. 24×7 Internet, IoT, network of authorized doctors using video chat, smartphones, and electronic medical records (EMR) cloud time is the solution to the one-hour need of the 21st century health. This is a new example in the healthcare industry [13, 14].

18.3.4.1 SOME OF THE TELEHEALTH SERVICES

1. **Telemedicine:** Providing professional advice to patients in remote areas or help your primary care physician diagnose. The American Medical Association (AMA) was able to handle 78% of emergency care using telemedicine efficiently.
2. **Telemonitoring:** Uses IoT to collect patient data and transmit healthcare Monitoring agency for remote testing and diagnosis. Tele monitoring service Include personalized alerts to inform patient healthcare providers about the bar Physical/mental injury.
3. **Remote Surgery:** Allows surgeons to perform surgery on remote patients' location using telerobotics technology.
4. **Healthy Distance Treatment:** Provide medical education for medical services Communities and target groups according to geographically different locations.

5. **Telehealth Data Services:** Share specific health information with other healthcare Service providers, education industry, research institutes, government, etc.

18.3.4.2 BENEFITS OF TELEHEALTH SERVICES [15]

- Taking care of treatment immediately, especially in emergencies and natural times disaster;
- Don't have to wait in long lines to see a doctor;
- Physically eliminates the need to take any medical benefits;
- Telehealth declines distance limitations, less documentation and paperwork;
- Reduces cost-effective-increasing telehealth space mass insurance and reduces premiums and in some cases reduces the amount patients have to leave work;
- Everything abolishes, equal, and provisions related to health geographical barriers;
- Care better communication with primary care and specialists. It happens at the same time because everyone lives in virtually the same room diagnosis.

18.3.5 CHALLENGES OF IOT [15]

18.3.5.1 DATA SECURITY AND PRIVACY

One of the most important threats to IoT is data security and privacy. Devices based on IoT technology detects and transfers the data in real time. Some of the IoT devices lack data protocols and standards. Also, there is considerable ambiguity about data ownership control. All of these factors make the data even more risky for cybercriminals, who can hack the system and endanger the personal health information (PHI) of the patient and the physician.

Cybercriminals can create fake identities using patient data and buy drugs and medical devices that can then be sold. Hackers can also claim fake insurance in the name of the patient.

18.3.5.2 INTEGRATION: MULTIPLE DEVICES AND PROTOCOL

Multiple device integration creates a barrier to the generation of IoT in the medical care sector. The reason behind this limitation is that device manufacturers have not reached a consensus on communication standards. Hence, different communication protocols complicate and hinder the process of data collection even when different types of devices are connected. This uniformity of connected device standards reduces the process and the chances of IoT scalability in medical care.

18.3.5.3 DATA OVERLOAD AND ACCURACY

Data integration is tedious as it uses different communication protocols and standards. But IoT devices still collects a huge amount of data. The data acquired by IoT equipment is used to gain important insights. But the large volume of information has made insights very difficult for physicians to achieve and ultimately affect the quality of making decisions. This concern is growing as more devices are connected to record more data.

18.3.5.4 COST

The cost of treatment is a sign of concern for everyone, especially in developed countries. Acute patients can avail medical facilities in developing countries and "medical tourism" has been born, costing less than one-tenth. IoT is an interesting and promising concept as a concept about healthcare.

18.4 CONCLUSION

Healthcare is one of the most essential sectors of human existence. Hence the advancement of healthcare is very much needed. At the present world scenario automation of healthcare using IoT has made this sector more advanced. Introduction to IoT in the present healthcare and medical sector has made this handier and more user-friendly. One can monitor their health using a simple device by sitting and home without traveling a long distance. Also, this has reduced the physical labor and the IoT devices are mostly cost-effective which can be affordable by common people. In the near future IoT in healthcare would reach in certain platform that cure and diagnosis of various serious diseases would become much easier.

KEYWORDS

- **American Medical Association**
- **electronic medical records**
- **healthcare**
- **Internet of medical things**
- **Internet of things**
- **medical devices**
- **m-health**

REFERENCES

1. Babu, B. S., Srikanth, K., Ramanjaneyulu, T., & Narayana, I. L., (2016). IoT for healthcare. *International Journal of Science and Research, 5*(2), 322–326.
2. Yeole, A. S., & Kalbande, D. R., (2016). Use of internet of things (IoT) in healthcare: A survey. In: *Proceedings of the ACM Symposium on Women in Research 2016* (pp. 71–76).
3. Kodali, R. K., Swamy, G., & Lakshmi, B., (2015). An implementation of IoT for healthcare. In: *2015 IEEE Recent Advances in Intelligent Computational Systems (RAICS)* (pp. 411–416). IEEE.
4. Selvaraj, S., & Sundaravaradhan, S., (2020). Challenges and opportunities in IoT healthcare systems: A systematic review. *SN Applied Sciences, 2*(1), 1–8.
5. Haghi, M., Neubert, S., Geissler, A., Fleischer, H., Stoll, N., Stoll, R., & Thurow, K., (2020). A flexible and pervasive IoT-based healthcare platform for physiological and environmental parameters monitoring. *IEEE Internet of Things Journal, 7*(6), 5628–5647.
6. Gope, P., Gheraibia, Y., Kabir, S., & Sikdar, B., (2020). A secure IoT-based modern healthcare system with fault-tolerant decision-making process. *IEEE Journal of Biomedical and Health Informatics*.
7. Chacko, A., & Hayajneh, T., (2018). Security and privacy issues with IoT in healthcare. *EAI Endorsed Transactions on Pervasive Health and Technology, 4*(14).
8. Mathew, P. S., Pillai, A. S., & Palade, V., (2018). Applications of IoT in healthcare. In: *Cognitive Computing for Big Data Systems Over IoT* (pp. 263–288). Springer, Cham.

9. Adhikary, T., Jana, A. D., Chakrabarty, A., & Jana, S. K., (2019). The internet of things (IoT) augmentation in healthcare: An application analytics. In: *International Conference on Intelligent Computing and Communication Technologies* (pp. 576–583). Springer, Singapore.
10. Banka, S., Madan, I., & Saranya, S. S., (2018). Smart healthcare monitoring using IoT. *International Journal of Applied Engineering Research, 13*(15), 11984–11989.
11. Panchatcharam, P., & Vivekanandan, S., (2019). Internet of things (IoT) in healthcare–smart health and surveillance, architectures, security analysis and data transfer: A review. *International Journal of Software Innovation (IJSI), 7*(2), 21–40.
12. Yassein, M. B., Hmeidi, I., Al-Harbi, M., Mrayan, L., Mardini, W., & Khamayseh, Y., (2019). IoT-based healthcare systems: A survey. In: *Proceedings of the Second International Conference on Data Science, e-Learning and Information Systems* (pp. 1–9).
13. Dauwed, M., & Meri, A., (2019). IoT service utilization in healthcare. *Internet of Things (IoT) for Automated and Smart Applications.*
14. Martínez-Caro, E., Cegarra-Navarro, J. G., García-Pérez, A., & Fait, M., (2018). Healthcare service evolution towards the internet of things: An end-user perspective. *Technological Forecasting and Social Change, 136*, 268–276.
15. Nausheen, F., & Begum, S. H., (2018). Healthcare IoT: Benefits, vulnerabilities, and solutions. In: *2018 2nd International Conference on Inventive Systems and Control (ICISC)* (pp. 517–522). IEEE.

CHAPTER 19

DESIGN AND PROTOTYPING OF A CLOUD-BASED PREDICTIVE MODEL FOR THE ENRICHMENT OF A NUTRITION PLAN

NANDITA SANJAY PAL,[1] JAI PRAKASH VERMA,[1] and MANOJ KUMAR KHINCHI[2]

[1]*Institute of Technology, Nirma University, Ahmedabad, Gujarat, India, E-mail: jaiprakash.verma@nirmauni.ac.in (J. P. Verma)*

[2]*Mody University, Laxmangarh, Rajasthan, India*

ABSTRACT

In today's rapidly growing world, people are so busy and careless about their health that they tend to neglect what they are eating. Fast-food consumption is increasing day by day, resulting in an unhealthy lifestyle. This causes minor to severe health issues, including diabetes, high blood pressure, obesity, thyroid, and many more. And these are prevailing these days. Many applications related to monitoring and improving health conditions are developed. Research done in this chapter deals with the lifestyle and eating habits of individuals, and based on that, it predicts about a person's health. A cloud-based machine learning (ML) model is proposed to predict an individual's health and recommend a nutrition plan for a healthy lifestyle. By this, people could be aware of their health and can improve it.

IoT and Cloud Computing-Based Healthcare Information Systems. Anand Sharma, PhD, Hiren Kumar Deva Sarma, PhD & S. R. Biradar, PhD (Eds.)

19.1 INTRODUCTION

This chapter mainly emphasizes a predictive analysis generated from the system, which will provide the nutritional plan of an individual, who should follow to have a healthy lifestyle. The nutritional plan that is generated through the model will be clinically useful to determine any health-related issue or disease that may occur following the given lifestyle [1]. It will be helpful in monitoring and tracking health from time to time. Through ML, we can make predictions for an event and plan the action against the same. The only thing it needs is appropriate "data" to train the model. After a model is trained, it can predict the output by giving a test input. Nowadays, many such applications for predicting the health issues of an individual and recommending a proper nutrition diet plan are developed [7]. Many people are familiar with it. Before doing anything, first, we have to prepare data. Data is a fundamental need to train a ML model, whether it is supervised, unsupervised or reinforcement. The supervised ML technique is generally used when we have labeled data. In the essence, when we have output matched with the inputs. While Unsupervised ML technique is used when we don't have labeled data. Many such applications are readily available in the market that monitors a person's health and keep them updated about their health. In this project, we are trying to develop a model that is capable of predicting health-related things for users [6].

To understand the nutritional model, we first have to understand the different sub-components involved in it. The first thing is the user model that includes, personal information about users like their lifestyle and eating habit. The second one is a food item that includes all nutritional information (macronutrients) that a food item has. These two components are essential while developing any health model. A balanced diet refers to the intake of each necessary nutrient meets its adequate demand and total caloric intake balances with total calories burnt. Not only eating habits but also various other factors take part in predicting an individual's health. Other factors include age, gender, disease (if any), food items that are not recommended or are allergic, their exercising habit, etc. Not only do we have to keep the calorie goals in mind while developing such a health-related system but also the nutritional values of the food items. Because some food products have more calories, but their nutritional benefits are more as compared to a food item that has less amount of calories but is less nutritional.

19.1.1 CASE STUDY: WOMEN NUTRITION PLAN PREDICTION MODEL

Women are a central entity of the family. They play many roles at different stages of life, in all fields, and at various parts of society, be it rural or urban. Nowadays, due to a lot of responsibilities as well as a modern lifestyle, it is becoming very challenging for women to keep track of their nutrition [10]. The government of India has been taking various steps in the context of women's health such as National Nutrition Policy (NNP) [14], Indira Gandhi Matritva Sahyog Yojna (IGMSY) [15], Janani Suraksha Yojana (JSY), etc. [16]. Even though women especially those who are working are not able to take proper nutrition due to various societal and household responsibilities. While some have access to good life needs, others do not. This leads to less accessibility of the food products, environment, and lifestyle, eventually not making it to nutrition needs. This may be also due to various socio-economic aspects like financial, medical, or physical lifestyle, which will consequently result in a lot of deficiencies, non-consumable diseases, mental illness, and others [11]. Now due to rapidly increasing all above issues it needs to take initiative for making them aware of nutrition issues and providing solutions based on their lifestyle [12]. The proposed project will survey mobile applications and smart devices, analyze them, and based on survey data developing a system using ML which will provide an efficient nutritional plan [13].

Figure 19.1 is the complete system architecture for the proposed project. Here, women-centric nutrition requirements are identified from the different states of the nutritional status of women. Pathophysiology suggests women disordered physiological processes that are either caused by any disease or injury to an individual. Physiology provides the status of women's normal functions of living organisms and their parts. Metabolic provide information relating to or deriving from the metabolism of a living organism of women. Social context describes about the social environment of an individual. It mainly includes family behavior, whether she is happy in her life or not. The features are selected from the data generated, and a predictive analytical model is designed and developed for a recommendation of women's nutrition plan.

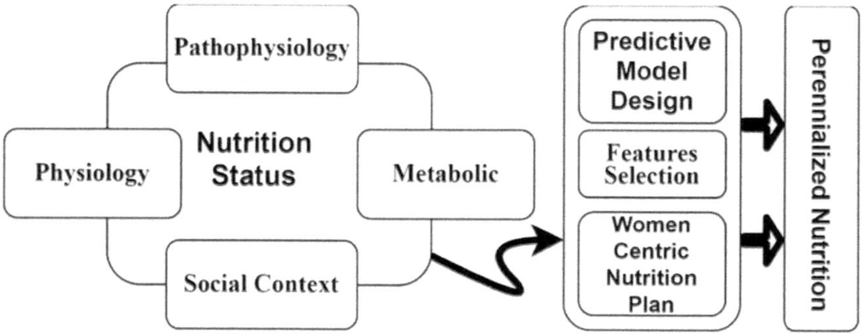

FIGURE 19.1 Women nutrition plan prediction model.

19.2 RELATED WORK

This section describes the work done by other researchers in the area of individuals health prediction and nutrition diet recommendation. Mahmoud et al. [2] proposes healthy food habits and eating patterns so that anyone can know the number of calories burnt, the intake of macronutrients, and so on using data mining tools. The main goal behind this is to predict a healthy diet for an individual and nutritionist to design a diet plan as per the patient's need. They used KDD (knowledge discovery database) model for a better understanding of the model. Weber et al. [3] talks about taking data from food diaries and then applying a ML model to predict calorie goals. Motive behind this chapter is to train a model that can tell whether a person can achieve their diet goal or not. The author collects data from MyFitnessPal App, preprocesses it then applied the SVM algorithm to get an output. This chapter contributes to advances in this field by exploring how public food diaries can be used to understand differences in unsuccessful and successful diets with the help of data mining.

Áine et al. [4] demonstrates how a programming system can be used in order to improve a person's health. The main objective behind this is to define some important parameters related to food and then using it to predict a person's health. Artificial neural networks (ANNs) and decision trees algorithms were used to predict HEI (healthy eating index) based on the food consumed. Schäfer et al. [5] integrates general nutritional theories into information systems and certain user-specific nutritional measures for evaluating the utility of a given nutritional model. The objective is to reflect on different error sources concerning nutrition and consider how such issues can be tackled in future systems. They discussed the quality assessment of the nutritional model. They also talked about uncertainties in modeling.

Table 19.1 refers to certain pros and cons for each one and started to work upon own ideas. The future work mentioned in Ref. [5] chapter is selected as the base paper for this research and tries to build, implement, and evaluate the same. Since it is an unsupervised ML model, it will try to build some relation between given data, and based on that, it will classify whether a person is healthy or not.

TABLE 19.1 Comparison of Research Work Done by Various Researchers

References	[5]	[2]	[4]	[3]
Approach	Integrates general nutritional theories into information systems and certain user-specific nutritional measures for evaluating the utility of a given nutritional model.	This chapter is proposing various ways in which we can improve our lifestyle by predicting about the health using data mining tools.	This chapter demonstrates how a programming system can be used in order to improve a person's health.	Taking data from food diaries and then applying a machine learning model to predict calorie goals.
Objective	To reflect on different error sources with respect to nutritional systems and how they can be overcome via certain ways in future systems.	Prediction of a healthy diet for any individual and nutritionist to design a diet plan as per patient's need.	To evaluate the usability of food-based coding system in order to predict correctly the health of an individual.	To train a model that can tell whether a person is able to achieve its diet goal or not.
Methodology	They have discussed about user model and food items. Then they access the quality of nutritional model. They also talked about uncertainties in modeling.	Systematic way of preparing data and using it has been described. They have used KDD (knowledge discovery database) model for better understanding.	Artificial neural networks (ANN) and decision trees algorithms were used to predict HEI (healthy eating index) based on the food consumed.	After collecting data from MyFitnessPal App, they preprocessed data and then applied the SVM algorithm on it.

TABLE 19.1 *(Continued)*

References	[5]	[2]	[4]	[3]
Pros	Reflected uncertainties in nutritional models and way to quality assessment.	Data mining process is applied in a systematic way.	In order to predict the health of an individual, ANN, and decision tree performed well.	This chapter contributes to advances in this field by exploring how public food diaries can be used to understand differences between successful and unsuccessful diets with the help of data mining.
Cons	Complexities related to food and cultures are yet to be addressed.	Decision Tree algorithm will give accuracy only when non-repeated values are there.	Applicable to current dataset only.	The percentage of false positive and false negative is higher.
Future Work	Real implementation of nutritional model that overcomes uncertainty issues.	Model could be able to predict correctly based on particular disease and lifestyle of an individual.	Validation can be done on the models.	Variations in food recipes can be incorporated.

19.3 TOOLS AND TECHNOLOGIES

This section describes the tools and technology applied during the implementation of the proposed ML-based predictive model in a cloud environment.

19.3.1 CLOUD-BASED COMPUTING: GOOGLE COLAB

Collaboratory is abbreviated as "Colab." It is a product from Google research team. It allows people to write and execute python code through the browser. Its main use cases include ML, data analysis, and education. Also, it supports GPU (Graphical Processing Unit). It also allows you to save your work to Google Drive as well as to your GitHub repository. It allows working as a team too, by sharing your work with other team members on Google Drive. It also allows plotting various graphical representations for analytical purposes. The best thing is no need to install any library or packages because collab offers all those. We just have to import it.

19.3.2 PYTHON API APPLIED

Python is a general-purpose coding language that can be used for programming and software development, web development. It can be used to develop front end, backend, in data Science. It is easy to learn, read, and maintain, provides broad standard libraries, is portable, extendable, provides an interface for various databases, supports various GUI applications. It can be used on a server to create web applications, software to create workflows, can connect to database systems, to read and modify files, it is efficient to handle big data and perform complex mathematical problems, can be used for rapid prototyping, or production-ready software development. No semicolons or parentheses are there as compared to other programming languages. It uses indentation, i.e., whitespace, to define the scope of methods and classes. While other programming languages use curly braces for the same.

19.4 PROPOSED SYSTEM

A data ingestion tool helps to integrate data generated from different sources into a repository with a uniform data structure. The proposed data ingestion tool in this research proposal will support a uniform data structure that will simulate a cloud-based storage environment and computing capability on Cloud. A cloud-based repository will enhance the usability of the system for all the stakeholders. As per Figure 19.1, the proposed data ingestion tool will be work as the composition of the middle layer with the capability of APIs, Web Interface, and Data Submission. The APIs will be responsible for all the negotiations required for data integration from different data sources. Here a robust and interactive Web Interface is proposed which helps users to submit data in a Cloud-based repository that supports a cloud computing environment.

Figure 19.2 shows a comprehensive infrastructure for a cloud-based Big Data Analytics environment for proposed research for the health prediction of an individual. All data will be a cloud-based network differentiated with their data types. Data source nodes will include the clinical data, Nutrition Data, and experimental data. Plans include nodes which support other research modalities such as clinical data, Nutritional data, and prediction models. Through a secure authentication and authorization channel, all stakeholders like biomedical researchers, tool developers, computer scientists, informaticians, clinicians, and patients will be able to access the system easily and host their own tools via GUI web interface. Users can also be able to access elastic compute capabilities for computational analyzes, visualization of results, and data queries in the cloud [17]. This ML model takes data from users. Apply ML algorithm on it and then gives output. Here, the K-mode algorithm is used as a clustering technique. Important parameters are taken into consideration while taking data from users. That all data is sent into the model for further processing. Since the data is of categorical type, the K-mode algorithm is used for clustering. The motive behind this presented work is to identify and alert the user of their health.

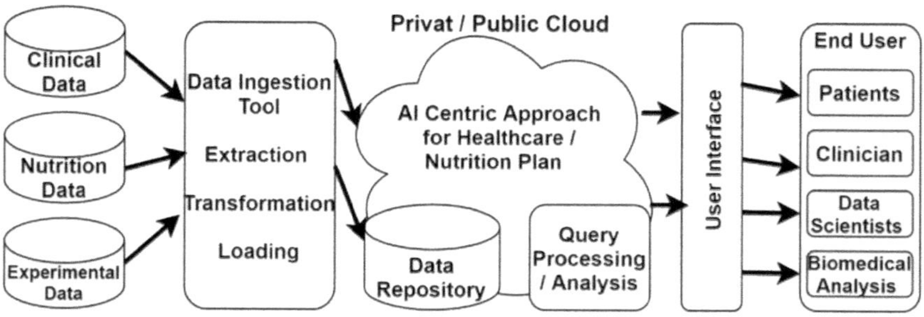

FIGURE 19.2 Proposed comprehensive system architecture.

19.4.1 DATA ACQUISITION AND COLLECTION

As per the study, the Government of Gujarat has surveyed women's nutritional status for women including both urban and rural types. The study indicated the presence of obesity and under-nutrition in different regions of Gujarat. Results show that nutritional health problems are mainly in urbanizing areas of our country. This project aims to facilitate the same thing most easily and appropriately using technology. This project will consider challenges faced by women and providing solutions based on those problems. Figures 19.3–19.6 show the data analysis performed based on the women's habit and behavior on the data collected (the sample is shown in Figure 19.7).

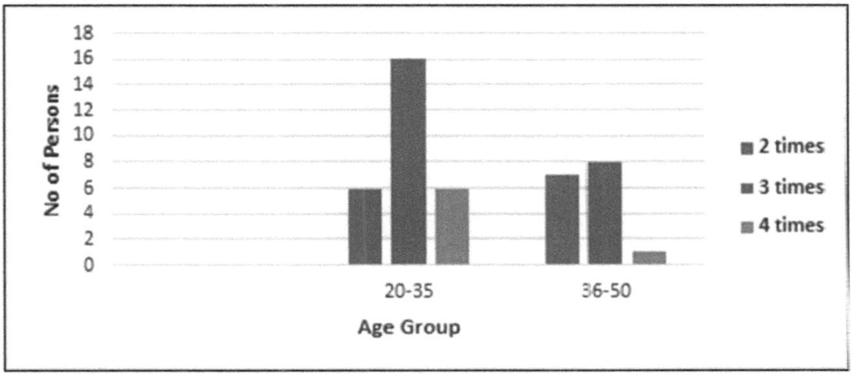

FIGURE 19.3 Frequency of meals taken by women of different age groups.

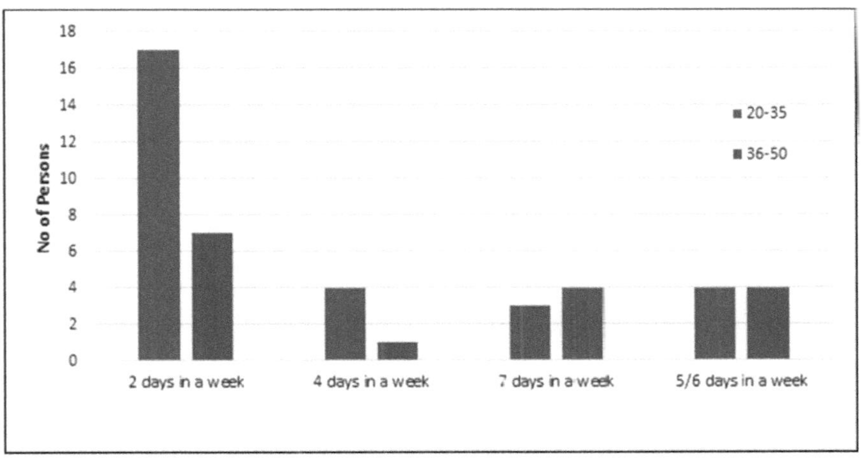

FIGURE 19.4 Frequency of exercise done by women of different age groups.

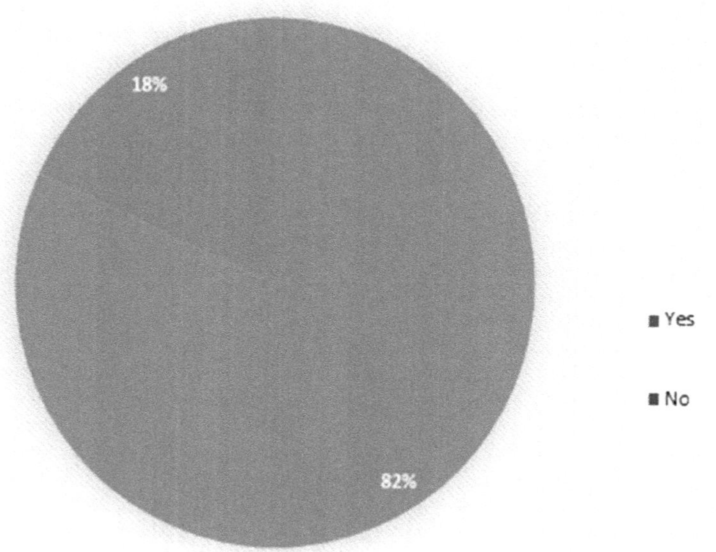

FIGURE 19.5 Women suffering from health problems due to lack of nutritional knowledge.

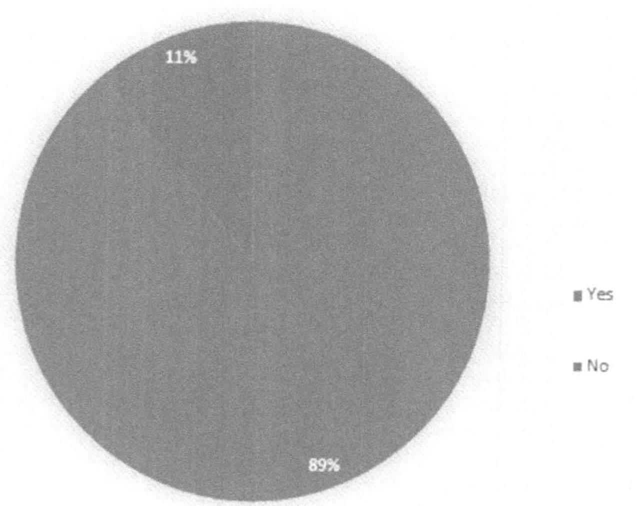

FIGURE 19.6 Women require nutrition management system to track their nutrition intake.

Since data is a crucial part of any ML project, the process of data collection has to be done precisely. Here the data is taken from the user through a google form (as shown in Figure 19.7). The form includes parameters like age, gender, Disease (if any), Allergic food item (if any), How are your eating habits? How many times do you take a meal in a day? Type of Job, How many hours in a day did you usually work? Exercise related questions. These data are essential in order to determine the health of an individual. Since data are restricted to be entered in a particular format only, no preprocessing step is done.

Gender	Age	Disease (if any)	Allergic food item (if any)	How is your eating habits?	How many times do you take meal in a day?	Type of Job	How many hours in a day did you usually work?	How often do you exercise?
Female	between 20 to 35	no	no	home made food	4	more mental work	less than 4 hours	often
Male	between 20 to 35	no	no	home made food	3	more mental work	between 4 to 8 hours	daily
Female	between 20 to 35	Anxiety	no	mix of both	3	mix of both	less than 4 hours	often
Male	between 20 to 35	no	no	mix of both	3	more mental work	more than 8 hours	often
Female	between 20 to 35	Anxiety	no	mix of both	2	mix of both	more than 8 hours	not at all
Male	between 20 to 35	no	no	mix of both	3	more mental work	between 4 to 8 hours	often
Male	between 20 to 35	no	no	mix of both	4	more mental work	more than 8 hours	not at all
Female	between 20 to 35	no	no	home made food	3	more mental work	between 4 to 8 hours	often
Female	between 20 to 35	Migrane	no	mix of both	3	mix of both	less than 4 hours	often
Male	between 20 to 35	Stress	no	home made food	2	more mental work	more than 8 hours	daily
Male	between 20 to 35	no	no	home made food	3	more mental work	between 4 to 8 hours	not at all
Male	between 20 to 35	no	no	mix of both	2	more mental work	between 4 to 8 hours	often
Male	between 20 to 35	Migrane	no	home made food	3	more mental work	more than 8 hours	daily
Male	between 20 to 35	no	no	mix of both	3	mix of both	between 4 to 8 hours	not at all
Female	between 36 to 50	no	no	home made food	2	more mental work	more than 8 hours	daily
Male	between 36 to 50	no	no	home made food	3	more mental work	more than 8 hours	often
Female	between 36 to 50	no	no	home made food	2	mix of both	more than 8 hours	often
Male	between 20 to 35	no	no	home made food	2	more mental work	between 4 to 8 hours	often
Female	between 20 to 35	no	no	home made food	2	more mental work	between 4 to 8 hours	not at all
Male	between 20 to 35	no	custurd apple	mix of both	2	more mental work	less than 4 hours	not at all
Male	between 36 to 50	no	no	home made food	1	more physical work	between 4 to 8 hours	not at all
Male	between 36 to 50	no	no	home made food	2	mix of both	less than 4 hours	often
Female	between 36 to 50	no	no	home made food	3	more mental work	more than 8 hours	often
Male	between 20 to 35	no	no	home made food	1	mix of both	less than 4 hours	often

FIGURE 19.7 Sample dataset preview.

19.5 METHODOLOGY

The proliferation of web applications and the internet has driven exponential growth of users and information over the web. Such a plethora of information is available in every domain of life, education, lifestyle, science, health, and nutrition, shopping, and many others. In such excessive information, it is difficult to locate and operate on the information of interest. In this context, information retrieval systems are essential tools to guide one to the information they are seeking. This demands the need for ML techniques that can process such enormous data and provide relevant information [2]. Those techniques will help to build the model, need to be trained, validated, and tested to achieve the required performance accuracy and efficiency.

Looking into the current context of health and nutrition, the various options of food and dietary plans are available over the internet. In such an abundance of information, it is a challenging task to fish out the relevant information that can benefit the user to satisfy their nutritional needs [8, 9]. Even if the relevant information is found, it may or may not suffice the needs, as the nutritional requirement changes from person to person based on their body type. So, this demands the necessity of a system that can cater to a varied audience, eventually leading us to the use of ML-based models. The ML-based models will go through the stages shown in Figure 19.8.

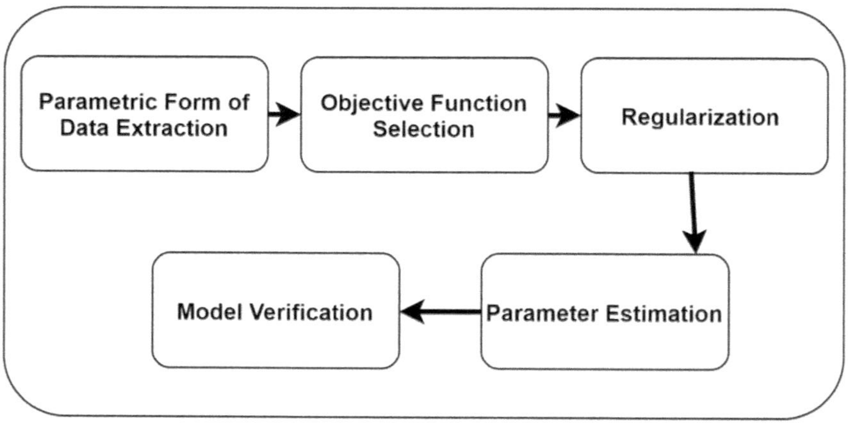

FIGURE 19.8 Execution flow of machine learning based prediction model.

The developed model with the collected nutritional data will help us build a system that provides nutritional recovery plan. The model will be trained and tested based on the user parameter and appropriately optimized to achieve better accuracy and efficiency.

19.5.1 STEP BY STEP EXECUTION

An individual faces different challenges like societal pressure, financial stability, cultural issues, and non-availability of resources. Lack of awareness about nutritional requirement and improper diet plan is the main reason for the deterioration of women's health which includes deficiencies, mental illness, fatigueness, obesity, anemia, menstruation, and pregnancy related problems. So, this chapter aims to spread awareness amidst socio-cultural norms.

As shown in Figure 19.9 the developed model with the collected nutritional data will help us build a system that provides nutritional recovery plan. The model will be trained and tested based on the user parameter and appropriately optimized to achieve better accuracy and efficiency.

Steps:

1. **Collection of data**
   - **Data Integration**
   - **Data Cleaning**
   - **Data processing**
     - **Classification and Clustering**
     - **Feature Selection**
2. **Model Formation**
   - **Parametric form**
   - **Finding parameter**
3. **Designing mobile application using ML**
4. **Implementation of Nutritional management system**
5. **Model Validation**

FIGURE 19.9 Model learning and execution flow.

19.6 RESULTS ANDDISCUSSION

K-modes is used for clustering categorical variables. It defines clusters based on the number of matching categories between data points. This is in contrast to the well-known k-means algorithm, that clusters numerical data based on Euclidean distance. K-modes is an extension of k-means. Instead of distances it uses dissimilarities. Here, modes are similar to clusters centroids in K-means. So, we can have as many modes as per our need (as shown in Figures 19.10 and 19.11). From a user point of view, most food items are recipes, not individual items. So, for that we have to study some pre-built databases that have details of all Indian food recipes. Portion sizes are also a big concern in this. Because in recipes also, everyone has a different method and taste. That's why till now no realm AI model is developed in the nutrition domain. Also, human's biological behavior changes with the time so, it is a tedious task to do. But if both, a healthcare expertise, and a ML expertise work together to make some incredible growth in this domain, would surely make a change.

```
import pandas as pd
from google.colab import drive
drive.mount('/content/drive')
df = pd.read_excel('/content/drive/My Drive/Colab Notebooks/Nutritional Survey.xlsx')
shape=df.shape
print("Size of dataset:",shape)
df.head()
```

```
Mounted at /content/drive
Size of dataset: (55, 9)
```

	Gender	Age	Disease (if any)	Allergic food item (if any)	How is your eating habits?	How many times do you take meal in a day?	Type of Job	How many hours in a day did you usually work?	How often do you exercise?
0	Female	between 20 to 35	no	no	home made food	4	more mental work	less than 4 hours	often
1	Male	between 20 to 35	no	no	home made food	3	more mental work	between 4 to 8 hours	daily
2	Female	Female	Female	Female	Female	3	mix of both	less than 4 hours	often

FIGURE 19.10 Importing libraries and dataset.

```
pip install kmodes

Collecting kmodes
  Downloading https://files.pythonhosted.org/packages/9b/34/fffc601aa4d44b94e945a7cc72f477e09dffa7dce888898f2ffd9f4e343e/kmodes-0.11.0-py2.py3-nor
Requirement already satisfied: scikit-learn>=0.22.0 in /usr/local/lib/python3.7/dist-packages (from kmodes) (0.22.2.post1)
Requirement already satisfied: joblib>=0.11 in /usr/local/lib/python3.7/dist-packages (from kmodes) (1.0.1)
Requirement already satisfied: numpy>=1.10.4 in /usr/local/lib/python3.7/dist-packages (from kmodes) (1.19.5)
Requirement already satisfied: scipy>=0.13.3 in /usr/local/lib/python3.7/dist-packages (from kmodes) (1.4.1)
Installing collected packages: kmodes
Successfully installed kmodes-0.11.0
```

FIGURE 19.11 K-means and K-modes python API.

19.7 CONCLUSION

This chapter is mainly based on the analysis and study done for improving one's health. Also, how modern-day technology like machine learning is helpful to achieve this. The main goal of this chapter is to demonstrate the use of artificial intelligence (AI) for the well-being of humans. How AI can help us to make our life better. Also, some evaluation process should be generated for evaluating such models. Since the importance of a healthy diet plan is increasing day by day, demand, and need for such smart systems are also increasing. By keeping user's lifestyle and eating habits in mind, automated software can be developed, to make a healthy lifestyle. Here, ML-based algorithm is used to predict the health of an individual. Since data is the main focus while designing any ML models, it is suggested to choose data wisely. And accordingly, algorithm. After having the domain knowledge, the design of a model is started. But when not finding a proper dataset, it has been decided to make own dataset by circulating a google form that has all the parameters that are needed. The type of data is categorical and unlabeled. So, it is identified an algorithm that suits well with this type of data. K-modes clustering has been used for that. Model evaluation is very much important task after training a ML model.

KEYWORDS

- **artificial neural networks**
- **diet recommendation**
- **graphical processing unit**
- **health prediction**
- **healthy eating index**
- **K-means and K-modes**
- **machine learning**
- **nutritional plan**
- **predictive analytics**

REFERENCES

1. Marta, S., Mafalda, R., Olga, V., Zita, E. M., Miguel, F., Susana, C., Edgar, P., et al., (2021). Exploring two food composition databases to estimate nutritional components of whole meals. *Journal of Food Composition and Analysis, 102*, 104070, ISSN 0889-1575.
2. Mahmoud, Y. S., Omar, M. E., Lobna, M. A., Aboul, E. H., Mohamed, A. E., & Hanaa S., (2021). HANA: A healthy artificial nutrition analysis model during COVID-19 pandemic, *Computers in Biology and Medicine, 135*, 104606. ISSN 0010-4825.
3. Weber, I., & Achananuparp, P., (2016). Insights from machine-learned diet success prediction. *Pac Symp Biocomput., 21*, 540–551. PMID: 26776216.
4. Áine, P. H., & Michael, J. G., (2008). Analysis of meal patterns with the use of supervised data mining techniques—Artificial neural networks and decision trees. *The American Journal of Clinical Nutrition, 88*(6), 1632–1642.

5. Schäfer, H., Elahi, M., Elsweiler, D., Groh, G., Harvey, M., Ludwig, B., Ricci, F., & Said, A., (2017). User nutrition modelling and recommendation. Adjunct Publication of the *25th Conference on User Modeling, Adaptation and Personalization.*
6. Gojiro, N., Shinichiroh, Y., Aya, K., Toshiaki, T., Kojiro, M., Hiroshi, N., Kazuhiko, O., & Hiromi, S., (2021). Supervised machine learning-based prediction for in-hospital pressure injury development using electronic health records: A retrospective observational cohort study in a university hospital in Japan. *International Journal of Nursing Studies, 119*, 103932. ISSN 0020-7489.
7. Verma, J. P., Agrawal, S., Patel, B., & Patel, A., (2016). Big data analytics: Challenges and applications for text, audio, video, and social media data. *International Journal on Soft Computing, Artificial Intelligence and Applications (IJSCAI), 5*(1), 41–51.
8. Jacob, M. H., Steven, J. P., Stephen, C. R., & Christopher, D. B., (2021). Diet composition: A proximate mechanism explaining stream salamander declines in surface waters with elevated specific conductivity. *Global Ecology and Conservation, 29*, e01719. ISSN 2351-9894.
9. Vatsala, L., Prakash, J., & Prabhavathi, S. N., (2017). Food security and nutritional status of women selected from a rural area in South India. *J. Food Nutr. Popul. Health, 1*(2), 10.
10. Mallikharjuna, R. K., Balakrishna, N., Arlappa, N., Laxmaiah, A., & Brahmam, G. N. V., (2010). *Diet and Nutritional Status of Women in India, 29*(3), 165–170.
11. Patel, P. A., et al., (2016). Nutritional status assessment of women from different occupations in urban and semi-urban regions of Gujarat. *Int. J. Food Nutr. Sci., 3*(6), 1–4.
12. Cacheda, F., Carneiro, V., Fernández, D., & Formoso, V., (2011). Comparison of collaborative filtering algorithms: Limitations of current techniques and proposals for scalable, high-performance recommender systems. A*CM Transactions on the Web (TWEB), 5*(1), 2.
13. Pouladzadeh, P., Kuhad, P., Peddi, S. V. B., Yassine, A., & Shirmohammadi, S., (2016). Food calorie measurement using deep learning neural network. In: *2016 IEEE International Instrumentation and Measurement Technology Conference Proceedings* (pp. 1–6). IEEE.
14. Wcd.nic.in. (2020). *Home | Ministry of Women & Child Development* | GoI. [online] Available at: https://wcd.nic.in/sites/default (accessed on 13 June 2022).
15. Anon, (2020). [online] Available at: http://niti.gov.in/writereaddata/files/document_publication (accessed on 13 June 2022).
16. Nhp.gov.in. (2020*). Janani Suraksha Yojana (JSY)* | National Health Portal of India. [online] Available at: https://www.nhp.gov.in/janani-suraksha-yojana-jsy-_pg (accessed on 13 June 2022).
17. Lekha, R. N., Sujala, D. S., & Siddhanth, D. S., (2018). Applying spark-based machine learning model on streaming big data for health status prediction. *Computers & Electrical Engineering, 65*, 393–399. ISSN: 0045-7906.

CHAPTER 20

ROBOTICS IN THE HEALTHCARE INDUSTRY

ANAND SHARMA,[1] VIBHA OJHA,[2] AADITA SONI,[1] and ARIN SONI[3]

[1]*Mody University of Science and Technology, Laxmangarh, Rajasthan, India*

[2]*Government Engineering College, Ajmer, Rajasthan, India, E-mail: vibha.ojha@gmail.com*

[3]*Indian Institute of Technology, Mumbai, Maharashtra, India*

ABSTRACT

Changing applications in a public domain with restricted capabilities of healthcare structures has cleared the way for robots to move out of industrial environments and into conditions that are more human-centered, for example, healthcare. Commercial and research interest in medical and healthcare robots has seen tremendous progress over the past decade. Telerobotic fractures are used for surgery, which comes with short recovery times and powerful effects on some systems. Robotic rehabilitation agencies successfully deliver physical and occupational therapies, allowing for outstanding flexibility and flexibility in the patient's needs. The robots' social networking devices are designed for moderate and home use in training and monitoring physical, mental, and social exercise.

Advances in robots have the potential to promote the development of treatments for various ailments and diseases, to improve openness of care,

IoT and Cloud Computing-Based Healthcare Information Systems. Anand Sharma, PhD, Hiren Kumar Deva Sarma, PhD & S. R. Biradar, PhD (Eds.)

and to improve patient health outcomes. Straight forward and independent than at any other time in recent memory, and equipped to help, but complex medical procedures themselves are performed. Instead of industrial robots, they began to create 50 years back, making awesome, fragile, and dangerous machines, current health and healthcare robots designed for a variety of situations and activities – including direct contact with theater clients, community rescue, and family room.

The purpose of this chapter is to highlight some of the most important skills and special achievements of the medical and healthcare robots needed to improve human health and prosperity. We define application regions, provided management, transformation challenges, and other activities that should be considered in the health and health robots system.

20.1 INTRODUCTION

Unless everyone seems to understand what a robot is, it is difficult to give a precise explanation. The Oxford English Dictionary gives the same meaning: "A machine equipped to perform complex tasks as a result, especially one designed by a PC." This description includes some of the attractions:

Perform "performing tasks naturally." This is a critical part of robots, but in addition to many other simple machines called automata. The difference between a robot and a straight machine like a dishwasher lies in the definition of "unexpected operation." Is washing done in anticipation of an unexpected action or not? Is flying a self-help plane a confusing task? Is baking complicated? In all these settings, there is a balance between automatics and robots.

The program "computer program" is another sensitive aspect of robotics because some automatics are precisely modified and do not really change. Then PCs are everywhere, so it's hard to use this foundation to find a robot in another machine.

The emergency part of the robots is not indirectly described in the definition of sensory use. Most automata have no sensors and cannot convert their functions to their current state. Sensors are the key to the robot's ability to detect and perform complex tasks in the brain.

Robots can be programed with a fixed input field and with their commitment. A description of the robots by system is shown in Figure

20.1. We refer to industrial robots operating in the most visible conditions. The first robots were industrial robots because extreme weather conditions disrupted their system. App robots, too, help people in their assignments. These include home deployments such as vacuum cleaners, self-driving vehicles, and security systems, for example, detection drones. Medical professionals have also seen an increase in the use of robots in medical, recovery, and preparation processes. These are late applications that require advanced sensors and close relationship with the client.

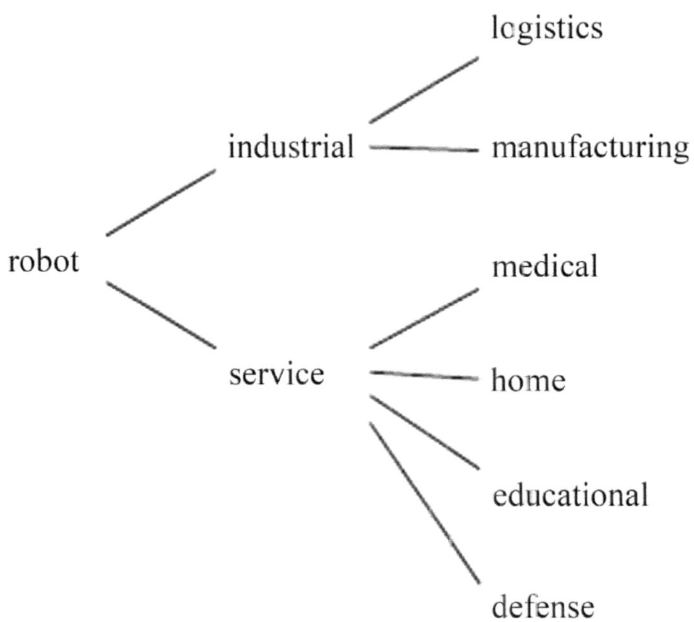

FIGURE 20.1 Robot classification as per application

20.2 APPLICATION OF ROBOTICS

Robotics is a broad concept and every day there is alien construction in the field. Robots have been developed by us not only for entertainment but are now being used to guide people in various fields. Humans are better prepared for integrated, creative, interactive, and robotic tasks that lead to unexpected, repetitive tasks, allowing people to perform complex mental tasks, and robots are used to replicate repetitive tasks or to make money.

In recent years, robots have come up with an incredible variety of functions, and the number of robots sent by them has increased dramatically. The best way to distinguish robots from species is to classify them by their function.

Robotic is a broad field and consistently there is a leading nature in the field. Manmade robots are now being used to help people in various places. Humans are better equipped with a variety of positions, art, various activities, and robots that are useful for repetitive, repetitive robots, allowing humans to perform complex mental tasks, whether the robot is used to replicate or entertain to make life much easier.

Currently, robots play a wide variety of roles in a variety of fields, and the rate at which robots are being made is increasing. The best way to differentiate robots from species is through their system.

20.2.1 INDUSTRIAL ROBOTS

These robots went into operation at an industrial assembly site. Often these descriptive arms are specifically designed for applications such as facing, welding, painting, and more. If we experimented with programming, such a robot could have a variety of targeted vehicles and various robots.

20.2.2 HOME OR DOMESTIC ROBOTS

Robots for home use. Such robots contain various pinion wheels such as robotic pool cleaners, robotic cleaning robots, robotic sweepers, robotic cleaners, and various robots that can perform a variety of household tasks. In addition, testing a few telepresence robots can be considered home-grown robots whenever they play in such an environment.

20.2.3 MEDICAL ROBOTS

Robots are used in medical and rescue organizations. Most important is the careful handling of the robots. Also, a few cars are connected to cars and perhaps even to their counterparts.

20.2.4 SERVICE ROBOTS

Robots cannot be separated by training. These could be different robots for collecting information, robots designed for new displays, robots used for research, and so on.

20.2.5 MILITARY ROBOTS

Robots are played in armed forces and in battle. Such a robot contains grenade launchers, different transport robots, and probe drones. The first standard robots installed by armed forces with military objectives can be used in legal, investigative, rescue, and other related fields.

20.2.6 FUN ROBOTS

These types of robots are used for entertainment. This is the most active category. It starts with model robots, for example, Robosapien or an active image frame, and then closes with heavy metals such as arms of used robots that are used as advanced testing systems.

20.2.7 SPACE ROBOTS

We like to remove robots that have undoubtedly been used in space as a variant. This type of robot will include robots used in the Canadarm that was played at Space Shuttles, the International Space Station, as well as Mars explorers and various robots used in space exploration and various exercises.

20.2.8 COMMUNICATION AND COMPETITIVE ROBOTS

Deer robots are designed. Fans of the line, Sumo-bots, robots designed for fun, learning, and robots designed for challenges.

Currently, as we see, a few models fit well in at least one of these methods. Theoretically, there may be a deep-sea revelation robot that can collect a few important details that can be used for naval or military purposes.

20.3 ROBOTICS APPLICATIONS IN HEALTHCARE

Robots are beginning to influence drugs (the use of science and innovation to treat and prevent injuries and infections) and healthcare (access to treatment and anticipation of illness). Telerobotic frameworks are used to make provision, deliver limited recovery times and powerful effects on specific programs [1–3]. Robotic structures are increasingly improving occupational and physical therapy [4, 5] and replacing lost function [6]. Studies have also shown that robotic properties can provide therapeutic, educational, and regenerative drugs that add to one's mind almost without human intervention and can continue home treatment for a long time after hospitalization [7–11]. Creating a robotic framework that enables the biology of accurate biology has been used as a means of studying and studying how the human brain and body function [12]. In addition, robots can be used to capture information from natural phenomena with astonishing accuracy, enabling us to acquire more information about physical and social behavior.

Globally, the healthcare industry is under intense pressure for better openness, productivity, and price charts as it seeks to support (or improve) the type of healthcare delivery. Providing healthcare to rapidly matured people who use small items has become increasingly important in this century. Similarly, tailors, and citizens have raised the level of development that can be met – or if not limited – to this category [13].

Robots capture certain interests such as self-deception and gadgets that have been modified to meet human needs [14]. The power of robots to help support and care for human beings in the future is reflected in the novels and has similarly embraced the elements of broader communication at a growing rate 'presented examples of overcoming adversity [15, 16].

Following Ref. [17], a service robot is a machine that can perform tasks in unpredictable, human-centered weather. Essentially, the International Standardization Organization defines a robot used as a machine that "performs important human functions or gears, blocking the industrial applications of the robot" [18]. In contrast to industrial robots, which often operate in controlled or potentially dangerous environments (for example collecting lines, mines, outdoors), used robots often operate close to humans and in truly uncontrolled weather.

Following Ref. [19], the domain of use is also a good reference for increasing segregation. In healthcare, we can distinguish between robots designed for 'health land' (or used in care facilities) and 'non-clinical world' (or for use in patients' homes) [20]. As we investigate health workers' concerns related to the introduction of robots in their organizational areas, we are reducing our size to devices designed for use in hospitals and specialized care centers.

20.3.1 IN THE BODY

Robots can aid recovery and aid in recovery. For example, the removal of Cyberdyne's hybrid assistive limb (HAL), which uses nerve implants on the skin to detect small electrical signals in a patient's body and respond to joint movements, is intended to help patients recover from debilitating conditions, including spinal cord injuries.

We've seen them in movies, abused them in computer games, and now they're very sick: exoskeletes. These robotic designs will create a sense of insecurity for certain people by helping people to move and lift heavy loads – or themselves. Later, it is not hard to imagine how the soldiers, soldiers, specialists, or cell staff and nurses who accompanied patients could use the floodwaters regularly to increase their muscle strength, endurance, and weightlifting.

They are currently assisting clinical specialists in finding a long-term course of treatment, and, in some of its latest information, the BBC is talking about a French man who had the opportunity to deliver all four of these ineffectively controlled brain products. In 2019, ReWalk Robotics, an organization that builds outdoor buildings, announced that the office had removed the fragile organizational structure available for purchase and relocated throughout the United States.

Such gadgets are immodest – HAL's monthly suit hire costs up to $ 1,000 – and costs should be reduced as scales and upgrades, including sensors, hardware, and power generation are reduced.

The exoskeleton market is one of the fastest growing parts for robots. Includes bio-input lumbar assistance with air conditioners and stockbrokers, now in Japan. Advances in the acquisition of equipment in the brain will affect the formation of exoskeletons. Major organizations in the sector are Ekso Bionics, Cyberdyne, and ReWalk Robotics.

20.3.2 INSIDE THE BODY

We have to change gears from large metal arms to minus, capsule-sized robots that lead to the acceptance and treatment of infection. The procedure known as "capsule endoscopy" received approval from the Food and Drug Administration (FDA) years ago, but the current invention could eventually pass all the guarantees.

Capsule endoscopy requires the patient to swallow a small camera so that doctors can take pictures of the abdomen-related tract. This camera helps to identify signs of illness or disability that may need treatment. The problem with existing efforts is that the case cameras move perhaps as the patient's body retains its normal energy.

Although we are not yet in the age of nanotechnology, the patterns that point to a new look are growing. With the increase in digestible and computer pills, we are slowly approaching the nanorobots. At the same time: analysts from the Max Planck Institute have been experimenting with a variety of microscopic robots that are much smaller than a millimeter – that in a literal sense absorb your natural fluid and can be used to transfer drugs or other medical devices to a concentration. These tiny scallop-like insects are designed to swim using non-Newtonian fluids, such as your circulatory system, around your lymphatic structure, or across the invisible goo outside your eyes.

An origami robot, no matter how large, is as impressive as a powerful transmitter. When reached, the contained contents penetrate the patient's abdomen and open. Obstructed by a specialist with the help of a magnetic field can repair stomach or intestinal injuries or safely eliminate abnormal objects, for example, restricted toys.

20.3.3 ARTIFICIAL LIMBS

Bones protect, support, or enhance the strength of the various limbs, limbs, foot, knee, and spine. Unlike robotic gadgets, traditional orthoses are professionally smoked, and as a result, they are unable to adjust the level or type of assistance as the patient grows and his or her flexible energy. Robotic orthoses are usually an external mirror, which protects the active part of the body. They should allow free movement of appendages while providing the necessary assistance. Most of the existing outdoor robots that are research devices that emphasize military use (e.g., allowing heroes to carry heavy loads on their backs) return to the facility. However, these structures are not yet economically viable and strong enough to be used as organs. Prosthesis is a counterfeit supplement that alters the support of a body part (often lost through injury or environmental deformity) by mixing gadgets with bones, human muscles, and nerve systems.

Existing commercial filling gadgets are very limited in power (usually only allowing the opening/closing of the holder) because they are driven by precision or electromyography (EMG), which is a record of the electrical activity of a body part without defect). Robotic Input Gadgets fully expect to fully replicate a lost attachment or other body part by the repetition of multiple organs and fragments, as well as a constant neural combination that provides natural control of the appendix as a touch detector. Over the past few years there has been significant progress in the development and development of nerve endings that will drive these high levels of input. Further research into robots is expected to improve the interaction and simplicity of artificial limbs.

20.3.4 SURGERY

Surgery is an unbalanced joint. Emerging records may depend for a long time on the jobs and assets available. In this way, alert robots are a marvel of surgery. With each market test, the business will explode.

The development of surgical robots is fueled by the desire to improve the performance of the system by integrating data and activity into the workplace or intervention area and ascending beyond the actual operating limits and other intervention strategies, while still managing human costs on the road. Around 20 years after the first robotic surgery was announced, alert robots are now widely used in the operating room or in the intervention area.

Leading manufacturers have expanded their R&D efforts within the robotic monitoring framework. The mainstream market is currently frustrated by Intuitive Surgical, but the situation is changing rapidly. The passing of major manufacturers, for example, Johnson, and Johnson and Medtronic are support the robotics market.

The robot most commonly introduced by the DaVinci Surgical System, and honestly, was successfully launched 15 years back! It includes a high-resolution viewing frame of a magnified notch top and small twisted instruments and turns at a level that is more visible than the human hand. While a robotic robot engineer, he can perform more precise tasks than expected recently.

Some are interested in the field of surgical robots, too. Google reported in 2015 that it began working with pharma monster Johnson and Johnson on building a robotic design for the Verb Surgical system. In mid-2018, Google's biggest supporter Sergey Brin used a robot to sew some synthetic tissue. From then on, J&J bought Auris, which has been causing robots to transform into lung cells and acquired Orthotaxy, a privately held program developer that makes new discoveries. In mid-2019 you saw a previously reported example of distance surgeons using robotic devices and the 5G web organization. Remote surgery has been a bad thing with the establishment of the network in the past, because 5G has the low bandwidth needed to maintain the balance between technological advances and arm robots.

There is a clear supply of products from each organization in each studyable region for unpopular robotic surgery. For example, the Da Vinci System is a complete diagnostic robot equivalent to several surgeries in urological, bariatric, and gynecological surgery. In addition, the MakoSurgical System from Stryker spends a lot of time on muscle surgery, which obviously balances and replaces the knees. One up-and-comer focused on MakoSurgical muscle robot guidance. Inside the modular loop, the robot transmits the necessary equipment for a CT scan to the patient's knee, 3D drawings of a straight limb model and assists with preoperative surgery performed for each patient. The robot has a point-keeping arm and a straight monitoring device and is followed by both measurements throughout the operation.

The coming years will assume that this will be further enhanced as the required development grows. That includes the 5G network, which is not yet widely available, and the power of robots to show you independently with a small human attraction.

A way to show good governance would be a repetition of an item, as each organization tries to add its own outstanding points. Disclosure organizations have surprisingly hidden operational strategies, for example, identified by Intuitive Surgical compared to TransEnterix. The two companies offer robots to provide robots with a clear connection, but Intuitive has a few characters to determine the use of their commercially available decorations, and TransEnterix communication also works. The cost of robotic surgical technology within the healthcare business is declining.

20.3.5 REMOTE HEALTH CENTER

You may have been in a situation where before, in the event of a serious incident, medical professionals would not have had the option to contact you as expected. For the few of us in the created world, it is a rare event. However, even by 2019, millions live without a standard of problem-solving management in Vanuatu or the Inuit group in Northern Canada.

Through InTouch Health, Health Tap, Doctor on Demand, Teladoc, American Well, Avizia, or Babylon Health, patients in remote areas approach meetings for stroke, heart, skin problems, or other complaints. On the patient side, it is often available on tablets or computers, and doctors can also use the same types of gadgets depending on their needs.

20.3.6 CARE

Drawing blood and disinfecting robots during the clinic stay, patients are in close contact with medical providers. Like Shiva, the eight-year-old Indian goddess, they are there, as a rule in 12 hours, to draw blood, check your vital signs, check your status, and take care of your hygiene if necessary. They are often overwhelmed by their professional and intellectual activities and the result is often an unpleasant encounter for all involved.

Robotic staff will help reduce these problems over time. They are designed to have the option of doing horrible and unpleasant things, so human employees have a lot of potential to deal with problems that require human motivation, thinking, and a big part of it all, care, and empathy. In some cases, blood-sucking robots can prevent healthcare providers from doing this tedious task, and they can perform laboratory tests without human intervention.

A TUG-compatible transport robot can also be a top choice for medical providers. It can be close to a large number of trucks, trucks or containers weighing 453 kilograms as instructions, examples of research institutes or other fragile items – so that medical clinic staff can perform other important tasks. The TUG is sent or spoken using the touch interface and after completing its "main goal," it returns to the charging port to taste power while being reserved for the next position. TUG has received evaluations at emergency clinics and makes more than 50,000 referrals each week to more than 140 clinics in the United States.

However, healthcare robots mean more than just drawing blood or circulating rats. For example, with remote-controlled health robots, those created by Anybots, managers can communicate with their patients; pay attention to their daily environment and the need for additional arrangements. This will aid the execution of the order by taking a tedious home visit. Another organization, Luvozo, made Sam, work with robots, and tried for the first time in a large residential area in Washington DC A robotic, human-sized robot incorporates the best in new blood and human touch to provide continuous and thoughtful registration for passengers in long-term care facilities. Thus, it reduces the cost of care, while increasing the list of peaceful achievements by regular presence of the elderly.

With the highway of robots and artificial intelligence (AI), social partner robots are beginning to come true: these human or artificial creatures, the most modest or professional creatures can create a variety of ways and adapt to humans and their current state. Later, they can become a little personal helper for each parent in the kitchen, they can support a housekeeping guard canine, they can show children and be their friends and support adults by reminding them to take their medication until they feel abandoned.

Buddy, Zora, Paro, Pepper, and Jibo are all available models for social care friend robots. Some of them even have contact sensors, cameras, and oral nails, so their owners can contact them, ask them to get an unusual show at night or simply remind them of their medication.

Big and small, smiles, and anonymity, pharma, and surgery: robotics move everything together with structures that seriously question healthcare. That may scare some, but they can make good progress: taking clinics to districts where they are not available; making the manufacture and distribution of drugs less expensive and more efficient; relieving the burden of clinical specialists; to help people get back on track.

The number of robots used to care for and support elderly and infirm patients is currently very low but is likely to rise sharply in the next decade, especially in countries like Japan, which is facing an expected shortage of available caregivers. Initial cases of use of these items are usually straightforward, for example, to help people wake up, but they will most likely be asked to perform unexpected tasks, ranging from reminding patients when to take medication to provide emotional support and communication with those who lack contact.

Another common cause of the use of care robots is to help medical providers with a large number of tasks they perform per hour. A large number of these assignments are straightforward but important, for example, taking blood, recording temperature, or improving patient hygiene. If robots had the opportunity to help with these critical issues, it would provide more opportunities to get individual patient consideration and to develop treatment strategies. Things like Robear Japanese, made by research organization Sumitomo Rikoa.

20.3.7 HOSPITAL ASSISTANCE

Hospital robots, such as Aethon's TUG robots, can be used to transmit drugs, laboratory specimens, or other sensitive material inside a hospital climate. Drag you can explore using the included guide and various sensors in the valley. Also, it uses Wi-Fi to talk about elevators, scheduled access, and alarms.

Among the major clinical tool manufacturers, McKesson, Nokia, and GE are similarly making hospital robots. The industry-based Robot has partnered with InTouch Health to create a transparent robot-made robot.

Robots are designed to clean machines and hospitals. The only organization that shows great assurance in this market is Xenex, which developed a reproductive robot using Xenon light and can clean the entire patient's room in less than 20 minutes. Currently, more than 400 hospitals work with Xenex.

Hospital-acquired infections (HAI) are some of the leading causes of death in the US. The CDC data used by Xenex show that in the United States, one in 25 patients will receive HAI. Of those, one in nine will die.

Apart from personal expenses, it causes significant financial damage. This pollution costs more than $ 30 billion dollars every year. Xenex, a Texas-based organization, introduced a novel robot. It uses bright light to clean any area in the healthcare office quickly and effectively. Xenex Robot has more power to make cells that damage microorganisms than any other gadget intended for cleaning, and thus reduce the amount of HAI. And it is just another example of how robots in healthcare help the hospital with a reduction in staff to reduce the remaining burden and greatly facilitate an infected climate.

20.3.8 ROBOTS ARE IN A SUPPLY CHAIN

Robots can try scary and boring assignments, but they can also be dangerous to humans – for example, moving heavy boxes or exploration arrangements. For example, one of Boston Dynamics' robots, Petman, was designed to test U.S. military uniforms. It is even more important in the worst situations that are most dangerous to humans.

Past robots can be placed in unsafe conditions for humans, and robots can also have devastating effects on drug supply chains. Clinical distribution facilities, physician administration arrangements, for example, PharmASSIST ROBOTx assists any office given the status of "correct size" by its volume. In addition, it is a well-established practice for these robots to be designed with solid data mining skills, so drug stores can obtain valuable pieces of information about the road and their regular operation. If robots are not used to do this work, drug specialists will have the opportunity and momentum to participate in the social rehabilitation phase: teach people how to protect themselves, provide effective leadership and thus ensure that healthcare is truly remembered.

20.4 ADVANTAGES AND SERVICE IN HEALTHCARE

Robotics development and AI development continue to support professionals, providers, and clinics by making equipment and facilitating sustainable thinking.

There are a few benefits to healthcare providers and patients where robots become part of the advertised management. These preferences include:

- Provide assistance or comfort to patients or visitors;
- Eliminate human error in critical, dangerous ways;
- Reduce the time required for treatment procedures;
- Improve continuous recovery time;

- Short the health clinic remains;
- Create a focus on custom medicine.

The opportunity for robots to improve healthcare is not new – in early 1985 there was an arrangement to turn modern robots into more accurate medical devices. The emergence and growth of the DaVinci robot in the mid-2000s and this video of popular vintage processes show how far we have come with the mechanics.

However, strangely enough, healthcare robots are still human. The real magic of the 21st-century robo-specialist will emerge from man-made imaginative frameworks that can change so much that they will surpass leading professionals by joining all the information found in all clinical literature. In any case, most experts agree that AI will not replace trained clinical staff but will make them more effective in a number of areas which are discussed in subsections.

20.4.1 IMPROVES ACCURACY

Robotic frames are emotional, unpredictable, and never have a thought slip. In the event that this looks like the right professional, it was the same thinking behind the many robots now used in top clinics around the world. Called Waldo's experts, these can overcome any obstacle between humans and machines and perform tasks with astonishing accuracy, increased power, and the absence of earthquakes. Regardless of how long a product has been successfully developed, a human scientist takes over the work of his or her own choice.

Amazing accuracy also comes as small robots that focus on sight, direct where needed and transmit peace to your area or perform minor surgeries, for example, to close arteries.

20.4.2 REMOTE TREATMENT

The plan to use the robot for therapeutic purposes came a long way from DARPA in the 1990s, but communication networks at the time were unable to provide much-needed administrative support on the front line.

Current 4G and future 5G styles have made this a problem of the past. DARPA continues to support these efforts, but so far it seems that the robotic treatment system actually needs human partners for the purpose of hygiene and various other roads, which, frankly, makes things very confusing and financially unreasonable.

Especially as time has passed, the US Study Division of Defense has funded Carnegie Mellon University and the University of Pittsburgh to develop a self-regulatory framework for self-propelled robots to manage invading armies in remote areas.

Other AI, along with some augmented reality (AR) skills, can help specialists in building a continuous, modified overhaul during a medical procedure, consisting of arteries and other affected areas. If it is possible to use the arm of the robots, the library may suggest various tools to be used according to current accepted practices.

Another type of remote healthcare robot is a basic pill that plays endoscopy more flexibly than previous methods. This 'complex pill' sends pictures of your digestive organs as they go along, and you use them regularly.

20.4.3 TO DEVELOP HUMAN SKILLS

Some clinical robots help patients' more than clinical staff. For example, outdoor robots can help patients who are unable to work to move around without monitors.

Another use of new materials is intelligent AI technology. These bionic machines have nerves that make them replicate and accepted and more precise than the original organs, which increase the chances of attaching themselves to bionic skin and connecting them to human muscles.

20.4.4 UP SUPPORT MENTAL HEALTH ACTIVITIES AND DAILY ACTIVITIES

Service robots can make a person's power, such as making disabled or elderly patients feel lost. Talking about robots with friends can help these patients stay positive, remind them to take their medication and make general registers such as temperature, circulatory difficulty, and blood sugar levels.

This is very similar to individual participants and is associated with working with character testing skills and assessment skills, which is very helpful for depressed patients.

20.4.5 HELPFUL ROBOTS

There is a lot of work in the medical clinic, not just specialists who can use a particular aid. Medical providers and emergency clinic skills can benefit from the help of robots, for example, the Moxi Diligent Robotic robot. The robot is concerned with reusing, delivering, and cleaning so that guards can invest more energy in patients and provide human touch while leaving the granulating machine.

Another amazingly useful robot is the UV Light anti-microbial robot, which enters the emergency room and does not leave until it is infected.

20.5 ENABLING TECHNOLOGIES

The critical development of the robotics specialists is important to understand the skills demonstrated in the "Required System Skills" area. This section briefly identifies areas considered to be the best in robots and clinics.

20.5.1 ROP STRUCTURES AND REPRESENTATION

The robot approves buildings with the correct sequence of project projects that control robotic structures. The development of robotic control systems has also reached a point where it is becoming increasingly difficult with medical and healthcare systems, as those structures have to deal with continuously, complex, and reassuring conditions, ranging from human communication and human interaction. To address this challenge, designs should be created to promote a spry-based system, flexible frameworks for uncertain conditions that include direct physical contact and non-physical communication with one or more human clients.

20.5.2 STANDARD METHODS

Legal strategies are a form of numerical information, development, and framework testing. For clinical robots that directly interact with parent and patient statistics, control systems, facilitators, applications, and equipment should be tested and approved as protection using legal methods. From now on, much of the work with appropriate techniques does not include uncertainty about the level required for clinical and health robots. The purpose is linked to the implementation of formal strategies in the system and to indicating the formation of human resources.

20.5.3 CONTROL AND PLANNING

Control is the basic foundation of every real robot. For clinical robots, the most important part of managing is communication/power control. Maintaining consistent, secure connections tests the postponement of powerful innocent models. All of these problems need to be addressed through the use of enhancements in robotic configuration, display, and control. The readiness of robots in clinics and health requires new ways of working in uncertain conditions and human knowledge.

20.5.4 THINKING

Robot perception, which uses sensory information and models to create assignment understanding of an environment or environment or client, is an integral part of all clinical and health robots. In image-oriented surgery, image details should be categorized and converted into important data about specific highlights, for example, organs, obstacles, and objectives. Another type of understanding that works in healthcare is to specify details, power, and sensory data to create human models, robots, and conditions, and communication between them. Finally, an important test of a customer-focused framework is a progressive understanding and understanding of customer action to empower an effective human resource organization. Common, uncontrolled human habits are complex, notoriously inexpensive, and full of uncertainty.

20.5.5 ROBUST, SENSORS OF HIGHER INTEGRITY

Sensors, as well as cognitive calculations, are always important to give a person/doctor status to the parent, patient, and (often) environment. Incompatible/embedded sensors can have an unusual effect on important pathways in this field. Real-time interactions between robots and patients require formation that will not damage body tissues or stop working when in contact with them. At a time when robots are operating in an undisturbed environment, especially where humans are meeting, the use of a sense of touch is essential for performing precise, efficient, and secure operations. Essentials, strengths, and contact details are needed to control the teaching of critical issues, from human organs to covers and variables in the family field. The latest sensors are limited in resolution, power, size, and paralysis.

20.5.6 WRITING METHODS AND ACTUATORS FOR HIGH PERFORMANCE

With features ranging from small surgical robots to human-sized fingers, robots require small actuators and systems with advanced weight-bearing systems. These programs will allow us to build robots that are much smaller, less powerful, and less expensive. In surgery, novel devices are expected to allow the handling of very small, cheap robots, and those (or rotting) robots that can be treated outside the body. Imaginative surgery relies on robots that emit electromagnetic devices. Advanced installation enhances the design of hand-made robots with robes and arms and robust artificial limbs that look at the issues of volume and weight requested for human construction. The average power rating of conventional (electromechanical) actuators is very small compared to other possible modes, for example, the most flexible memory/combination of materials and materials in power conversion.

20.5.7 READING AND ADAPTING

As previously examined, the ability of the framework to improve its delivery over time and to improve customer engagement is essential for clinical and health robots. With this, dedicated work is required for the realization of AI in the true clinical and health information anonymously. Such statistics should ensure established standards of quality (well-being and reliability) while learning new methods, practices, and skills. Efforts in the field of acquisition and skills acquisition through teaching, demonstration, and impersonation should be directed to the realities of clinical and health fields and use unconfirmed data to validate the technology.

20.5.8 HYMN HRI

Such collaboration is a feature of many clinical applications. Demonstrating and improving the simulation of human structure and energy is the reason for the development of human-made robots.

20.6 ROBOTICS ADOPTION CHALLENGES AND OPPORTUNITIES IN HEALTHCARE

The need for framework changes and training is particularly evident in the HRI areas. All clients have clear characteristics, needs, and tendencies where the framework needs to be adjusted. In addition, similar characteristics, needs, and tendencies may change over time as the client becomes accustomed to the structure and health status of client changes, short-term (rehabilitation), intermediate (recovery), and health (lifestyle changes, aging). Adoption, efficiency, and usability, robots that interact with human customers should have the option to adjust and teach in new settings and extended time scales for various scenarios and settings.

Difficulties in long-term teaching include a combination of long-term information about the client, negative thoughts and behavioral changes, and surprising experiences. Machine learning (ML), including robotic learning, has become the subject of progressively more advanced techniques. In any case, the work has not yet gone to verified data (audible, deficient, and contradictory), more customer-specific information (from signal-level data from tests, tests, anodes, and wearable gadgets to represent data from drawings, studies, and patient meetings), and withdrawal details long-term (over months and long periods of treatment).

The ability to communicate with a customer through natural signal signals (wands, and speech) and benefit from the show and impersonation are powerful experimental lessons. They represent the novel test of long-term home interaction where the framework depends on customer learning and familiarity, as well as minimizing the consequences of unfamiliarity and tolerance. Robotic learning frameworks have not been tested in very long tests, and very focused learning is not this point beyond comprehension. Because learning frameworks are often difficult to self-evaluate and break down, it is important that innovations like these are designed to give the organ's natural perspective as a consumer health government. Due to these difficulties, the flexible healthcare robot framework will have the option to experience changes in the client/persistent health status and modify the delivery of its management; accordingly, will transform its customer delivery, empowerment, and training strategies on a regular basis in order to capture its appeal and performance in support of long-term customer commitment. Such a framework will have measures set to reflect positive health outcomes based on rehabilitation/intervention/treatment and health measures.

While there are encouraging advances in healthcare robots, it is important that you take a look at some of the problems that come with healthcare robots and explore ways to beat them. Robots can allow for real change in the world, but in health, that country is the foundation of well-being, full of people who cannot fight injury due to powerlessness, chaos, injury, or illness. Partners are faced with five important considerations when considering sending robots to healthcare: Usability and acceptance, Safety, and reliability, Strength, and performance, Clinical efficiency, and cost-effectiveness.

20.6.1 USABILITY AND ACCEPTANCE

Robots that are difficult to use for key partners have a high chance of being abandoned. This miracle was recorded by the Assistive Technology Community [21, 22]. For example, a recent report revealed that 75% of such robots have never been tried by end-users, making them unable to speak and completely discarded [23].

An important difficulty is that physicians, even people who are knowledgeable and have benefited from their orders, often have lower levels of new education [24]. Next, in the event that, at the end of the day, they find an unused robot, the likelihood that they will be better prepared for the client or robber who will use the robot is greatly reduced. Another challenge is that DRUs are often rejected in relation to the configuration of robots, making the technology unusable and unacceptable. Robots with varying degrees of probability, for example, wearable armor or armchairs, require an undeniable level of mental control [25]. In any case, many people who need such robots develop co-dreariness (e.g., in some cases), which can lead to another disabling process. There are many different ways to deal with this issue. Another way to make robots creators reduce the weight of robots.

Forlizzi and Zimmerman suggested that there may be a certain level of resource focus, when compared to the thinking and structure of each client, the editors considered incorporating a more comprehensive biological system [26]. This is very helpful in the healthcare of the robot. Sometimes there will be one DRU and one robot; rather, there are complex social structures involved in the provision of considerations that should be considered as protections in the construction of robots. Another major obstacle to the distribution of health robots is their acceptance. The morphology, function, and use of the robot play a major role in its adoption and use. At a time when the DRU is openly using a robot, they quickly identify their disability, confusion, or illness. DRUs currently face significant cultural discrimination, so it is common to use anything that continues to express their differences, even if it offers health benefits [27, 28].

Shinohara and Wobbrock said that although the creators were concerned about the availability of the framework, they were also looking at its openness to the public, using the "design for social acceptance" (DSA) method. Robotic makers are often concerned about the useful abilities of robots, e.g., a robot can perform its function safely and reliably given the operating environment, environment, and stage requirements. In addition, the above-mentioned document suggests that there may be unusual stimulus in similar behaviors to help enable new discoveries.

20.6.2 SAFETY AND RELIABILITY

When robots and individuals are available, safety, and reliability are paramount. This is especially important for DRUs who may be heavily dependent on robots to help them execute physical and mental commands, and who may not be able to recover from the frustrating effects of robots like DRUs. There has been little work to do and secure communication made by robots, especially in improving crash speeds, unrestricted control methods, and new developments in soft robots to promote critical interaction [29]. There is also the steady development of algorithmic evidence for robots operating in unknown operating environments [30].

However, there has been little work so far in the safe interaction of human robots. People with intellectual disabilities and adolescents tend to be deceived by robots [31]. For example, ensuring the presence of a robot is largely controlled by its volume (e.g., avoiding missing objects), allowing it to understand how the robot determines, and maintaining the safety and confidence of DRUs [32].

20.6.3 ABILITY AND PERFORMANCE

Its robot nest seems to be intensifying as it eventually did, a few of which have been used in healthcare. In any case, apart from this development, robots are currently a surprisingly problematic problem. For example, many new robotic exhibitions have left the demo, going beyond the most binding situations [33]. This is especially dangerous when new healthcare systems are being developed: many issues are open, and there is no provision for "all-inclusive" [34]. Individually, the delivery, and maintenance care is amazing, and they expect robots to have the opportunity to gain power and adapt to the aircraft.

Indeed, even the same type of care, for example, to solve problems or to help a residential office, has significant comparisons to their current and cultural circumstances. In our new health data planning activities, we have shown that these divisions can be overcome by regulating multiple institutional systems, and by developing mechanisms that are consistent with different perspectives. [35] The same approach can be taken from robots. Real understanding of the earth, consistent, and emotional in human conditions, is another important test for robots. In addition, more in-depth learning methods and long-term diagnostic methods have given the physician the ability to overcome some of these cognitive problems. Demonstrating the nature of the object and the object and the natural concepts within them can also help to overcome these problems [36].

Reading, too, is a test. It is important that key partners, who have a lot of real strengths, cognitive skills, and new levels of education, can undoubtedly revive robots without the existing RM. This wide band opener list gives robots makers a frustrating and special social test. As has already been said, directly without a doubt it is better; it helps to force the problem space and reduce the complexity of the structure. Another important guideline will be a testing ground that continues to build new data, test standards, and standard categories; they have proven to be useful in some areas of processing, so they will be useful here.

20.6.4 EFFECTIVE OPERATION

While robots are available in healthcare, it is important that their cost-effectiveness is considered to transfer, purchase, and adjust the cost of the framework. For example, when electronic health records (EHRs) are available for a period of time, they are promoted as a way to save doctors and patients' time. In any case, due to the fact that the EHR structures were not working properly, were difficult to implement, and were less likely to be found, they ended up working with greater confidence. This has led to "unintended consequences," including increased costs and trauma in patients [37]. It is basic that these traps are equally blocked by robots. The Agency for Healthcare Research and Quality (AHRQ) has developed a guide to reduce these unintended consequences of EHRs; the same process can be applied to robots. In the model, when testing the detection and repair of a robot in front of everyone.

Are you assembling a robot (and is the robot set up for you)? They should carefully consider the availability of robots on their base. Robots can face many challenges, but they can also increase some. For example, consider the stock that brought a purchased robot to help security guards save time. However, it feels stressed at times during large periods of daytime due to neurological disturbances, so the shutdown closure is postponed. This results in educational outcomes, increasing the remaining burden of medical caregivers. Situations like these can be treated by carefully examining the performance of a live unit, as well as a complete understanding of the strengths and barriers of current robots.

Why do you need a robot? It is important for partners to accurately explain why a robot is important in making something original. What are the intentions of the partners? What is the process of transmitting robots, and how can success be measured? These questions can also be investigated using an exercise program to assess performance and institutional status.

How do you choose a robot? As mentioned earlier, being useful is just one aspect of robots; there are similarities: ease of use, safety, acceptance, incomparable quality, and adequate clinical practice. Although there are no authoritative laws to assist HAs in this process, a scientific strategy is being developed within this space. The CCC hosted a conference called "Discovery and Innovation in Smart and Pervasive Health," which brought together more than 60 analysts from all over the world of education, industry, and government, most of the robots working in health. These efforts will begin to provide rules over time.

To distance you from the consequences of an error, it is important to:

- The level of the robot is surrounded by all the obvious objectives;
- Detailed plans are currently not overly complicated.
- There are various ways to collect, investigate, and track feedback:
- The main partners are integrated and accountable from the outset;
- Quality improvement must be maintained on a regular basis;
- Success rates should be resolved in advance and evaluated regularly.

Towards the end of the year, IEEE submitted an archive to "Ethically Aligned Design" containing natty suggestions on how to get involved in the proper process of focusing on construction, which will be useful to all developing partners.

20.6.5 THERAPEUTIC PERFORMANCE

Clinical adequacy answers the question "does it work?" directly, does the mediation provided provide an opportunity for the significant participant? This question is answered by directing a comprehensive, evidence-based science. For robots directly influencing DRUs, this evidence comes from practical clinical research (CER), "made from therapeutic hypotheses, clinical gadgets, tests, treatment procedures, or methods of transferring healthcare." CER may recall both clinical adequacy tests, or may incorporate current writing into specific studies.

All portable robots and most physical robots must pass administrative authorization before they can be promoted and sold. In the United States, this approval is granted by the FDA, which always requires strong evidence of clinical and health gadget satisfaction. Out-of-body robots do not need to go to a gadget testing level to provide a cross within existing arrangements;

for example, the Paro robotic marker is marked by the FDA a useful sensory gadget, and in this way was not included in previous audits.

Simshaw et al. [38] states that the lack of a healthcare robots guide can harm both participants with integrity and knowledge and should be responsible for pre-testing standards for measures that include safety, security, ease of use, and reliability.

At the same time, while the local strategy competes with innovation, the local robots can and should participate in clinical trials testing the adequacy of robots in all settings.

20.7 FUTURE MARKET GROWTH AND MOVING FORWARD

Many people use online media, Netflix, Alexa, Siri, and other "sharp" frameworks without realizing that many of these frameworks are controlled by AI. With all these AI developments and robots advances in healthcare, it would be better for authorities to clarify the benefits of these developments, not new ones, to help promote selected curves and reduce feelings of fear of using AI and robots in the clinic space. Admittedly, existing discussions of the acceptance of robotic applications in healthcare reflect high expectations and goals, and often mimic the experiments of professional designers and experts.

The robot has officially joined a long list of healthcare skills and vocabulary strategies for development in the coming years. The other half includes drug specialists, registered doctors, dentists, and lab staff, among others. Internally and externally, elsewhere in the period 2016 and 2026, healthcare aims to add 2.4 million new openings.

The global market for healthcare robots could be estimated at $ 11.44 billion by 2025, according to a few speculations. All products emphasize the fact that it is another industry that makes its mark as new requirements are made sufficiently and appropriately enough for testing and widespread use.

20.8 CONCLUSION

Aside from the differences in staff changes, we acknowledge that there is something more in favor of restructuring. Robots don't have to worry about rest or food, they don't discriminate, and will no doubt not work out why they need to finish the same tedious tasks for 1,000 years – for example, cleaning the floor at the clinic or bringing medicine up. To embrace the rewards and avoid the potential dangers of new conflicts, we need to keep up with scientific measures so that we can easily prepare for and adapt to a truly unimaginable future when clinical robots play an urgent role and work closely with us.

There has been a remarkable development in the emergence of robots since ancient times, highlighting a brighter future. How these robots will eventually be connected to the existence of an important receiver remains a matter of doubt, but it is not uncommon for robots to be agents for enabling (and disrupting) life.

Robots are ubiquitous: in plant production, in homes and in emergency clinics, even in space. Most of the installation work involves resources in building robots that interact directly with humans. Robots are used in healthcare organizations to build offices for health workers and the prosperity of patients.

In this way, we can see how healthcare robots can perform the authoritative and intimidating tasks of people who want to escape at any time while health managers, staff, and directors can give their most valuable opportunity to the work they pursue – focusing on the weak and weak. With a little planning and reflection, we can ensure that the human touch remains medically important while using our metal partners. Some drivers of robotic health promotion markets are investing in creating new types of fast-growing samples and trying to think better in new and unused savvy markets.

As a conclusion we can explain that robots can be something different in healthcare: better health and success, filling care holes, supporting parental statistics, and assisting healthcare workers.

KEYWORDS

- **artificial intelligence**
- **augmented reality**
- **design for social acceptance**
- **electromyography**
- **healthcare**
- **medical assistant**
- **robotics**
- **therapeutic performance**

REFERENCES

1. Kazanzides, P., Fichtinger, G., Hager, G. D., Okamura, A. M., Whitcomb, L. L., & Taylor, R. H., (2008). Surgical and interventional robotics: Core concepts, technology, and design. *IEEE Robot. Automat. Mag., 15*(2), 122–130.
2. Fichtinger, G., Kazanzides, P., Okamura, A., Hager, G., Whitcomb, L., & Taylor, R., (2008). Surgical and interventional robotics: Part II, surgical CADCAM systems. *IEEE Robot. Automat. Mag., 15*(3), 94–102.
3. Hager, G. D., Okamura, A. M., Kazanzides, P., Whitcomb, L. L., Fichtinger, G., & Taylor, R. H., (2008). Surgical and interventional robotics: Part III, surgical assistance systems. *IEEE Robot. Automat. Mag., 15*(4), 84–93.
4. Hogan, N., & Krebs, H. I., (2004). Interactive robots for neurorehabilitation. *Restor. Neurol. Neurosci., 22*(3–5), 349–358.
5. Guglielmelli, E., Johnson, M., & Shibata, T., (2009). Guest editorial special issue on rehabilitation robotics. *IEEE Trans. Robot., 25*(3), 477–480.
6. Micera, S., Carrozza, M. C., Beccai, L., Vecchi, F., & Dario, P., (2006). Hybrid bionic systems for the replacement of hand function. *Proc. IEEE, 94*(9), 1752–1762.
7. Matari_c, M. J., (2006). Socially assistive robotics. *IEEE Intell. Syst., 21*(4), 81–83.
8. Matari_c, M. J., Eriksson, J., Feil-Seifer, D., & Winstein, C., (2007). Socially assistive robotics for post-stroke rehabilitation. *J. Neuroeng. Rehabil., 4*(5).
9. Bers, M. U., Ackermann, E., Cassell, J., Donegan, B., Gonzalez-Heydrich, J., DeMaso, D. R., Strohecker, C., et al., (1998). Interactive storytelling environments: Coping with cardiac illness at Boston's children's hospital. In: *Proc. ACM Conf. Human Factors in Computing Systems* (pp. 603–610). Los Angeles, CA.
10. Kidd, C. D., Taggart, W., & Turkle, S., (2006). A sociable robot to encourage social interaction among the elderly. In: *Proc. IEEE Int. Conf. Robotics and Automation.* Orlando, FL.
11. Lathan, C., Vice, J. M., Tracey, M., Plaisant, C., Druin, A., Edward, K., & Montemayor, J., (2001). Therapeutic play with a storytelling robot. In: *Proc. Conf. Human Factors in Computing Systems* (pp. 27, 28).
12. Wada, K., Shibata, T., Saito, T., & Tanie, K., (2002). Analysis of factors that bring mental effects to elderly people in robot assisted activity. In: *Proc. Int. Conf. Intelligent Robots and Systems*. Lausanne, Switzerland.
13. Hedberg, A., & Morosi, M., (2015). *Keeping Health High on the EU Agenda: Role for Economic Governance*? European Policy Centre, Brussels, Belgium.
14. Oborne, Barrett, M., & Darzi, A., (2011). Robots and service innovation in health care. *Journal of Health Services Research & Policy, 16*(1), 46–50.
15. The Economist, (2014). *New Roles for Technology: Rise of the Robots.* http://www.economist.com/news/leaders/21599762-prepare-robot-invasion-it-will-change-waypeople-think-about-technology-rise (accessed on 13 June 2022).
16. The Wall Street Journal, (2012). *The Robots are Coming to Hospitals.* http://www.wsj.com/news/articles/SB10001424052702304459804577281350525870934 (accessed on 13 June 2022).

17. Haidegger, T., Barreto, M., Gonçalves, P., Habibe, M., Ragavanf, S. K. V., Li, H., Vaccarella, A., et al., (2013). Applied ontologies and standards for service robots. *Robotics and Autonomous Systems, 61*(11), 1215–1223.
18. International Standardization Organization, (2016). *Robots and Robotic Devices—Vocabulary.* http://www.iso.org/obp/ui/#iso:std:iso:8373:ed-2:v1:en:term:2.10 (accessed on 13 June 2022).
19. Prestes, E., Carbonera, J. L., Fiorini, S. R., Jorge, V., Abel, M., Madhavanb, R., Locoro, A., et al., (2013). Towards a core ontology for robotics and automation. *Robotics and Autonomous Systems, 61*, 1193–1204.
20. Mettler, T., & Raptis, D., (2012). What constitutes the field of health information systems? Fostering a systematic framework and research agenda. *Health Informatics Journal, 18*(2), 147–156.
21. Brose, S. W., Weber, D. J., Salatin, B. A., Grindle, G. G., Wang, H., et al., (2010). The role of assistive robotics in the lives of persons with disability. *Am. J. Phys. Med.*
22. Dawe, M., (2006). Desperately seeking simplicity: How young adults with cognitive disabilities and their families adopt assistive technologies. In: *Proceedings of the SIGCHI Conference on Human Factors in Computing Systems.*
23. Balasubramanian, S., Klein, J., & Burdet, E., (2010). Robot-assisted rehabilitation of hand function. *Curr. Opin. Neurol.*
24. Lluch, M., (2011). Healthcare professionals' organizational barriers to health information technologies-a literature review *International Journal of Medical Informatics.*
25. Tsui, K. M., Kim, D. J., Behal, A., Kontak, D., & Yanco, H. A., (2011). "I want that": Human-in-the-loop control of a wheelchair-mounted robotic arm. *Applied Bionics and Biomechanics, 8*(1), 127–147.
26. Forlizzi, J., & Zimmerman, J., (2013). Promoting service design as a core practice in interaction design. In: *The 5th IASDR World Conference on Design Research.*
27. Riek, L. D., & Robinson, P., (2011). Using robots to help people habituate to visible disabilities. In: *IEEE International Conference on Rehabilitation Robotics (ICORR).*
28. Shinohara, K., & Wobbrock, J. O., (2011). In: The shadow of misperception: Assistive technology use and social interactions. In: *Proceedings of the SIGCHI Conference on Human Factors in Computing Systems.*
29. Trivedi, D., Rahn, C. D., Kier, W. M., & Walker, I. D., (2008). Soft robotics: Biological inspiration, state of the art, and future research. *Applied Bionics and Biomechanics*
30. Lahijanian, M., Maly, M. R., Fried, D., Kavraki, L. E., Kress-Gazit, H., & Vardi, M. Y., (2016). Iterative temporal planning in uncertain environments with partial satisfaction guarantees. *IEEE Transactions on Robotics.*
31. Riek, L. D., (2015). Robotics technology in mental health care. In: Luxton, D., (ed.), *Artificial Intelligence in Behavioral and Mental Health Care*. Academic Press.
32. Hartzog, W., (2015). Unfair and deceptive robots. *Maryland Law Review, 74*(785).
33. Christensen, H. I., Okamura, A., Mataric, M., Kumar, V., Hager, G., & Choset, H., (2016). *Next-Generation Robotics*. arXiv preprint arXiv 1606.09205.
34. Gonzales, M. J., Cheung, V. C., & Riek, L. D., (2015). Designing collaborative healthcare technology for the acute care workflow. In: *9th Int'l Conference on Pervasive Computing Technologies for Healthcare (Pervasive Health).*

35. Gonzales, M. J., Henry, J. M., Calhoun, A. W., & Riek, L. D., (2016). Visual task: A collaborative cognitive aid for acute care resuscitation. In: *10th Int'l Conference on Pervasive Computing Technologies for Healthcare (Pervasive Health).*
36. Riek, L. D., (2013). The social co-robotics problem space: Six key challenges. *Robotics Challenges and Vision (RCV2013) Workshop at Robotics: Science and Systems (RSS).*
37. Jones, S. S., & et al., (2011). *Guide to Reducing Unintended Consequences of Electronic Health records*. Agency for Healthcare Research and Quality.
38. Simshaw, D., Terry, N., Hauser, K., & Cummings, M., (2016). Regulating healthcare robots: Maximizing opportunities while minimizing risks. *Richmond J. of Law & Tech.*

INDEX

B

F

T

U

V

W

X

Z